Brain Imaging:
Applications
in
Psychiatry

Brain Imaging:
Applications
in
Psychiatry

Edited by

Nancy C. Andreasen, M.D., Ph.D.

Department of Psychiatry,
The University of Iowa College of Medicine,
Iowa City, Iowa

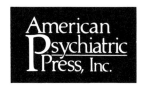

American
Psychiatric
Press, Inc.

1400 K Street, N.W.
Washington, DC 20005

Copyright © 1989 American Psychiatric Press, Inc.

ALL RIGHTS RESERVED

Manufactured in the United States of America

88 89 90 91 92 93 5 4 3 2 1

First Printing

Library of Congress Cataloging-in-Publication Data

Brain imaging: applications in psychiatry / edited by Nancy C. Andreasen.
    p. cm.
    Includes bibliographies.
    ISBN 0-88048-229-X
    1. Mental illness—Diagnosis.   2. Brain—Imaging.
    I. Andreasen, Nancy C.
  RC473.B7B73 1988
  616.89'07572—dc19   88-16775
                                          CIP

Contents

Contributors

Nancy C. Andreasen, M.D., Ph.D.
Department of Psychiatry
University of Iowa College of Medicine
Iowa City, Iowa

Jeffrey A. Coffman, M.D.
Department of Psychiatry
Ohio State University Hospital
Columbus, Ohio

Michael D. Devous, Sr., Ph.D.
Nuclear Medicine Center
The University of Texas
Health Science Center at Dallas
Dallas, Texas

Henry H. Holcomb, M.D.
University of Maryland
Psychiatric Research Center;
Johns Hopkins University
School of Medicine
Division of Nuclear Medicine
Baltimore, Maryland

Jonathan Links, Ph.D.
Johns Hopkins University
School of Medicine
Division of Nuclear Medicine
Baltimore, Maryland

John M. Morihisa, M.D.
Professor and Chairman, Department of Psychiatry
Georgetown University School of Medicine
Washington, D.C.

Caroline Smith, Ph.D.
National Institute of Mental Health
Laboratory of Cerebral Metabolism
Rockville, Maryland

Dean Wong, M.D.
National Institute of Mental Health
Laboratory of Cerebral Metabolism
Rockville, Maryland

Introduction

Understanding the brain offers us the hope that we may be able to understand ourselves as human beings. Since its origins psychiatry has recognized that the brain is its principal province. As psychiatrists, we are fortunate to have the most interesting and complex organ of the body as our area of specialization. From the brain derive most functions that characterize us as human beings: the capacity to speak, to think creatively, to develop abstractions, to form loyalties and attachments, to plan for the future, and a host of other functions. Unfortunately, hating, destroying, and killing with forethought and malice also appear to be primarily human characteristics that derive from the brain. Many symptoms of mental illness appear to represent distortions of normal brain functions or loss of such functions. For example, hallucinations are abnormal auditory, visual, or tactile perceptions, while delusions are abnormalities of inferential thinking. Affective blunting or poverty of speech and thought (alogia) represent a diminution of such normal brain functions as the capacity to express emotions freely or to think and speak fluently. Understanding the brain offers the hope that we may eventually understand the mechanisms of major mental illnesses and ultimately develop methods for treating them or perhaps even preventing them.

During the 19th century psychiatrists were heady with excitement over the possibility of learning more about the brain, for at that time techniques for studying neuropathology were being developed, using new stains such as the Nissl or Golgi stains. It soon became clear, however, that examining neuronal structure alone would not suffice. Examining brain structure, even at the cellular level, did not yield adequate power to resolve such difficult functions as thinking, feeling, and believing. Further, postmortem techniques have many inherent limitations, such as artifactual effects of the death process, the necessity to study predominantly elderly individuals, and a scarcity of informative samples of brain tissue. Consequently, during most of the 20th century, psychiatry retreated from the study of the brain because suitable techniques were not available.

Within the past several decades, the situation has changed dramatically. The development of brain imaging is one major reason for this change.

Brain imaging refers to a related group of techniques that permit us to study the structure and function of the human brain in people while they are still living. These techniques are not invasive. Some, such as computed tomography (CT) or nuclear magnetic resonance imaging (NMR or MRI) are similar to a simple x-ray from the patient's point of view, although NMR does not even require the use of ionizing radiation. Positron emission tomography (PET), the most complicated and demanding, still only requires an intravenous injection. The oldest of these techniques to enjoy wide clinical use, CT, was first performed in 1971 and became available clinically over the next decade. Techniques and applications for the others are still in their infancy. Prior to CT, we were able to see only the skull with x-ray techniques, or at best to obtain an outline of the ventricles to make inferences about the brain through the complicated process of pneumoencephalography. Now we can actually obtain clear pictures of the structures of the brain and observe it as it thinks and solves problems.

Brain-imaging techniques are divided into two broad categories: structural techniques, and dynamic or functional techniques. CT and MRI are the two major structural techniques. Both are useful in visualizing brain anatomy. CT is still the most widely available and best understood, but in many centers it will be supplemented with MRI during the coming years. CT is useful for observing cortical atrophy, ventricular enlargement, tumors, and strokes. Because CT is limited to visualizing structures seen in a transverse plane, its applications for reconstructing three-dimensional anatomy are limited. MRI has some advantages over CT, in that it does not use ionizing radiation, permits visualization in a variety of planes (including coronal and sagittal in addition to transverse), and is exquisitely sensitive for detecting white-matter lesions such as multiple sclerosis plaques. CT has already proved useful in exploring brain abnormalities in the major psychoses, and MRI promises to have similar, and perhaps better, applications as well.

CT and NMR permit only the study of structure and anatomy, but the dynamic or functional techniques allow us to observe the brain in action. The three major functional techniques are computerized mapping of the electrical activity of the brain (sometimes referred to as brain electrical activity mapping or BEAM), regional cerebral blood flow (rCBF) which is based on single photon emission computerized tomography (SPECT), and positron emission tomography (PET). Each of these techniques permits us to examine brain metabolism and regional variations in brain activity. The electrical activity mapping techniques are limited to observing changing patterns in the frequency of brain waves, but both SPECT and PET permit a direct observation of cerebral performance and metabolic activity. In addition, PET currently permits study of neurotransmitter systems and the effect of drugs on chemical activity, and SPECT has promising potential for this as well. These functional techniques permit the observation of cognitive activation, especially through stimulation with tasks designed to activate such cognitive functions as verbal memory. Clearly, these techniques have great promise for mapping cognitive function in normal individuals and observing abnormalities in patients suffering from mental illness.

This book has been designed to make brain-imaging techniques more accessible to a broad range of readers, including both clinicians and researchers. Heretofore, no single book existed which provided in-depth coverage of all existing brain-imaging techniques. Readers were required instead to read a book on a single technique, such as NMR or PET, or to go to articles found chiefly in radiological journals in order to understand these techniques.

This book consists of five chapters designed to explicate each of the major brain-imaging techniques: CT, MRI, BEAM, SPECT, and PET. Each chapter begins with a brief introduction to the specific technique and thereafter provides a more detailed description of its basic principles and applications in psychiatry. The section on basic principles will provide detailed technical information for those who want it, such as how the scanners are constructed, how they produce images, how the images can be interpreted, how the scanning techniques can be modified, and the kinds of scanning equipment available (including a discussion of cost, relative strengths and weaknesses of commercially available systems, access and availability within university and non-university settings, and so on). This section on basic principles should be particularly useful to individuals who want to undertake research or to have an in-depth understanding of it.

Individuals interested primarily in clinical aspects of brain imaging may wish to scan the section on basic principles relatively quickly and to focus primarily on the second section, which deals with applications in psychiatry. This section will provide a critical overview of the research conducted to date with each of the brain-imaging techniques, and discuss when and if it is appropriate to order such procedures. In the case of technologies not yet widely available, such as PET, the chapters will describe opportunities for referring patients elsewhere. This section will assist in answering questions such as: When should I order a scan? What will it tell me? Is it diagnostically useful? In addition, each chapter will discuss strengths, limitations, and cost of the particular technique covered in the chapter and will compare it to other techniques. Finally, each chapter will discuss technological advances likely to occur in the future, future applications in research, and future clinical uses.

Each chapter has been written as an independent unit, so that readers interested in a single technique can study it in depth without referring to other chapters. While this may produce some redundancy in the book (for example, PET studies will be discussed in both the SPECT and PET chapters), it also makes study easier for readers with limited time. Each technique can be studied as a separate module.

It is hoped that a broad range of readers will find this book to be a useful map in exploring one of the most exciting frontiers in psychiatry— the localization of cognitive activities in the brain and the study of the mechanisms that govern them. This book includes a substantial amount of technical information about how the various brain-imaging methods actually work, because we wish to permit an in-depth coverage of each topic for those readers who wish it. Yet our goal has also been to make these techniques clear and accessible and clinically informative. At present, brain imaging is a collection of techniques used primarily for research. But as this field advances during the next decade, these techniques will be more frequently used clinically as well. This book is intended to help readers keep in touch with the progress that is occurring in our knowledge and understanding of the brain.

Nancy C. Andreasen, M.D., Ph.D.

Chapter 1

Computed Tomography in Psychiatry

Jeffrey A. Coffman, M.D.

Computed tomography (CT), although not the first radiologic technique to allow visualization of the brain in living persons, rapidly superseded its predecessors, due to the greatly enhanced quantity and quality of information afforded through the computerized processing of x-ray transmission data. CT and other imaging techniques described in this book allow a wide variety of structural and functional information to be collected from living human beings in a way scarcely imaginable a few decades ago. Perhaps if psychiatrists in the 1940s and 1950s had known such techniques would shortly become available, they would not have despaired of finding anatomical and physiologic bases for mental disorders.

This chapter will explore the technical underpinnings of computed tomography from its early theoretical bases to initial practical applications and the ultimate development of rapid, high-resolution scanners. The rapidity with which these developments occurred is in itself a fascinating story. In addition, this chapter will summarize the many studies of psychiatric patients that have been made using this technique. Studies in computed tomography of psychiatric patients are still being conducted and published. Consequently, this chapter should not be considered the final word on computed tomography in psychiatry.

TECHNICAL ASPECTS OF COMPUTED TOMOGRAPHY

Development of Computed Tomography

The mathematics of reconstruction imaging, which provide the basis for many of the recent innovations in medical imaging, were derived around

1917 by an Austrian mathematician, J. Radon (1917), who was working at the time on problems related to gravitational fields. Further developments of reconstruction techniques as an imaging tool came in solar astronomy (Bracewell 1956) and electron microscopy (DeRosier and Klug 1968). Oldendorf (1961) was the first to recognize the clinical imaging potential of reconstruction tomography and constructed a prototype CT scanner. In the early 1960s Kuhl and Edwards (1963) adapted the technique of image reconstruction to problems in nuclear medicine and developed a crude version of emission CT.

Parallel to these early developments, in 1956 a South African medical physicist, Cormack, became interested in correcting for tissue inhomogeneities as they affected dosage requirements of patients undergoing radiation therapy. Such corrections required accurate knowledge of whether the radiation had attenuated in tissue across anatomic planes through the patient. Cormack realized that a cross-sectional matrix of attenuation coefficients could be determined if measurements of the amount of x-ray radiation transmission could be obtained at multiple angles and projections through the body. He also recognized that these coefficients could be displayed as an image of internal anatomy. He reported two experiments, in 1956 and in 1963, the second of which involved study of a nonsymmetrical phantom and use of a computer to process the transmission data obtained by passing ^{60}Co gamma rays through 7.3-degree angular increments. The results were greeted with nothing more than a yawn, though Cormack later shared the 1979 Nobel Prize in physiology or medicine with Hounsfield for this early work. Its further development awaited availability of better, less expensive computers.

Although a number of investigators were, in the late 1960s and early 1970s, exploring various approaches to reconstruction tomography, the principal breakthrough in reconstruction imaging was the work of Hounsfield, an engineer at the Central Research Laboratories of Electro-Musical Instruments (EMI), Ltd., in England. In 1967, while investigating pattern-recognition techniques, he became convinced that there were many areas of endeavor where large amounts of data were lost due to inefficiency in data retrieval. He deduced, independently of Cormack, that images from the body's interior could be reconstructed from measurements of x-ray transmissions taken from all possible directions through the body, with the most convenient approach being a tomographic one. Hounsfield's preliminary calculations led him to the conclusion that measurements of the x-ray attenuation in a slice could be made with an accuracy of 0.5% without excessive radiation dosage, nearly 100 times better than was possible with conventional methods, due to the greater sensitivity of photomultiplier tubes over radiographic film.

The first laboratory device consisted of an americium gamma ray source and a sodium iodide detector mounted on a lathe bed which provided rotation in 1-degree steps at the end of each linear scan. The device produced useful reconstruction data, although a complete study required 9 days, and accuracy was only 4%. To improve accuracy and shorten data-acquisition time, a conventional x-ray tube and a crystal/photomultiplier detector were brought into play, providing accuracy approaching 0.5%, requiring a scanning period of 9 hours, and allowing images of biological specimens to be obtained.

The first computed tomographic scanner for clinical scanning of the human head was installed in 1971 at the Atkinson Morley's Hospital in Wimbledon. The scanner used simultaneous translation of the x-ray source and detector, with each translation occurring in a separate angular increment of 1 degree over a 180-degree arc. A water bag was placed around the patient's skull to make the transmission path length of the x-rays equal in all directions. Over a period of 4½ minutes, 28,800 transmission measurements were obtained, with a later period of 20 minutes required for image reconstruction.

Clinical data were first published in 1973 (Hounsfield 1973a, 1973b), and in the same year the first commercial CT scanners were installed. In the four years that followed, CT technology proceeded through four generations of scanners, with progressively improved mechanical design yielding shorter scan times. A brief discussion of these mechanical features follows.

In the first scanner marketed by EMI, whose basic features are shown in Figure 1, the x-ray beam is collimated (focused) into two thin parallel beams directed toward two sodium iodide scintillation detectors on opposite sides of the patient, allowing collection of data for two adjacent images of the patient's head. The x-ray source and detectors are attached to a common frame that allows them to move in a synchronous linear scanning motion across the patient, obtaining 240 measurements of x-ray transmission. At the end of this linear motion, the frame rotates 1 degree and the process repeats as data are accumulated. Altogether the frame is rotated by one degree 180 times, providing 43,200 transmission measurements which are delivered to a computer. From these measurements, using 43,200 simultaneous equations, a series of CT numbers is computed to be stored and displayed as a gray-scale image on the display unit. The first CT scanner display utilized an 80×80 matrix of 6,400 picture elements or pixels, though the available 43,200 data points would have allowed a 160×160 matrix with 25,600 pixels, which was in fact later substituted.

In early first-generation scanners, the patient's head was surrounded by a water-filled rubber bag so that the x-rays passed through no air,

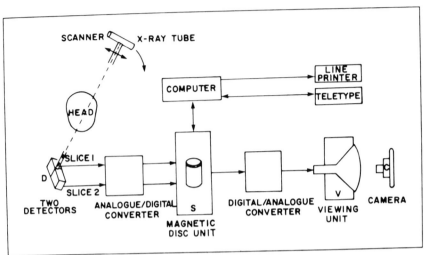

FIGURE 1. Diagram from the first Hounsfield publication on computed tomography. This diagram shows how signals from two detectors are digitized, stored in a magnetic disc, processed by computer, and displayed on a viewing unit or printed on a line printer. Reproduced with permission from Hounsfield GN: Computerized transverse axial scanning (tomography), 1: description of system. British Journal of Radiology 46:1016, 1973.

minimizing the potential changes in x-ray transmission and the need for wide-ranging detectors, simplifying computations and improving accuracy. These early scanners required 4½ minutes for data collection and 5 minutes for computation of CT numbers to make up a single image. Though computations could be performed while the scanner accumulated data for the next image, a total of 35 minutes was needed for accumulation and processing of a 6-image study. Although adequate for studies of the head, the lengthy motionlessness required provided an impetus toward development of faster scanners.

Second-generation CT scanners introduced minor modifications that reduced data collection times for a single plane section to around 20 seconds, and later to 5.3 seconds. However, respiratory movements still interfered with abdominal scans, and further efforts to shorten scan time led to a third generation of CT scanners. By simplifying scanner motion from the combination of translation and rotation that had characterized first- and second-generation scanners, to an exclusively rotational motion with the x-ray tube and detectors synchronously rotating around the patient, scan times were reduced to 5, and even as little as 2.5, seconds. Extending the search for faster scans still further to the fourth generation brought stationary detector rings, a rotating x-ray source, and scan times of

1.5 seconds. Fifth-generation scanners use multiple x-ray sources and reduce scan times to as little as 16 milliseconds.

Physical Principles of Computed Tomography

Computed tomographic imaging systems measure the attenuation of x-ray beams passing through target tissue. This attenuation is the result of various absorption and scattering processes, three of which are important in the energy range of x-rays utilized in CT: coherent scattering, photoelectric absorption, and Compton scattering.

In coherent scattering, which occurs only rarely with the high-energy, highly filtered x-ray beams used in CT, an x-ray is diverted from its original path with little loss of energy, as shown in Figure 2. In photoelectric interactions all of the energy of an x-ray is transferred to an electron in an inner orbital of an atom within the target medium. The x-ray disappears as a result and the electron is ejected from the atom, as shown in Figure 3.

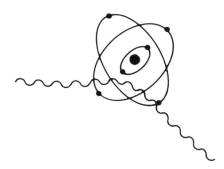

FIGURE 2. Coherent scanning in which an x-ray is scattered with negligible energy loss after interaction with the cloud of electrons in an atom. Reproduced with permission from Hendee WR: Interactions of x and gamma rays, in Medical Radiation Physics: Roentgenology, Nuclear Medicine and Ultrasound (2nd Edition). Chicago, Year Book Medical Publishers, 1979.

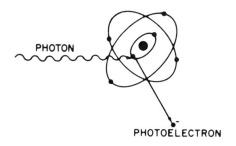

PHOTON

PHOTOELECTRON

FIGURE 3. Photoelectric interaction in which the energy of the x-ray is transferred completely to an electron. The electron (termed a photoelectron) is ejected from the atom with a kinetic energy $E_\kappa = E_x - E_\beta$. Reproduced with permission from Hendee WR: Interactions of x and gamma rays, in Medical Radiation Physics: Roentgenology, Nuclear Medicine and Ultrasound (2nd Edition). Chicago, Year Book Medical Publishers, 1979.

In Compton scattering, the x-ray interacts with an outer electron of an atom in the target and part of the x-ray's energy is transferred to the electron, which is then ejected from the atom, and a new x-ray of different energy careens off in a new direction. The probability of Compton scattering increases with increasing electron density (electrons per gram) and physical density (g/cm^3) of the target medium. A principal influence on electron density is the hydrogen content of the medium, since hydrogen has two or more times the electron density of any other element.

For a high-energy, filtered x-ray beam such as that found in CT, almost all scattering in soft tissues is due to Compton interactions. Only in materials with high atomic numbers and densities, such as bone and contrast media containing iodine, are photoelectric scatterings important.

The number of x-rays attenuated in a medium can be expressed in the following relationship: $P = \mu I$, where P is the removal rate of x-rays from the incident beam by absorption and scattering, I is the number of incident x-rays, and μ is the attenuation coefficient of the medium for the x-rays. If P is expressed as a function of path length, then μ becomes known as the linear attenuation coefficient. If all the x-rays in the beam were of the same energy, narrowly focused and unscattered, then the number I of x-rays penetrating a target of thickness x is $I = Io \, C^{-Mx}$ where Io is the number of incident x-rays. In this case the transmittal x-ray intensity would yield a straight line when plotted semilogorithmically.

In CT, x-ray tubes provide the incident x-rays yielding a spectrum of x-rays with a transmission of:

$$I = \sum_{k=1}^{n} Io \, (E_k)e^{-M(E_k)x}$$

In general the linear attenuation coefficient $\mu(E_k)$ is greater for lower energy x-rays. Therefore, the average energy of an x-ray beam increases with depth in the medium as lower energy components are gradually peeled off. This nonlinear change in beam energy with depth leads to the beam-hardening artifact characteristic of CT images, which will be discussed further below.

During the CT image-reconstruction process, the CT number computed for a material is related to the linear attenuation coefficient μ of the material for the effective energy of the beam (a corrected value allowing for beam hardening). This relationship given in Hounsfield units (Hu) is as follows:

$$Hu = 1000 \, \frac{\mu - \mu_v}{\mu_w} = 1000 \, \frac{\mu}{\mu_w} - 1000$$

where μ_w represents the attenuation coefficient of water. In Hounsfield units, air has a value of $-1,000$ and water a value of 0. CT numbers do not vary greatly with changes in x-ray beam energy or filtration, and they remain relatively constant from one scanner to another because they are derived as the ratio of attenuation coefficients of various materials and water. The physical characteristics of the absorbing materials then become the primary influences on CT numbers, particularly the physical density of the materials in g/cm[3]. For most soft tissues, CT numbers should vary closely with the mass density of the absorbing substance. The tight correlation between CT number and mass density for various soft tissues is shown in Figure 4.

Image Reconstruction in Computed Tomography

In a single CT scan across one section in a patient, thousands of x-ray transmission measurements are obtained along many transmission rays through many different angular projections. From these measurements, utilizing a variety of mathematical paradigms, a matrix of CT numbers can be computed for the cross-sectional plane through the patient and later displayed as a gray-scale image. There are three major paradigms for image construction: 1) simple back-projection, 2) filtered back-projection, and 3) iterative reconstruction (Hendee, 1983).

Simple Back-Projection

If a series of x-ray transmission measurements were made at different

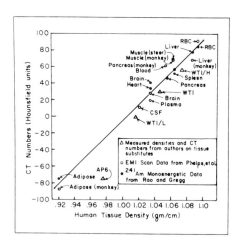

FIGURE 4. CT numbers measured for excised tissue samples and tissue-simulating plastics, plotted against best estimates of tissue and tissue-substitute mass densities. Reproduced with permission from Fullerton GD: Fundamentals of CT tissue characterization, in Medical Physics of CT and Ultrasound: Tissue Imaging and Characterization. Edited by Fullerton GD, Zagzebski JA. New York, American Institute of Physics, 1980.

orientations across a single plane through the cube shown in Figure 5, the x-ray transmission data shown on the axes would result.

For simple back-projection, each transmission ray is divided into 10 parts. On the x axis each ray shows either 30 or 40% transmission or, conversely, 80 or 60% attenuation. Transmission is presumed to be linear, with each portion of the ray absorbing equally. Therefore, each tenth provides 6% attenuation along the 40% transmission rays and 8% along the 20% transmission along both axes. In Figure 5 these attenuation figures are added along the single plane to show the effect of back-projecting the transmission data. In the cross-hatched area, projected attenuations of 8% per element from each axis combine to provide a total attenuation of 16%. In the diagonally hatched elements, a projected attenuation of 8% from one axis adds to an attenuation of 6% from the other axis to provide a total attenuation of 14%. Attenuation totals 12% for the clear elements. Differences in shading similarly combine to provide a gray-scale reproduction of the plane through the cube; with more rays and views the reproduction comes to more nearly resemble the object.

Images constructed using this simple method are less than satisfactory, since the projected attenuations are averaged for the entire path length of the ray. As a result a star or spoke pattern can result in the reconstructed image if dense regions are present in the scanned object.

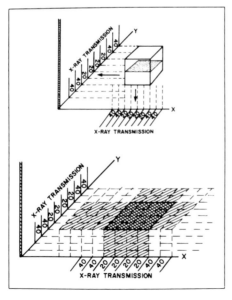

X-RAY TRANSMISSION

X-RAY TRANSMISSION

FIGURE 5. Conceptual mathematics of simple back-projection. *Top:* x-ray transmission across a single plane of the cube measured from two orientations at right angles to each other. The measurement plane is indicated by closely spaced dots. *Bottom:* The percent attenuation is divided equally among each of 10 parts of each ray, and the attenuations are added in each intersecting element to yield values of 16% (8% + 8%) in each cross-hatched element, 14% (6% + 8%) in each diagonally hatched element, and 12% (6% + 6%) in each clear element. Reproduced with permission from Hendee WR: Physical Principles of Computed Tomography. Boston, Little, Brown, and Company, 1983.

Filtered Back-Projection

To minimize the spoke artifacts and fuzziness of back-projected images, the x-ray transmission data can be modified prior to image generation. This modification adds negative components to the back-projected data so that the spokes are significantly minimized, and proper selection of the modifying filter functions reduces image blurring. The process is illustrated in Figure 6.

    With this method of combining projection data with a filter function, the convolution method is rapid, accurate, and can be implemented during data acquisition, with the result that it has become the most widely used method of image reconstruction in CT scanning.

Iterative Reconstruction

In applying an iterative reconstruction technique, values for the matrix of attenuation-coefficient numbers are initially assumed. As transmission data are obtained, the assumed coefficients are found to be inaccurate and corrections are made to produce better agreement with the actual transmission data. This process is repeated many times, or iterated, with successive corrections becoming progressively smaller until a satisfactory set of CT numbers is obtained.

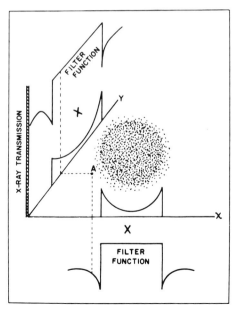

FIGURE 6. x-ray transmission data from Figure 5 convolved with a filter function to improve the sharpness of the reconstructed image. The point A outside the object received a positive contribution from the filter function on the y axis and a negative contribution from the filter function on the x axis. Reproduced with permission from Hendee WR: Physical Principles of Computed Tomography. Boston, Little, Brown, and Company, 1983.

When iterative techniques are used, all the x-ray transmission data must be collected prior to reconstruction. This adds delay to scanning, and so this method is infrequently used for newer, faster third- and fourth-generation scanners.

Image Display and Recording

The attenuation-coefficient numbers are stored as an array of values by a computer. In order to provide an image, this matrix of values must be converted into a suitable display form such as video monitor. Three major considerations arise regarding proper display and storage of CT images. They are 1) adjustment of the video display parameters of contrast and brightness; 2) selection of level and window settings to optimize the display of anatomic structures of interest within the video gray scale; 3) image recording for long-term storage.

Every video device possesses its own gray scale, ranging from its darkest to its brightest illumination. Contrast controls determine the degree of change, as is the case with any video monitor.

One major advantage of CT viewing is the ability to *window* anatomic tissues of interest. Windowing (window width) refers to the process of assigning to a certain discrete range of attenuation values, characterizing certain tissues, the entire distribution of the monitor's gray scale. For instance, the level setting assigns the middle of the video gray scale to a certain CT number, while the window setting defines the total gray-scale range. By way of example, a head CT could be viewed at a level of +50 and a window of 200 CT units. As +50 corresponds to the vicinity of CT numbers for gray and white matter, these tissues will be displayed at mid-gray illumination. With a window of 200 CT units, the range of CT numbers displayed will be from −50 to +150. All tissues with CT numbers greater than 150 will appear white while those below −50 will appear black. At these settings, bone, calcifications, and pooled blood will appear light, and cerebrospinal fluid dark. If the full tissue range of −1000 to +1000 would be displayed, particular tissues of interest (i.e., gray and white matter) would be limited to a relatively small range of grays with little illumination difference.

Image Storage

By tradition and for convenience and economy, CT images have been recorded on film. However, there are advantages to also storing the actual attenuation-coefficient numbers on computer tape, since these values can be subsequently manipulated to enhance features of interest other than those originally recorded on film. Commonly available modification features include magnification or various other image-enhancement routines.

Interpretation of Computed Tomographic Data

Artifacts in Computed Tomography

There are a number of artifacts that affect the performance of CT scanning and the quality of available data. These artifacts can be of sufficient severity to lead to streak patterns on image display or may, more subtly, appear in the form of CT number inaccuracies. Though classification of these artifacts has proved troublesome (Joseph 1981), one proposed approach involves subdivision according to the stage in data collection when the artifacts are introduced (Villafana 1983). These are summarized in Table 1 and will be discussed in turn.

Patient Motion

As previously noted, the measurements of x-ray transmission that go into the process of CT scanning result from passage of rays along different angles around the patient. If the ray paths do not always intersect the same volume units of tissue such that attenuation data are consistent (or, in other words, if variations in ray paths contribute to assignment of different values to the same pixel), streak artifacts result. The most common cause of such inconsistencies is patient motion. Patient motion was a particular problem in early, slow scanners. When motion during the scan occurs, the computer is unable to determine where a given tissue volume element or

TABLE 1. Major CT Artifacts

Generation Step	Source
x-ray transmission phase	Patient motion
	Polychromatic effects
	Equipment misalignment
	Faulty x-ray source
x-ray detection and measurement	Detector imbalance
	Detector nonlinearity
	Scatter collimation
Data acquisition	Slice geometry
	Profile sampling
	Angular sampling
Data processing	Algorithm effects

voxel is in space or which attenuation data sums belong in which column or row of the data matrix. The result is streaking, which is increased by the presence of high-density structures such as bone within the scan field. Motion also introduces potential losses in spatial and density resolution though these are overweighed by streaks. Faster scan times have progressively reduced the significance of motion as a source of artifact.

Polychromatic Effects

The spectral or polychromatic nature of the x-ray source in CT leads to a number of artifactual changes in CT data due to a process labeled *beam hardening*. An attenuation-coefficient value is provided for each voxel. Attenuation coefficients vary with the energy of the incident x-ray photon, and x-ray beams are made up of a population of x-ray photons with a distribution of energys. As the beam traverses the patient, the lower-energy photons are more readily absorbed, and the average beam energy increases as a result, or it "hardens." The effect is one of generally lowering the set of attenuation values for each beam path. As measurements are made, a given voxel will have a variable attenuation value assigned depending on the particular path of a particular beam. The result is a pattern of dark streaks as the assigned lower attenuation values imply lower tissue density. The effect is greatest in the vicinity of dense bony structures, giving rise to the dark streaks commonly seen in the anterior and posterior cranial fossae.

Beam hardening also produces a consistent increase of CT number values for soft tissues adjacent to bony structures such as the edge of the skull. This increase in values was at first interpreted as the cerebral cortex (Hounsfield 1973b), though its artifactual nature was soon discovered (Gado and Phelps 1975). The basis for this change, also referred to as *cupping*, is that rays passing through the periphery of a structure are less hardened than those passing through the center. Therefore the central regions are assigned relatively lower, and peripheral regions relatively higher, CT values than they would be if hardening did not occur. A number of alterations in reconstruction algorithms have been proposed to deal with this effect (Brooks and DeChiro 1976; Duerinck and Macovski 1978). Although current CT scanners include some corrective measures in their reconstruction algorithms, further correction (using bone-correction algorithms) often requires time-consuming off-line processing and is therefore only rarely used.

Equipment Misalignment

Mechanical misalignment of the x-ray source and detectors can lead to another form of streak artifacts (Shepp and Stein 1977). Another misalignment problem occurs in 180-degree view, leading to a vertical streak along the edges of the object. A sweep greater than 180 degrees will minimize this artifact.

Faulty X-Ray Source

When x-ray source output varies, data inconsistencies result because detectors cannot separate changes in radiation level due to changes in output from changes due to increased or decreased absorption along the x-ray path. In spite of corrections made for single-angular views by reference detectors, variations between views lead to crisscrossing streak artifacts (Joseph 1981).

Detector Imbalance

Each detector in an array must be matched in response to the others. When imbalance occurs, ring artifacts result. This imbalance can result from individual detector gain shifts, with shifts of as little as 0.1% causing visible artifacts. Automatic detector calibration during examination corrects for these difficulties in first-, second-, and fourth-generation scanners.

Detector Nonlinearities

Ideal detector response would be directly proportional to the amount of x-radiation striking it. Factors contributing to nonlinear response include dark current (response in the absence of radiation), saturation (detector output maximal at a point where incident energy is increasing), and hysteresis (continual output after irradiation ceases). All these can produce data inconsistencies and lead, again, to streak formation.

Scatter Collimation

X-Ray scatter can occur around a very dense object where, although x-ray intensity behind the object should be low, scattering of the x-rays striking the object will provide detectable radiation levels higher than actually transmitted. These spurious elevations around the object are inconsistent with data obtained from ray paths not intersecting the dense object, producing streak artifacts.

Partial Volume Effect

The interposition of linear slice geometry on the CT representation of nonlinear anatomic structures leads to an artifact that is less immediately obvious. This artifact can be explained by recalling that the pixel on the CT screen represents a CT number assigned to a particular voxel or volume element of the slice, which is determined by its area and the slice thickness. A voxel may intercept more than one tissue type, such as gray matter and cerebrospinal fluid, but the assigned CT number will represent an average attenuation parameter for the entire voxel. For example, if half of a voxel contains tissue with a CT number of 50 and the remainder of the voxel contains tissue with a CT number of 0, the voxel is assigned a CT number of 25. The voxel will be displayed as a pixel with value 25, which is invalid. The partial volume artifact then leads to a loss of spatial and tissue resolution.

Another artifact results from the divergence of the x-ray beam as it passes through the patient. The slice is therefore not uniformly thick but varies through the scan volume. The size of partial volume effect then becomes a function of position, with greatest artifact at the periphery of the slice.

Profile Sampling

During the detection process, each detector intercepts and averages that portion of the x-ray transmission information (or profile) which occurs over its face. This sampled profile, as transmitted to the computer, is then only a somewhat degraded representation of the actual profile. The averaging smooths out peaks and valleys in the data, leading to a lessening of spatial and tissue resolution. Moreover, some information passes undetected in the spaces between detectors. These effects are a function of detector size and spacing, with increases in either leading to signal degradation and a special form of streak artifact known as *aliasing* that results from bogus features introduced by the averaging process. Closely packed, small detectors would obviously minimize this particular problem.

Angular Sampling

Sampling can be deficient in a given profile as well as in the number of angular views sampled. Angular undersampling leads to streaks separated some distance from small dense objects, although profile undersampling appears the more important of the two sampling effects (Brooks et al. 1979).

Algorithm Effects

The algorithms used to process the data acquired in computed tomography may also contribute artifactual information to the final image data not previously caused by the sampling factors discussed above. One such algorithmic effect involves the use of an edge-enhancement algorithm that can lead to a false subarachnoid space. Another has been described by Joseph (1981) and involves scanning long, straight-edged, bony structures. Approximations applied in reconstruction algorithms lead to streaks along the edges. In first- and second-generation scanners these can be lessened by narrower collimators, while smaller detectors are helpful in third- and fourth-generation units. Additional help comes from filtering to provide a more monochromatic x-ray beam.

CT Number Accuracy

Several factors limit the absolute accuracy of CT numbers. These include x-ray beam energy (kilovoltage) and spectral distribution, tissue location and structure, partial volume effect, and algorithm and calibration shifts. Since CT numbers reflect the x-ray attenuation, tissue density, and therefore, inferentially, tissue structure, considerable effort has been applied to the study of these data. However, there is the question about the validity of the numbers.

First of all, CT numbers are dependent on the incident x-ray energy. In general the CT number of any material having a lower atomic number than water rises with x-ray energy increases, while substances of higher atomic number than water show decreases in CT number (Zatz 1976). Correlation of CT numbers from different units therefore depends on close calibration of incident x-ray energy in kilovolts.

Beam hardening also plays a significant role in determining the accuracy of "density" numbers, particularly since differing tissue thicknesses lead to differing beam paths and degrees of beam hardening. As noted previously, beam hardening tends to artificially lower CT numbers in the center of a homogeneous object and to produce elevations or spillover of CT numbers adjacent to very dense portions of inhomogeneous objects. Tissue thickness-induced changes in beam hardening lead to the apical artifact, in which the progressively small tissue sections of the head toward the apex have progressively higher CT numbers (DiChiro et al. 1978). Partial volume effect and algorithm functions also affect CT number accuracy. All these factors require caution in comparing CT numbers from place to place, from scanner to scanner, and even from scan to scan.

CT Imaging: Further Performance-Related Issues

Beyond artifact-related difficulties, three major areas of concern arise regarding the information available from computed tomography: spatial resolution, contrast resolution, and image noise.

Spatial resolution refers to the ability of an imaging system to display two closely associated small structures as distinct objects. The spatial resolution of CT images is in the range of 1–2 mm for the x–y dimension of the slice with the slice thickness determining the third. In CT this resolution factor is determined primarily by the focusing or collimation of the x-ray beam as it strikes the detectors. Another factor is the reconstruction algorithm of the system. As noted above the trend in CT design has led to smaller collimators and more detectors being added to the detector ring. More space is occupied by collimators, and less x-ray energy reaches the detector, causing an increase in image noise.

It is important to note that in modern CT units the video display may offer greater "resolution" than is actually possible with CT. For instance, the display of a 300 × 300-mm section of tissue on a device having a 512 × 512-pixel image matrix provides that each pixel displays a 0.59 × 0.59-mm area of tissue. This implies a spatial resolution of about 0.6 mm, much finer than the 1–2-mm resolution defined by the x-ray data itself. It is apparent that the display must interpolate to provide image information which does not exist.

Slice thickness also influences the quality of image data, as it is varied from 2 to 15 mm by controlling the thickness of the x-ray beam. As the beam is narrowed, fewer x-ray photons contribute to the image data and noise increases. This can only be overcome by increasing the x-ray energy delivered. On the other hand, increasing slice thickness leads to added difficulty with partial volume effect. Again, a trade-off ensues.

Contrast resolution refers to the discrimination possible between regions of differing physical density. With CT this resolution is 0.5 to 1%, meaning that 0.5 to 1% differences in x-ray transmission are discernible. Noise in the image is the primary detractor in contrast resolution. Image noise reflects the number of photons absorbed by radiation detectors, which provide the data used to form an image.

Image-noise imprecision is referred to as *quantum mottle* and remains one of the major limitations to contrast resolution in computed tomography (Joseph 1978; Riederer et al. 1978). A simple illustration of quantum mottle follows (Hendee 1983). If a structure has an x-ray transmission that differs by 2% from that of the surrounding medium, how many x-rays would be needed to form a distant image with 95% confidence?

A 95% confidence level corresponds to a 200 $\sigma/N = 2\%$, 100 $\sigma/N = 1\%$ of 0.01. The statistics of x-ray transmission follow a Poisson distribution where $\sigma = N$. Therefore,

$$\sqrt{N}/N = 1\sqrt{N} = 0.01$$
$$\sqrt{N} = 100$$
$$\text{and}$$
$$N = 10,000$$

Thus, 10,000 x-rays must be transmitted and detected if a 2% transmission difference is to be revealed with 95% confidence. By inference, 100 x-rays would produce a noisier image, and a 20% difference would be needed for detection to occur with the same confidence.

The above example, although it shows the influence of quantum mottle on conventional radiography, fails to account for CT images due to the multiple angular source of absorption data. It is illustrative of the relationship between x-ray dose and image noise. Other noise-related factors are contributed by the radiation detectors and round-off errors in the reconstruction algorithm.

CT STUDIES IN PSYCHIATRIC PATIENTS

Not long after the application of Roentgen's rays to the observation of skeletal structures, attempts to apply various means to enhance visualization of the soft-tissue structures of the brain began. The method used, pneumoencephalography, involved entering the lumbar cistern in the subarachnoid space and withdrawing sufficient cerebrospinal fluid (CSF) to allow the injection of air which filled the cerebral ventricles and spaces surrounding the surface of the cortex (Dandy 1918). The application of the technique to the study of psychiatric disorders, particularly schizophrenia, began shortly thereafter (Jacobi and Winkler 1927) and continued until the early 1970s, when computed tomography became the established technique for evaluating intracranial structures. Due to the inconvenience and discomfort associated with the procedure, pneumoencephalography never became a widely applied technique in the clinical study of schizophrenia. However, as summarized by Weinberger and Wyatt (1982), pneumoencephalography contributed a number of observations: that schizophrenics appeared to possess enlarged lateral cerebral ventricles, enlarged third ventricles, and widened cortical sulci. Interestingly, these findings were also sometimes found to be associated with negative symptoms such as apathy or flattened affect and with cognitive impairment and poor outcome. The technique also posed many limitations, however, and consequently a noninvasive technique such as CT was greeted with open arms by psychiatric researchers and clinicians. The availability of this practical technique opened the way for a broad range of research.

Schizophrenia

The severe and chronic disability associated with schizophrenia has made it the focus of a variety of investigations designed to expand our understanding of the neuropathologic processes underlying the disorder. When computed tomography became a feasible clinical research tool, it was quickly applied to a sample of chronic schizophrenics, who showed significantly more ventricular enlargement than did control individuals of similar age (Johnstone et al. 1976). Thereafter the field developed rapidly.

Lateral Ventricular Enlargement

The lateral cerebral ventricles are CSF-filled spaces which are in close proximity to central forebrain structures such as the thalamus, hypothalamus, limbic system, and basal ganglia. Abnormalities in development or pathological atrophy of the structures adjacent to the cerebral ventricles or more distant structures can lead to lateral ventricular enlargement, since any decrease in brain tissue leads to replacement by fluid in the ventricular system. Ventricular enlargement is a nonspecific finding (Snyder 1982; Nasrallah et al. 1982a). In spite of the difficulty of pointing to pathology in a specific structure when one finds lateral ventricular enlargement, it seems clear some change in brain structure invariably must lead to a change in the anatomy of the ventricular systems, since the ventricular system has no structure of its own other than that imposed by the surrounding brain.

Many of the cases of ventricular enlargement noted in psychiatric patients, including schizophrenics, would be considered subtle, and in fact most CT scans of schizophrenic patients are read as "within normal limits for age" by neuroradiologists. Therefore, special techniques of measurement have emerged to allow comparison with control populations. The first measurement methods used were closely related to the linear measurement of ventricular size which had been applied to pneumoencephalograms. The indices developed for CT included the Huckman Index, which was the ratio of anterior horn span over the width of the brain at the same point; the cella media index, the ratio of the anterior horn span over the width of the brain at the same point; and the cella media index, the ratio of the maximum width of the anterior horns of the lateral ventricles and the width of the brain (Huckman et al. 1975; Meese et al. 1976). These linear measurements, though readily determined, were found to lack sensitivity to subtle changes and not to correlate well with ventricular volume (Penn et al. 1978).

Due to the problems with these linear measurement techniques, Synek and Ruyben (1976) promulgated the idea of computing a ventricular brain ratio (VBR). As first described, an area of measurement was determined with a planimeter, a mapping device used to measure closed two-dimensional areas. With this technique the outline of the lateral ventricles and brain on the CT films (see Figure 7) is traced, and the ratio

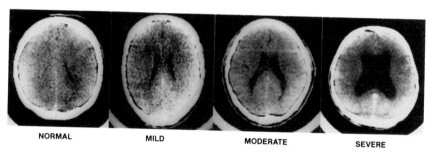

| NORMAL | MILD | MODERATE | SEVERE |

FIGURE 7. Increasing degrees of cerebral ventricular enlargement are shown looking from left to right.

of these areas is usually expressed as a percentage. Similar techniques include computer-based tracing (Andreasen et al. 1982b) and calculation of VBR by determination of the total number of picture elements represented by ventricle and brain using their relative density numbers (Jernigan et al. 1979). None of these ventricular measurement techniques is perfect, with the most common measurement error occurring in the assessment of structural boundaries, as discussed above in relation to partial volume effect. The determinations using density numbers are potentially less subjective, but affected by inaccuracies inherent in CT numbers themselves and algorithmic errors in assigning CT number values to specific structures.

A substantial number of studies of the lateral ventricular system in schizophrenia, using CT, have emerged. The results of some 40 of these studies will be discussed here. Of these studies, 31, or around 3/4, demonstrate a significant degree of ventricular enlargement in schizophrenic patients as compared to nonpsychiatric control samples. Many of the negative studies, such as those by Benes et al. (1982) and Jernigan et al. (1982a), differed from the other studies in methods of measurement, nature of control groups, and patient-selection criteria. The results of the studies are summarized in Table 2.

Several of the studies discussed here included linear measurements of ventricular size, which have limited sensitivity to subtle degrees of ventricular enlargement. Only four of seven studies using linear measures showed significant increases in lateral ventricular size in schizophrenics. This difference in results may reflect the diminished sensitivity of linear measurement to detection of ventricular enlargement.

Another source of variance in the results of studies of ventricular enlargement is that of the criteria used in selecting a control population. Many of the control populations used in studies of schizophrenics are patients scanned for a variety of reasons, and radiologically determined to

TABLE 2. CT Studies of Lateral Ventricular Enlargement in Schizophrenia

Study	Sample Characteristics	Method	Presence of Significant Enlargement
Johnstone et al. 1976, 1978	17 chronic schizophrenics (Feighner) 8 normal volunteers	planimetric VBR	+
Trimble and Kingsley 1978	11 schizophrenics (NR) v. literature control values	Evans Index	−
Weinberger et al. 1979a	66 chronic schizophrenics (RDC) 7 acute schizophrenics 56 normal volunteers	planimetric VBR	+ +
Moriguchi et al. 1981	55 schizophrenics (NR) 65 medical controls	volumetric reconstruction	+
Weinberger et al. 1981	10 schizophrenics (RDC & Feighner) 12 siblings 17 normal volunteers	planimetric VBR	+
Tanaka et al. 1981	49 schizophrenics (NR) 38 medical controls	width of anterior horns and cella media	+
Okasha et al. 1981, 1982	43 schizophrenics (NR) 39 medical controls	Cella Media Index	+
Takahashi et al. 1981	280 "nuclear" schizophrenics (IPSS) 234 volunteers and psychiatric controls	Cella Media Index	+

TABLE 2. *(continued)*

Study	Sample Characteristics	Method	Presence of Significant Enlargement
Pearlson and Veroff 1981	22 schizophrenics *(DSM-III)* 16 affective disorder 35 psychiatric controls	pixel count	+ +[a]
Johnstone et al. 1981	111 institutionalized schizophrenics (NR) 18 outpatient schizophrenics 10 institutionalized manic-depressives 22 outpatient manic-depressives 8 "neurotics"	planimetric VBR	+ + +[a] +[a]
Benes et al. 1982	10 schizophrenics (Feighner) 26 medical controls	Cella Media Index planimetric VBR	–
Frangos and Athanassenas 1982	70 schizophrenics (NR) literature controls	NR	+
Andreasen et al. 1982b, 1982c	52 schizophrenics *(DSM-III,* RDC) 47 medical controls	planimetric VBR (video cursor)	+
Reveley et al. 1982	7 schizophrenics (RDC) 7 discordant monozygotic twins	pixel counts	+
Nasrallah et al. 1982b	41 schizophrenics (Tsuang–Winokur) 40 medical controls	bifrontal ratio bicaudate ratio	–

TABLE 2. CT Studies of Lateral Ventricular Enlargement in Schizophrenia *(continued)*

Study	Sample Characteristics	Method	Presence of Significant Enlargement
Nyback et al. 1982	28 schizophrenics (RDC) 13 probable schizophrenics 2 schizoaffective 3 other psychosis 46 normal volunteers	bifrontal ratio	−
Jernigan et al. 1982a	29 schizophrenics *(DSM-III,* RDC) 13 normal volunteers	pixel counts planimetric VBR	−
Nasrallah et al. 1982b, 1982c	55 schizophrenics *(DSM-III,* Feighner) 24 manic depressives 27 medical controls	planimetric VBR	+ +[a]
Weinberger et al. 1982a	35 schizophreniform *(DSM-III)* 17 chronic schizophrenics 27 affective disorders 27 other psychiatric disorders 26 medical controls	planimetric VBR	+ + +[a]
Kling et al. 1983	26 schizophrenics *(DSM-III)* 13 alcoholics 9 neurological patients 20 medical controls	planimetric VBR	+ +
Reider et al. 1983	28 schizophrenics (RDC) 15 schizoaffectives 19 bipolar	planimetric VBR	−[a]

TABLE 2. *(continued)*

Study	Sample Characteristics	Method	Presence of Significant Enlargement
Woods and Wolf 1983	19 schizophrenics (RDC) 29 medical neurological controls	bifrontal ratio bicaudate ratio	+
Schulz et al. 1983a	8 schizophreniform 8 borderline	planimetric VBR	+
Pearlson et al. 1984, 1985	19 schizophrenics *(DSM-III)* 27 bipolars 19 controls *v.* schizophrenics 19 controls *v.* bipolars	planimetric VBR	+ +[a]
DeMeyer et al. 1984	8 schizophrenics 7 other psychiatric disorders 15 medical, neurological controls	planimetric VBR	–
Luchins et al. 1984	45 schizophrenics (RDC) 27 affective disorders 62 medical, neurological controls	planimetric VBR	+ +[a]
Pandurangi et al. 1984	23 schizophrenics *(DSM-III)* 34 normal volunteers and neurological controls	planimetric VBR	–
Schulsinger et al. 1984	7 schizophrenics 11 schizotypals 13 medical controls	planimetric VBR	+ +[a]

TABLE 2. CT Studies of Lateral Ventricular Enlargement in Schizophrenia *(continued)*

Study	Sample Characteristics	Method	Presence of Significant Enlargement
Largen et al. 1984	35 schizophrenics and schizoaffectives 17 medical, neurological controls	planimetric VBR (video cursor)	−
Carr and Wedding 1984	21 schizophrenics (RDC, *DSM-III*) 21 medical controls	planimetric VBR	+
Shelton et al. 1984	73 schizophrenics *(DSM-III)* 30 normal volunteers	planimetric VBR	+
Shima et al. 1985	46 schizophrenics *(DSM-III)* 46 normal volunteers and neurological controls	Evans Index Cella Media Index	−
Boronow et al. 1985	30 schizophrenics, schizoaffectives (RDC) 30 medically ill controls	planimetric VBR	−
Williams et al. 1985	31 schizophrenics (RDC) 9 schizoaffectives 40 neurological controls	Pixel Count	+
Owens et al. 1985	128 schizophrenics (institutionalized) 120 outpatient schizophrenics, affective disorders, and neurotics	planimetric VBR (video cursor)	+

TABLE 2. *(continued)*

Study	Sample Characteristics	Method	Presence of Significant Enlargement
Turner et al. 1986	30 schizophrenics *(DSM-III)* 26 normal volunteers	Pixel Count	+
DeLisi et al. 1986	26 schizophrenics *(DSM-III)* 10 well siblings 20 nonpsychotic controls	planimetric VBR	+
Nasrallah et al. 1986	11 schizophrenics *(DSM-III)* serving as own controls	planimetric VBR	+
Obiols-Llandrich et al. 1986	33 chronic schizophrenics *(DSM-III)* 25 medical controls	planimetric VBR	+

Key to Abbreviations:

NR = Method not reported

a = No difference between schizophrenics and psychiatric control group

RDC = Research Diagnostic Criteria

Feighner = Feighner Criteria

IPSS = Criteria of the International Pilot Study of Schizophrenia

DSM-III = *Diagnostic and Statistical Manual, 3rd Ed.*

Tsuang–Winokur = Tsuang–Winokur Criteria (Tsuang and Winokur 1974)

VBR = ventricle–brain ratio

have "normal" scans. As quite a number of medical conditions can lead to evidence of transient or permanent ventricular enlargement on CT scan, the use of such patients would tend to bias against the detection of a significant difference from the schizophrenic group, a potential type 1 error. This seems to be the case in the studies discussed here, where half of those studies comparing schizophrenics with neurologic patients revealed ventricular enlargement, whereas nearly 90% of those studies in which normal volunteers were used as controls revealed significant differences in ventricular size. Therefore, careful screening of potential controls for those medical and neurological disorders which can be associated with ventricular enlargement needs to be implemented in studies of ventricular size. It has been argued though that medically ill or institutionalized subjects provide better control comparisons with schizophrenic populations in that length of hospitalization and superimposed medical illness could occur in the schizophrenic population as well. However, as will be noted below, age, duration of illness, length of hospitalization, and other factors have not been correlated with ventricular enlargement in schizophrenics. So it may be that a normal control population does indeed provide a useful comparison.

The choice of patients is a third factor that may affect results of CT studies. Clinical and pathologic features of schizophrenia may have some relationship to degree of ventricular enlargement. Most studies of schizophrenic patients that show substantial differences in ventricular size from control subjects involve patients who are severely ill. Two negative studies, those of Jernigan et al. (1982a) and Benes et al. (1982), involved young, relatively unimpaired, often employed and married schizophrenic patients who tended to perform well on tests of cognitive performance. This suggests that patients with a more favorable initial presentation and "better prognosis" tend to show less evidence of ventricular enlargement. A study of young adolescent schizophrenics by Schulz et al. (1983a) indicates that ventricular enlargement in schizophrenia is not due to aging or chronicity, however, since these young patients showed prominent ventricular enlargement.

The meaning of ventricular enlargement in schizophrenia is unclear, but it has raised many questions about the relationship of the finding to a variety of clinical and demographic variables, such as the nature and extent of prior treatment and hospitalization, duration of illness, and age. Age has been shown to correlate strongly with ventricular size in a variety of populations including normal volunteers (Barron et al. 1976; Haug 1977; Earnest et al. 1979), control populations of CT studies of schizophrenia (Moriguchi 1981; Nyback et al. 1982; Andreasen et al. 1982a; Luchins et al. 1984; Shelton et al. 1984), and individuals with affective disorders (Rieder et al. 1983; Pandurangi et al. 1984). On the other hand, many studies have shown no clear relationship between age and ventricular size among schizophrenics either across the entire age range (Barron et al. 1976; Moriguchi 1981; Andreasen et al. 1982a; Nyback et al. 1982; Nasrallah et al. 1982a; Woods and Wolf 1983; Luchins et al. 1984; Schulsinger et al. 1984; Shelton et al. 1984; Owens et al. 1985; Williams et al. 1985; Nasrallah et al. 1986; Obiols Llandrich et al. 1986) or in young schizophrenics, who show ventricular enlargement very early in the course of their illness (Nyback et al. 1982; Weinberger et al. 1982a; Kling et al. 1983; Schulz et al. 1983a; Turner et al. 1986; Obiols Llandrich et al. 1986). All of these results, especially follow-up studies of the same individuals (Owens et al. 1985; Nasrallah et al. 1986), suggest that ventricular enlargement in schizophrenia tends to occur early in the illness and that it changes little over the course of time.

In addition, little relationship has been found between the degree of ventricular enlargement in schizophrenia and the extent and duration of treatment with neuroleptics, history of electroconvulsive therapy, duration of illness, or total duration of hospitalization (Johnstone et al. 1976, 1982; Trimble and Kingsley 1978; Nasrallah et al. 1982a; Schulsinger et al. 1984; Williams et al. 1981, 1985; Frangos and Athanassenas 1982; Owens et al. 1985; Jernigan et al. 1982a; Weinberger et al. 1979a; Andreasen et al. 1982c; Nyback et al. 1982; Golden et al. 1980b). The results of Weinberger et al. (1982b), Schulz et al. (1983b), and Nyback et al. (1982) showing that ventricular enlargement is present early and after little or no neuroleptic treatment. Those patients of Johnstone et al. (1976) who were treated only with institutionalization suggest that ventricular dilatation in schizophrenia does not stem from these clinical variables.

A number of studies of ventricular enlargement in schizophrenia have suggested that the finding might be used to subtype the disorder. The first suggestion that ventricular enlargement might relate to clinical parameters useful for subtyping came from the study of Johnstone et al. (1976), in which there was a significant relationship between increased ventricular size and cognitive impairment on the Withers and Hinton test (Withers and Hinton 1971). In a further study (Johnstone et al. 1978) the relationship continued to be apparent. Also these other tests of cognitive impairment showed a relationship between poor performance and the degree of "negative" symptomatology associated with the patient's illness. Johnstone and associates proposed that these individuals with large ventricles and poor cognitive performance represented a subgroup of patients with the "dementia of dementia praecox" as previously described by Kraepelin (1971) and Jaspers (1963). Following the lead of the Johnstone et al. group, Donnelly et al. (1980) used the Halstead–Reitan Battery (HRB), a standard neuropsychological test for cognitive impairment.

Those patients with enlarged lateral ventricles performed poorly. Using an average impairment rating of 1.55 or above across the subtests of the HRB, the investigators were able to predict in 12 of 15 cases whether a patient would fall within or outside the control range of ventricular size.

Two studies by Golden et al. (1980b, 1982) have also confirmed the relationship of ventricular enlargement to poor performance on neuropsychological testing in patients with schizophrenia. Some questions regarding the nature of the relationship of ventricular size to cognitive impairment in schizophrenics are raised by Owens and associates who found a curvilinear (inverted U) relationship (Owens et al. 1985). However, many studies have suggested that ventricular enlargement measured by CT and cognitive impairment seem to be related in many schizophrenics.

A number of other clinical findings have been found to be associated with ventricular enlargement. They include poor premorbid adjustment, persistent unemployment, a lower incidence of "positive symptoms" (bizarre delusions, hallucinations, and so forth), increase prevalence of "negative symptoms" (apathy, anhedonia, impoverished affect, social isolation, and so on), poor response to neuroleptic treatment, and an increased incidence of extrapyramidal side effects with neuroleptic treatment (Williams et al. 1985; Weinberger et al. 1980; DeLisi et al. 1983; Pearlson et al. 1984, 1985; Andreasen et al. 1982b; Luchins et al. 1984; Naber et al. 1985; Smith et al. 1983; Schulz et al. 1983a; Luchins et al. 1983a, 1983b).

Third Ventricular Enlargement

The third ventricle is the midline component of the cerebrospinal fluid system, which is connected to the anterior horns of the lateral ventricles through the foramina of Monroe and empties into the fourth ventricle through the aqueduct of Sylvius. Surrounding this ventricular space are the structures of the thalamus, hypothalamus, fornix, and habenula, all of which have been suggested as pathologically involved in schizophrenia (Neito and Escobar 1972; Stevens 1982).

Assessment of the size of the third ventricle is usually made by measuring its maximum width, since most pathologic conditions producing its expansion do so in its lateral extent. With the exception of situations in which the ventricle is too narrow to be seen, its diameter can readily be determined in transverse views. In addition to the studies which assess the size of the third ventricle by maximum width, two groups, Nyback et al. (1982) and Largen et al. (1984), have used a variation of the VBR method, tracing the outline of the ventricle and the perimeter of the brain in the slice in which the ventricle is seen, for a third-ventricular brain ratio. Both methods of assessing third-ventricular size have led to positive results in studies of schizophrenia.

To date there have been 15 third-ventricular studies of schizophrenia which are summarized in Table 3. Of these 15 studies, 13 showed a significant increase in mean third-ventricular size in schizophrenics as compared to controls. Nine of 11 studies using medical patients or neurological patients for controls showed a significant enlargement among schizophrenics, as did the 2 studies which used normal volunteers as controls (Nyback et al. 1982; Shelton et al. 1984). In a study by Boronow et al. (1985), where the control group consisted of medically ill patients, schizophrenics continued to show enlargement of the third ventricle even though there were no differences apparent in lateral ventricular size. This difference was present even though subsets of the medical control group such as those receiving chemotherapy for cancer showed third-ventricular enlargement. This suggests that perhaps the third ventricle is less often subject to enlargement from the various causes of lateral ventricular enlargement and is therefore less likely to be confounded than is the finding of lateral ventricular enlargement.

Relationships of other variables to third-ventricular enlargement have been studied less completely than have findings in regard to lateral ventricular enlargement. The age of the subject studied appears to correlate with third-ventricular size among normal volunteers (Nyback et al. 1982; Shelton et al. 1984; Meese et al. 1976). When medically ill controls were used this relationship did not appear (Moriguchi 1981). Among schizophrenic patients this relationship is unclear, with two studies demonstrating a correlation (Nyback et al. 1982; Schulz et al. 1983a). Several studies have demonstrated an association of third-ventricular enlargement with duration of illness and total number of hospitalizations (Rieder et al. 1983; Tanaka et al. 1981; Nyback et al. 1982; Gattaz et al. 1981). In contrast, Moriguchi (1981) could find no association with age of onset or duration of illness, and Boronow et al. (1985) reported finding no linkage to any of a wide variety of variables including length of illness, cumulative hospitalizations, nature of prior treatment, premorbid adjustment, symptom complex, subtype of schizophrenia, and so on. Although these findings suggesting an absence of a relationship do not convincingly demonstrate its absence, one possible explanation for such discrepant findings would be that third-ventricular enlargement simply occurs in a broad cross section of the schizophrenic population.

Widened Cortical Sulci

Another indicator of relative loss of brain tissue and displacement by cerebrospinal fluid is the presence of widened cortical sulci. It is pre-

TABLE 3. Third Ventricular Enlargement in Schizophrenia

Study	Sample Characteristics	Presence of Significant Enlargement
Gluck et al. 1980 Mundt et al. 1980	68 schizophrenics (NR) 68 medical controls	−
Moriguchi 1981	55 schizophrenics (NR) 65 medical controls	+
Takahashi et al. 1981	280 schizophrenics (IPSS) 234 medical controls	+
Tanaka et al. 1981	49 schizophrenics (NR) 38 medical controls	+
Okasha et al. 1981, 1982	43 schizophrenics (NR) 39 medical controls	+
Gattaz et al. 1981	40 schizophrenics (RDC) 40 medical controls	+
Nyback et al. 1982	28 schizophrenics (RDC) 18 psychiatric controls 46 normal volunteers	+
Dewan et al. 1983a	23 schizophrenics *(DSM-III)* 23 medical, neurological controls	+
Pandurangi et al. 1984	23 schizophrenics 23 neurological controls	+
DeMeyer et al. 1984	8 schizophrenics *(DSM-III)* 7 psychiatric controls 15 medical controls	+
Largen et al. 1984	30 schizophrenics (RDC) 5 schizoaffectives 17 medical, neurological controls	−
Shelton et al. 1984	73 schizophrenics *(DSM-III)* 30 normal volunteers	+
Boronow et al. 1985	23 schizophrenics (RDC) 7 schizoaffectives 30 medical controls	+
Nasrallah et al. 1985	55 schizophrenics 27 medical controls	+

Key to Abbreviations: NR = Not reported
RDC = Research Diagnostic Criteria
IPSS = Criteria of the International Pilot Study of Schizophrenia
DSM-III = Diagnostic and Statistical Manual, 3rd Ed.

sumed that the relative increase in CSF space over the surface of the cortex is due to shrinkage of the cortical gyri. This finding, like that of ventricular enlargement, is often associated with dementing illness, although it is not invariably present even in the face of severe cognitive deficits (Huckman et al. 1985; Fox et al. 1975; Roberts and Caird 1976; DeLeon et al. 1979; Jacoby et al. 1980a, 1980b). Figure 8 shows CT scans of the cortex displaying various degrees of gyral shrinkage.

It has proved difficult to develop a clearly superior method of rating sulcal widening; therefore, at least three approaches have been used. All of them are affected by partial volume artifacts and the beam-hardening artifacts referred to in the technical section of the chapter, to an even greater extent than in any of the other CSF-filled-space assessments previously discussed. One common method involves variations on the measurement of the widths of various sulci and fissures (Pearlson and Veroff 1981; Tanaka et al. 1981; Okasha et al. 1981; Okasha and Madkour 1982; Kling et al. 1983; Pandurangi et al. 1984; Gluck et al. 1980; Mundt et al. 1980; Dewan et al. 1983). The next most common method has been subjective visual evaluation of the degree of atrophy with or without use of a standard reference scale (Meese et al. 1976; Rieder et al. 1983; Turner et al. 1986; Takahashi et al. 1981; Nasrallah et al. 1982c; Oxenstierna et al. 1984). This method provides for gross judgment of the degree of atrophy present. Still another method of assessing an increase in CSF space at upper levels on the CT scan involves the use of a computer algorithm similar to that used for evaluation of the ventricular space filled with CSF, in which a criterion density number is used to correspond to tissue and one is also set for fluid values. Then for the entire slice the pixel counts for both tissue and fluid are summed for comparison. This method is typified by the work of Jernigan et al. (1982a).

Table 4 summarizes 21 CT studies of sulcal widening. Nearly two-thirds, or some 14 of the studies, revealed significant increases in the schizophrenics as compared to controls. This finding does appear to be

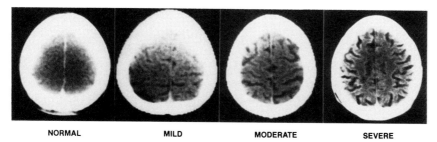

NORMAL   MILD   MODERATE   SEVERE

FIGURE 8. Increasing degrees of cerebral atrophy are shown moving from left to right.

TABLE 4. Studies of Cortical Sulcal Widening in Schizophrenia

Study	Sample Characteristics	Method	Presence of Significant Widening
Johnstone et al. 1978	17 schizophrenics (Feighner) 8 normal volunteers	total sulcal area	+
Weinberger et al. 1979b	60 schizophrenics (RDC) 62 normal volunteers	sum of widths of Sylvian, interhemispheric fissures and 3 largest sulci	+
Gluck et al. 1980	68 schizophrenics (NR) 68 medical controls	width of anterior horns and number of sulci 3 mm × 1 mm in top two slices	−
Mundt et al. 1980	68 schizophrenics (NR) 68 medical controls	number of sulci 3 mm × 1 mm in top two slices	−
Pandurangi et al. 1984	23 schizophrenics (DSM-III) 23 medical controls	width of Sylvian fissures, frontal, parietal, and occipital sulci	+
Tanaka et al. 1981	49 schizophrenics (NR) 38 medical controls	width of Sylvian fissures visual assessment of cortical surface	+
Pearlson and Veroff 1981	22 schizophrenics (DSM-III) 16 affective disorders 35 psychiatric controls	width of 3 largest sulci	+ +[a]
Okasha et al. 1981, 1982	43 schizophrenics (NR) 39 medical controls	sum of widths of Sylvian and interhemispheric fissures and 3 largest sulci	−

TABLE 4. *(continued)*

Study	Sample Characteristics	Method	Presence of Significant Enlargement
Takahashi et al. 1981	169 schizophrenics (IPSS) 169 volunteer and psychiatric controls	visual inspection	+
Nyback et al. 1982	28 schizophrenics (RDC) 18 psychiatric controls 46 normal volunteers	visual inspection 0–3 scale	+
Nasrallah et al. 1982b	41 schizophrenics (Tsuang–Winokur) 40 medical controls	visual inspection	+
Nasrallah et al. 1982a, 1983b	55 schizophrenics (*DSM-III* and Feighner) 24 bipolar disorders 27 medical controls	visual inspection 0–3 scale	+ +[a]
Jernigan et al. 1982a	29 schizophrenics (*DSM-III* and RDC) 13 volunteer controls	pixel counts	–
Kling et al. 1983	29 schizophrenics (*DSM-III*) 13 alcoholics 9 neurological controls 20 medical controls	Sylvian fissure width	–[a]
Rieder et al. 1983	28 schizophrenics (RDC) 19 schizoaffectives 19 bipolar disorders	visual inspection 0–2 scale	[a]
Dewan et al. 1983a	23 schizophrenics (*DSM-III*) 23 medical, neurological controls	Sylvian fissure width	+

TABLE 4. Studies of Cortical Sulcal Widening in Schizophrenia (*continued*)

Study	Sample Characteristics	Method	Presence of Significant Widening
Oxenstierna et al. 1984	30 schizophrenics (RDC)	visual inspection	+
Largen et al. 1984	30 schizophrenics (RDC) 5 schizoaffectives 17 medical, neurological controls	visual inspection 0–4 scale	−[a]
Shelton et al. 1984	73 schizophrenics (*DSM-III*) 30 normal volunteers	visual inspection parieto-occipital atrophy 0–3 scale prefrontal atrophy 0–3 scale	+
Boronow et al. 1985	23 schizophrenics (RDC) 7 schizoaffectives 30 medical controls	visual inspection 0–3 scale	−[a]
Turner et al. 1986	30 schizophrenics (*DSM-III*) 26 normal volunteers	Sylvian and interhemispheric fissures, cortical sulci 0–6 scale	+

Key to Abbreviations:

NR = Not reported
[a] = No difference between schizophrenics and affective disorder groups
RDC = Research Diagnostic Criteria
Feighner = Feighner Criteria
IPSS = Criteria of the International Pilot Study of Schizophrenia
DSM-III = *Diagnostic and Statistical Manual, 3rd Ed.*
Tsuang–Winokur = Tsuang–Winokur Criteria

somewhat affected when medical or neurologic patients are used as controls, since only 6 of 11 studies using such controls found differences between groups, whereas 5 of 6 studies using normal volunteers found a greater degree of sulcal widening among schizophrenics.

Among normal controls and patients with illness other than schizophrenia, both the presence and degree of cortical atrophy has appeared to correlate positively with age and degree of cognitive impairment (Huckman et al. 1975; Jacoby et al. 1981; Fox et al. 1975; Jacoby and Levy 1980; Naeser et al. 1980; Bondareff et al. 1981; Bird 1982). On the other hand, age did not correlate with degree of cortical atrophy in most studies of schizophrenics (Nyback et al. 1982), although two studies did demonstrate relationships between the degree of cognitive impairment and sulcal widening, compared with four matched schizophrenic controls without such widening, performance on the Halstead–Reitan Battery distinguishing the groups. All four individuals with atrophy were found to be "impaired" on the Battery. Nasrallah et al. (1983b) grouped patients into those with and without evidence of sulcal widening. Of the 22 subjects with such widening, 27% fell below the cutoff score of the Mini Mental Status Exam (Folstein and McHugh 1975), implying some degree of cognitive impairment, while none of the 33 patients without atrophy performed below the cutoff level. This relationship obviously requires further study.

Other clinical symptom correlates of sulcal widening have been studied only in very limited fashion, and therefore firm conclusions are difficult to reach. Weinberger et al. (1979b) reported no apparent connection between the presence of atrophy and the length or duration of illness but did find four of the patients in the study who had received ECT showed more atrophic changes than those who had not received ECT. Nasrallah et al. (1983b) also failed to find any differences in duration of illness, severity, premorbid adjustment and family history of schizophrenia, neuroleptic response, or positive and negative symptoms between those patients with and without sulcal widening. This absence of correlation differs markedly from that seen in studies of lateral ventricular size and suggests that cortical atrophy may bear a stronger relationship to cognitive impairment. However, since cortical atrophy occurs only rarely in isolation, samples examining this finding alone may as yet be too small to demonstrate significant relationships.

In considering sulcal widening in schizophrenics, most studies regarded the process as a diffuse one comparable to the changes induced by Alzheimer's disease, although a few studies have focused more selectively on certain regions of the brain. When measurements of the Sylvian fissure are reported, that region of the fissure measurable on CT lands primarily between the frontal and temporal cortices. Pandurangi et al. (1984) examined overall sulcal widening, the width of the Sylvian fissure, and reported differences only for the latter fissure. Takahashi et al. (1981), in comparing 169 schizophrenic patients and an equal number of controls, found highly significant differences in widening of the Sylvian fissure and sulci of the frontal cortex bilaterally; slight differences in sulci of the right temporal region; and no differences in comparing left temporal, parietal, and occipital regions. Tanaka et al. (1981) also found atrophy localized to frontal and temporal regions with no change apparent in parietal and occipital cortex, while Oxenstierna et al. (1984) found sulcal widening was limited to the dorsolateral prefrontal cortex in four of the ten patients with cortical atrophy. A further study by Shelton et al. (1984) evaluated schizophrenics in comparison with normal controls using scales delineating either generalized or prefrontal cortical atrophy and found no differences between groups on the generalized scale but marked differences between groups on the prefrontal atrophy scale with over half the schizophrenics showing some evidence of atrophy. Therefore, atrophy in schizophrenia may be more prominent in prefrontal and temporal regions than in other areas of the brain.

Cerebellar Atrophy

Atrophy of the cerebellum is not a particularly common finding among the general patient population undergoing CT scans, with only around 1% of routine CT scans in large surveys demonstrating findings consistent with cerebellar atrophy (Allen et al. 1979; Koller et al. 1981). CT evidence of atrophy can result from diminution in tissue volume of the cerebellar hemispheres, vermis, or nuclei. Such atrophy can occur in degenerative diseases primary to the cerebellum, cancer, alcoholism, and a chronic diphenylhydantoin treatment.

Due to its anatomical location, the cerebellum is not well seen on computed tomographic scanning. This occurs in particular because of the juxtaposition of the bony posterior fossa and related beam-hardening artifact and the inadequacy of the transverse plane of view for demonstrating the structures of the cerebellum. Atrophy has been assessed, however, with reasonable reliability through a variety of approaches. Methods involving assessment of the dimensions of the fourth ventricle, cisterna magna, and cerebellar vermis have been made, as have assessments of tissue density, presence of vermian folia, and qualitative visual inspection for the presence or absence of atrophy. Varying degrees of cerebellar atrophy can be seen in Figure 9.

The CT studies of cerebellar atrophy are summarized in Table 5. One can see that there are widely divergent findings reported, with the percentage of patients showing atrophy ranging from 0 to 50%. Given the

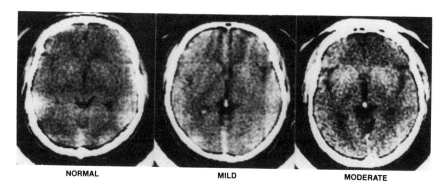

NORMAL   MILD   MODERATE

FIGURE 9. Increasing degrees of cerebellar atrophy are shown moving from left to right.

wide variability in measurement techniques, such differences in results seem to be explicable, although there may be some population differences which also account for the variety of results. However, in 7 of the 10 studies that made an attempt to assess the rate of cerebellar atrophy, these rates fall between 5% and 17%, suggesting that one could estimate the rate of atrophy at about 10% in the schizophrenic population. This is much greater than that noted in the population at large. However, it does not seem to differ from the rate observed in other psychiatric illnesses, particularly affective disorders.

The etiology of the atrophy demonstrated is not known and very little has been done to demonstrate any relationship to clinical variables. Dewan (1983) was unable to demonstrate any association of cerebellar atrophy with age or duration of hospitalization. Since the cerebellum and especially the cerebellar vermis is sensitive to chronic drug toxicity, examples being diphenylhydantoin and ethanol, one possibility is that the atrophy demonstrated in schizophrenics might be due to chronic exposure to neuroleptic drugs. In this regard it should be noted that the limited number of studies of first-episode patients have not demonstrated cerebellar atrophy.

Cerebral Asymmetry

Cerebral asymmetry refers to the anatomical asymmetry of homologous brain structures in the left and right cerebral hemispheres. Variations in the sizes of the paired structures have been known since the beginning of the 20th century, though significant controversy has surrounded them (Von Bonin 1962). With the advent of CT a number of commonly reproduced findings have emerged involving asymmetry of width or volume of

TABLE 5. Cerebellar Atrophy in Schizophrenia

Study	Sample Characteristics	Method	Results
Weinberger et al. 1979c	60 schizophrenics (RDC) 15 other psychiatric disorders	visual inspection	atrophy + 10/60 schizophrenics 0/15 other psychiatric disorders
Heath et al. 1979	85 schizophrenics (NR) 31 other psychoses	2 vermian folia visible	atrophy + 34/85 schizophrenics 9/31 other psychoses
Coffman et al. 1981	14 schizophrenics (DSM-III) 21 medical, neurological controls	vermis to brain ratio	atrophy −
Nasrallah et al. 1981	43 schizophrenics (DSM-III) 15 affective disorders 36 medical controls	hemisphere sulci > 1 mm presence of vermian folia enlargement of 4th ventricle or cerebellar cistern atrophy = 1 of 4 criteria	atrophy + 5/43 schizophrenics 4/15 manics 1/36 controls
Pearlson et al. 1981	22 schizophrenics (DSM-III) 16 affective disorders 35 psychiatric controls	NR	atrophy + 1/22 schizophrenics 0 affective 0 controls
Nasrallah et al. 1982b	41 schizophrenics (DSM-III, Tsuang–Winokur) 40 medical controls	visual assessment	atrophy + 4/41 schizophrenics significantly different
Nasrallah et al. 1982a	55 schizophrenics (DSM-III, Feighner) 24 affective disorders 24 medical controls	visual assessment 0–3 scale	atrophy + 5/55 schizophrenics 5/24 affective 1/24 controls

TABLE 5. *(continued)*

Study	Sample Characteristics	Method	Results
Lippman et al. 1982	54 schizophrenics *(DSM-III)* 18 affective disorders 79 unspecified controls	visual assessment 1–3 scale	atrophy + 16/54 schizophrenics 5/18 affective 4/79 controls
Heath et al. 1982	50 schizophrenics *(DSM-III)* 64 other psychoses 1586 psychiatric controls	size of cerebellar cisterns density assessment–vermis	atrophy + 25/50 schizophrenics 34/64 other psychoses 74/1586 psychiatric controls
Weinberger et al. 1982a	17 schizophrenics *(DSM-III)* 23 affective disorders 62 other psychiatric disorders 26 medical controls	presence of 2 vermian folia	atrophy + 2/17 schizophrenics 2/23 affective disorders 0 other groups
Dewan et al. 1983b	23 schizophrenics *(DSM-III)* 23 medical neurological controls	width 4th ventricle and vermis intermastoid ratio, density assessments	Atrophy + width 4th ventricle, vermis
Rieder et al. 1983	28 schizophrenics (RDC) 15 schizoaffective disorders 19 affective disorders	visual assessment	atrophy + 2/28 schizophrenics 1/15 schizoaffective 2/19 affective

Key to Abbreviations: NR = Not reported
RDC = Research Diagnostic Criteria
Feighner = Feighner Criteria
DSM-III = Diagnostic and Statistical Manual, 3rd Ed.
Tsuang–Winokur = Tsuang–Winokur Criteria

the frontal and occipital lobes. Among right-handed normal individuals there is a greater than expected incidence of larger right frontal and left occipital lobes, a finding confirmed through neuropathological studies (Weinberger et al. 1982b), CT (LeMay and Kido 1978), human cranial fossils, and nonhuman primate skulls (LeMay 1976). It has been suggested that this asymmetrical pattern is the result of lateralization of certain cerebral functions such as speech (Galaburda et al. 1978; LeMay 1977). Interest in the possibility of altered cerebral lateralization in schizophrenia has been spurred by findings such as increased frequency of left-handedness (Oddy and Lobstein 1972; Boklage 1977) and verbal intellectual deficits.

Computed tomographic assessment of these anatomical asymmetries can be done in a variety of ways. Some investigators have used a clear, millimeter ruler to measure the width of the frontal or occipital lobes on each side at the level of the third ventricle. Variants of this method have included projecting the image to actual scale in order to maximize potential width discrepancies, and measurement of the lobes on more than one slice. The relative difference in length of the two hemispheres, or *petalia*, can also be measured. In addition, some investigators have measured the individual lobes by planimetry. A significant source of error in these measurements involves incorrect positioning of the head in the CT scanner, producing a tilted image and secondarily producing spurious differences in the dimensions of structures providing inconsistent planes of section. This problem can be overcome by observing bony landmarks in other slices for symmetry and excluding scans which have been obtained at an angle. A summary of CT studies of asymmetry in schizophrenia can be found in Table 6. A few positive studies have appeared, although the majority have failed to demonstrate a significant difference between groups in the number of "reversed" anatomical asymmetries. It is not entirely clear why such differences have not been consistently established, but the problem does not seem to be one of patient sampling or clinical variables such as age, duration of illness, premorbid adjustment, neuroleptic exposure, and so forth (Luchins and Meltzer 1983). Therefore, it remains unclear as to whether there are any significant alterations in cerebral asymmetry in schizophrenics, although it seems that finding is not particularly robust.

Brain Density

Computed tomography, as previously discussed, is primarily a sophisticated method for comparing within-subject differences in tissue radiodensity. The processing of these data into a video and/or film image makes them more readily understandable and interpretable but limits the information available. Therefore a number of attempts have been made to peer more closely at CT density data in spite of the many sources of artifact noted earlier.

A variety of conditions affecting the brain reflect tissue damage in CT-density changes. Tissue damage following stroke produces areas of hypodensity which are often visible on plain radiographs. Williams and Walshe (1981) have shown that Wilson's disease produces damage to the basal ganglia visible as radiolucent areas on CT films which can resolve following treatment with penicillamine. In senile dementia, brain density abnormalities are less readily seen on film presentation. However, Naeser et al. (1980) demonstrated significantly lower CT density numbers in demented as compared to depressed elderly individuals. Bondareff et al. (1981) reported mean density values to be significantly lower in patients with senile dementia when compared with controls, with these changes being particularly notable in the medial temporal lobe, anterior frontal lobe, and head of the caudate. Brain density has also been examined in alcoholism and, in a single case reported, controlled dehydration (Mellanby 1982). Overall, one gains the impression that lower density numbers on CT scans reflect loss, absence, or abnormality of brain tissue.

The first attempt at evaluation of brain density in schizophrenia was reported in a series of three articles describing comparisons of patients to medical and neurological controls (Golden et al. 1980a; Lyon et al. 1981; Golden et al. 1981). The first of these studies (Golden et al. 1980a) compared 22 schizophrenic patients to 21 matched controls with regard to mean density values in left and right hemispheres at three levels. The patients were found to have lower densities overall at all levels, and in addition a difference in the pattern of densities between hemispheres emerged, with the controls showing a consistent left-greater-than-right difference in densities, while the schizophrenics showed no such difference. This altered asymmetry in brain density has been found in a number of subsequent studies. The second report of this initial series (Lyon et al. 1981) involved 16 patients and the same 21 controls. In this comparison the density data for each slice was divided into four quadrants for the slice including the lateral ventricles (that used for VBR measurement). In this study the primary group difference was diminished relative density in the left anterior quadrant among the schizophrenics. In addition, density in the posterior quadrants was correlated in the schizophrenic group with total neuroleptic exposure. The third study of the series compared 23 schizophrenics and 24 controls, sampling every fourth pixel at three levels and computing mean values for four separate regions in each hemisphere, particularly in its anterior aspect. Again the pattern of asymmetry in density among normals which was absent among schizophrenics appeared in this analysis.

TABLE 6. Studies of Cerebral Asymmetry in Schizophrenia

Study	Sample Characteristics	Method	Presence of Reversed Asymmetry
Luchins et al. 1979	57 schizophrenics (RDC) 80 literature controls	widths of frontal and occipital lobes	+
Nyback et al. 1982	28 schizophrenics (RDC) 18 other psychiatric 46 normal volunteers	widths of frontal and occipital lobes	+ +[a]
Andreasen et al. 1982a	43 schizophrenics (RDC, *DSM-III*) 40 medical controls	widths of frontal and occipital lobes	–
Nasrallah et al. 1982b	41 schizophrenics *(DSM-III)* 40 medical controls	widths of frontal and occipital lobes	–
Luchins et al. 1982	79 schizophrenics and schizoaffective disorders (RDC) 100 medical/neurological controls	width of occipital lobes	+
Jernigan et al. 1982b	31 schizophrenics *(DSM-III)* 32 normal volunteers	width of frontal and occipital lobes	–
Weinberger et al. 1982a	35 schizophreniform disorders *(DSM-III)* 17 chronic schizophrenics 23 affective disorders 27 other psychiatric 26 medical controls	width of frontal and occipital lobes	–

TABLE 6. *(continued)*

Study	Sample Characteristics	Method	Presence of Reversed Asymmetry
Luchins et al. 1983b	45 schizophrenics and schizoaffective disorders (RDC) 62 medical controls	planimetry of occipital lobes	−
Kling et al. 1983	26 schizophrenics *(DSM-III)* 13 alcoholics 22 medical/neurological controls	widths of frontal lobes	−
Tsai et al. 1983	55 schizophrenics *(DSM-III)* 27 affective disorders	widths of frontal and occipital lobes	+

Key to Abbreviations: [a] = No difference between psychiatric patient groups
RDC = Research Diagnostic Criteria
DSM-III = Diagnostic and Statistical Manual, 3rd Ed.

A variety of methodological criticisms were made of these initial studies. Foremost among the concerns raised was the inclusion of entire brain regions including ventricular, sulcal, and fissural spaces. This would imply that the density values reported reflect not only changes in brain tissue density but overall loss of brain tissue reflected in atrophic changes. In order to deal with some of these methodologic problems, attempts were made to assess brain density by sampling very limited tissue regions located by use of the CT scanner console.

Largen et al. (1983) examined the CT studies of 25 schizophrenic patients and 19 medical controls by outlining 0.25-cm^2 regions of interest on the CT console, a slice above the lateral ventricles bilaterally in gray and white matter both in the anterior and posterior portions of each hemisphere. Using this method they found no distinct differences from controls; however, there was a suggestion of increased density of gray and white matter in the right hemisphere of schizophrenic patients. This would again suggest a discrepancy in left–right density differences with the expected difference favoring the left hemisphere not being present in schizophrenics. In a follow-up study (Largen et al. 1984), the group again found no differences between patients and controls when they used the conservative Bonferroni inequality, although univariate statistical analysis suggested evidence of a relative increase in density in the anterior white matter on the right, again consistent with altered left–right asymmetry and density.

Again using a limited region of interest method of sampling density numbers, Kanba et al. (1984) measured the mean radiodensity in the parenchyma of the frontal, parietal, and occipital lobes at the level of the lateral ventricles. They discovered a bilateral relative diminution in density in frontal and occipital areas in both hemispheres of 40 schizophrenic patients as compared to poorly characterized controls. They noted no relationship of these density changes with age or neuroleptic exposure.

.Coffman et al. (1984), returning to a technique similar to that of Golden et al., found a pattern of asymmetry in controls, with the left hemisphere more dense than the right, and a reduction of this pattern among schizophrenics although a different scanner was used. In yet another study, Coffman and Nasrallah (1984) compared brain-density findings in 18 chronic schizophrenics and 11 manic males and found few significant interhemispheric differences in densities on the right versus left. They found that among the schizophrenic and mixed psychotic patients there were significantly more hemispheric density comparisons with the right values equal to the left, and significantly fewer left values greater than right, than noted in the medical control group.

Using again a region of interest methodology, Dewan et al. (1983a) examined densities of 0.1-cm^2 areas in the caudate and temporal lobes and 0.5-cm^2 in the thalamus in 23 male patients and matched medical controls. They found no differences in cortical measures but did find that the paraventricular nuclei of the thalamus showed greater density values in the schizophrenic group.

In a further recent study by Reveley et al. (1987) a group of monozygotic twins discordant for schizophrenia were examined with a CT-scan method that compared cerebral tissue density at all levels after excluding pixel values on the study incorporating CSF-filled spaces and skull. In this computer-based method, left-hemisphere densities were consistently higher than right-hemisphere densities among the nonschizophrenic co-twins and selected control monozygotic twin pairs. The reverse was found among the schizophrenic co-twins, where the left hemisphere was consistently less dense than the right. The results were felt to suggest that left-hemispheric dysfunction, though apparently present in schizophrenics and demonstrable by a variety of modalities, seemed to be occurring on an environmental rather than genetic basis.

Overall the studies of brain density in schizophrenia, although few in number, suggest a pattern of altered asymmetry in cerebral structure at the tissue level and therefore seem to be generally supportive of other CT findings suggesting abnormalities in schizophrenia, previously discussed. Methodologic differences have made it difficult to compare data from study to study, and even to compare density data from individual to individual, with all the variations in measurement of radiodensity imposed by various instrumental artifacts. However, it would appear that within-subject comparisons of tissue density lead to a conclusion of a further demonstrable deficit in schizophrenia. This interhemispheric density finding appears to hold even in the face of beam-hardening artifact (Coffman and Bloch 1984).

Affective Disorders

Mania

The presence of lateral ventricular enlargement in manic patients was originally reported by Rieder et al. (1981, 1983), and this was soon followed by reports from a variety of other investigators (Pearlson and Veroff 1981; Nasrallah et al. 1982b; Pearlson and Veroff 1981). Not all reports have been positive, however, with Tanaka et al. reporting absence of a difference in lateral ventricular size when manics were compared to controls, although they did find evidence of third-ventricular enlargement (Tanaka et al. 1982).

Nasrallah et al. (1981) reported the presence of sulcal widening and cerebellar atrophy in manic patients and this finding was later replicated by other investigators (Tanaka et al. 1982 and Standish-Barry et al. 1982). In manics little or no relationship was found between ventricular enlargement and sulcal widening (Nasrallah et al. 1982; Standish-Barry et al. 1982), although Nasrallah and associates did find that cerebellar atrophy was associated with the degree of ventricular enlargement.

There are two reports in the literature of the evaluation of cerebral asymmetry in mania. Tanaka et al. (1982) found a tendency toward an increase in a pattern of reversal of normal hemispheric asymmetry in patients with bipolar affective disorder as compared to a control group. On the other hand Tsai (1983) found that reversal of asymmetry was much less common in manics compared to controls.

Assessment of cerebral density has also been attempted in evaluating the CT scans of manic patients. Coffman and Nasrallah (1984) compared brain-density values in manics and schizophrenics and found that, for the highest slice, schizophrenics showed a reduction in overall density values, which was felt to reflect the higher degree of cortical atrophy found in this group. In addition they noted that both the schizophrenics and manics showed a lack of the interhemispheric differences that had previously been shown to occur in the density values of controls.

Few studies of the clinical correlations of the CT-scan findings in manics have been reported. Luchins et al. (1984) noted, in a combined group of manics and patients with depressive disorders, that there seemed to be an association between the presence of delusional symptoms and ventricular enlargement. Nasrallah et al. (1984) compared clinical features of manic patients with and without large VBR and found that the group with large VBR had fewer lifetime episodes of illness compared to the group with ventricular brain ratio measurements in the normal range.

Depressive Disorders

Jacoby et al. (1981) provided one of the first studies of ventricular enlargement in a group of elderly and depressed subjects compared with a normal control group. They noted that a subgroup of their elderly depressed patients with large cerebral ventricles had more "endogenous" clinical features, later age of onset, and increased mortality after two years of follow-up, compared to the depressed patients who showed no ventricular enlargement (Jacoby et al. 1980). In a later study they found that brain-tissue density in elderly patients was more similar to patients with senile dementia than to comparable healthy controls, and that this finding was also associated with ventricular enlargement.

Targum et al. (1983a) found that while there were no significant differences in mean ventricular size between patients with and without delusional symptoms, 25% of the depressed patients with delusions compared with none of the nondelusional depressives had ventricular brain ratios more than two standard deviations beyond the mean of 26 neurological controls. They found no demographic, clinical, or neuroendocrine differences between the groups with and without ventricular enlargement. In a later study which replicated most of the results of the previously noted investigation, Targum (1983b) noted that those depressive patients with delusions had significantly lower verbal and performance scores on the Wechsler Adult Intelligence Scale. Scott et al. have reported a larger mean VBR in depressed patients with psychotic symptoms (i.e., delusions and hallucinations) when compared to normal controls (Scott et al. 1983).

Kellner et al. (1983) found a positive correlation between urinary free cortisol levels and ventricular brain ratios in depressed patients. This finding is supported by studies showing increased cerebral atrophy following therapeutic steroid administration and in other cases of hypercortisolism (Bentson 1978; Okuno 1980). It may also be related to the reported association of electroconvulsive therapy (ECT) treatment with frontal cerebral atrophy (Calloway et al. 1982), since patients with severe depression and hypercortisolism may be more likely to receive ECT. However, in a follow-up study of 101 depressed patients and 52 normal controls, Dolan et al. (1985) found no association between ventricular size and course of illness, exposure to treatment, or electroconvulsive therapy. They did find that increasing age and male sex were associated with larger ventricular size in both patient and control groups, although when these effects were controlled the depressed patients had significantly larger ventricles than did the controls.

In a recent study Schlegel and Kretzschmar (1987a, 1987b) studied a group of 60 patients with affective illness (33 with major depressive disorder, 22 with bipolar disorder, 5 manic, 17 depressed, and 5 patients with either depression or mania and mood congruent psychotic features). In this sample no differences in brain ratio were detected, although linear ventricular values measuring the frontal horns and third ventricle showed increases in patients as compared to controls, particularly among older male and psychotic patients. They found no association between dexamethasone suppression test results and ventricular enlargement. Both patients and controls were found to have asymmetric density values, with higher values occurring in the left hemisphere. Patients with small ventricular size showed higher density values, while lower density values were found among psychotic as opposed to nonpsychotic patients. No other clinical differences related to density values were apparent.

Summary

Overall, findings of ventricular enlargement in patients with affective disorders demonstrate the lack of specificity of this CT finding in psychiatry. However, available data suggest that alternative mechanisms may be operative. Among depressed individuals ventricular enlargement is associated with positive psychotic symptoms, while in schizophrenics negative symptoms predominate in the enlarged-ventricle group. Additionally, hypercortisolism may be a major factor in producing ventricular enlargement in patients with affective disorder. This suggests a potential for reversibility, which remains to be investigated.

Dementia

Evaluation of psychiatric patients, particularly those who are elderly, often suggests that differential diagnosis of dementia. Various psychiatric syndromes often imitate dementia, and various dementing syndromes are often accompanied with psychiatric symptomatology. Computed tomographic assessment can be of some assistance in clarifying this diagnostic confusion, although, as has been already demonstrated, many psychiatric conditions which one would wish to distinguish from dementia seem to be accompanied by similar CT changes.

Senile Dementia of the Alzheimer's Type

Alzheimer's disease is a pathologic diagnosis which can only be made conclusively at autopsy; therefore, a presumptive diagnosis of Alzheimer's type dementia is made through a process of exclusion. One of the earliest studies of demented individuals with computed tomography (Huckman et al. 1975) suggested a correlation between a linear measurement of ventricular size and extent of dementia but found notable exceptions. This is probably related to the association of ventricular enlargement with age, which has been noted in a number of studies (Gyldensted 1977; Brinkman et al. 1981). Subsequent studies have shown a clear relationship between cognitive impairment and ventricular enlargement in demented patients. For instance when neuroradiologists visually ranked CT scans for progressive cerebral atrophy, it was found that impaired performance on psychometric tests correlated with increasing brain atrophy (DeLeon et al. 1979; Gado 1982).

A separate evaluation by Gado et al. (1983) used a variety of linear measurements (including the span of the frontal horns, septum caudate distance, width of the third ventricle and the width of cella media, as well as the maximum inner diameter of the skull) in 21 patients with neurologic diagnosis of Alzheimer's disease and 24 matched normal controls. In these measurements significant differences were found in the mean values of third-ventricular width or the total sum of all the linear measurements (the ventricular index) and a less substantial but still significant difference in frontal horn span.

Jacoby and Levy (1980a), using the Evans ratio, found a significant increase in lateral ventricular size in patients with Alzheimer's disease. When they further evaluated the patients by using planimetric measurement of VBR the Alzheimer's disease patients once again had a significant degree of enlargement. Attempts to confirm these findings with counts of all pixels with values corresponding to CSF have been confirmatory (Gado et al. 1982).

Assessments of brain density have also been made in patients with suspected Alzheimer's disease. Naeser (1980) reported differences in mean CT-density numbers between demented patients and depressed controls. Still others have found that, in severely demented patients and patients with increased ventricular size, density of the gray and white matter was significantly increased as compared to controls (George et al. 1981). Yet another study found no differences at all in density of gray or white matter (Gado et al. 1983), while a more recent study by Bird (1982) revealed an association between reductions in brain density in the region of the thalamus as well as frontal and occipital lobes which was correlated with cognitive impairment.

Multi-Infarct Dementia

It has been estimated that multi-infarct dementia accounts for nearly 20% of the dementing disorders occurring in elderly individuals. It is important to note that the simple presence of infarcts on CT scan in a patient with dementia does not adequately confirm an etiologic relationship. In one study, Glatt et al. (1983) found that patients with CT finding suggestive of multiple infarcts often did not show any clinical evidence of dementia. On the other hand, patients with clinical indications of multi-infarct dementia often did show evidence of multiple infarcts on CT.

Two patterns of abnormality are seen in multi-infarct dementia: multiple large infarcts and subcortical atherosclerotic encephalopathy. Large infarcts appear on CT as regions of low density that generally correspond to the distribution of cerebral artery branches. They generally involve the cerebral cortex and may involve the underlying white matter. The lesion often has a rather well-distinguished border that defines the vascular territory involved, and the lesions are often bilateral. The territories of branches of the middle cerebral artery are most often the ones involved, although lesions may appear in the distribution of any of the cerebral arteries. Computed tomographic findings in subcortical atherosclerotic encephalopathy involve two prominent features: lateral ventricular enlargement and diminished paraventricular white matter density (Bondareff et al. 1983). The lateral ventricles are enlarged out of proportion to any widening of the cerebral sulci. The third ventricle is often dilated as well, although the fourth ventricle is usually normal in appearance. In addition, the temporal horns of the lateral ventricles are usually not enlarged, and this factor as well as the presence of a reduction in density in the paraventricular white matter tends to distinguish this condition radiologically from normal pressure hydrocephalus.

Hydrocephalic Dementias

Disruption in the flow of cerebrospinal fluid may produce a marked degree of ventricular enlargement with normal to below normal CSF pressure. When the block to fluid flow is located at the level of the tentorial hiatus, the abnormal CT pattern seen involves enlargement of the lateral and the third ventricles with marked enlargement of the temporal horns and narrowing of the cerebral sulci. Leakage of fluid into the adjacent regions results in periventricular white matter lucency near the frontal horns and in other regions as well. These findings added together should suggest the possibility of such a diagnosis (Huckman et al. 1981; Gado et al. 1982).

Communicating hydrocephalus with increased CSF pressure can occur on a subacute basis following meningitis or intercranial hemorrhages secondary to trauma or ruptured aneurysms. Block to CSF flow can occur at the same level as that in normal pressure hydrocephalus and the CT appearance can be the same. It is the historical context in which the CT picture occurs which allows the diagnosis to be made. In addition, a more rapid evolution of symptoms of dementia often accompanies this clinical situation.

Uncommon Types of Dementia

In Pick's disease characteristic features on CT include extreme shrinking of relatively localized areas of cerebral hemispheres. This atrophy is most often frontotemporal in distribution, and the involved regions show prominent widening of the cerebral sulci due to loss of brain volume in the affected regions. On occasion other regions of the brain are involved, specifically the parietal lobe.

Huntington's disease can be diagnosed by comparison of caudate size to the size of the lateral ventricles. Often linear measurements are used for this, with the span of the frontal horns of the ventricles being compared to the separation of the caudates from ventricular margin to ventricular margin. The ratio of the two ranges is from 1.7 to 1, to 3 to 1 in normal individuals, with a mean of 1.3. In patients with diffuse cerebral atrophy and associated Parkinson's disease the ratio is similar to that in normal individuals (Terrence et al. 1977).

Alcoholism

Evidence of brain atrophy in alcoholics has been reported in the era of pneumoencephalographic examination (Courville 1966; Victor et al. 1959; Haug 1968; Brewer and Berrett 1971). With computed tomography it has become easier to investigate brain atrophy in alcoholics in comparison with a control group (Cala and Mastaglia 1981; Ron et al. 1982).

In reviewing seven controlled studies, Cala and Mastaglia (1981) reported that six showed greater degrees of brain atrophy among alcoholics than controls. In their own report accompanying the review, atrophy seemed even to be associated with heavy social drinking, with that group showing scores falling between those noted in control and alcoholic groups. Patients with Wernicke–Korsakoff syndrome showed a higher degree of cerebellar and brain-stem atrophy, which was also associated with some degree of cerebral atrophy. Overall the degree of atrophy even in advanced cases of alcoholism was much less than that noted in cases of dementia. Carlen et al. (1978) noted some reversibility of cortical atrophy in alcoholics. Ron et al. noted a reduction on follow-up in either ventricular size or cortical atrophy among the alcoholics she studied, which was significantly related to the amount of time during the follow-up period (1982). Preliminary assessments of brain-tissue density by CT have been undertaken by Golden et al. (1980c), and they noted a diffuse reduction in brain density seemed to be associated with alcoholism.

Computed Tomography in Child and Adolescent Psychiatry

Anorexia Nervosa

Evidence of cortical atrophy in anorexia nervosa prior to the availability of computed tomography has come from postmortem (Martin et al. 1955) and pneumoencephalographic (Heidrich and Schmidt-Matthias 1961) studies. With the development of computed tomography more reports have emerged. Enzmann and Lane found evidence of ventricular enlargement and widening of cortical sulci in four individuals with anorexia nervosa (1977). Nussbaum et al. (1980) also noted cerebral atrophy in seven patients, which constituted half of the patients admitted during the year. They also noted that total weight loss was less in the group not showing atrophy. Several authors have noted that the changes in brain volume seen in this disorder appear to be reversible (Heinz et al. 1977; Kohlmeyer 1983). Some relationship of these changes to dietary protein–calorie deficiency is suggested by findings of cerebral atrophy in marasmic infants (El-Tatawy 1983), in addition to apparent partial reversibility of changes in a 20-year follow-up of marasmic individuals (Handler et al. 1981), and the occurrence of reversibility of such atrophy among alcoholics who may also suffer from qualitative if not quantitative nutritional deficiencies.

Autism

Several studies have been performed in autistic individuals, with computed tomography. Hier et al. (1979) reported a higher incidence of reversed cerebral asymmetry in the occipital lobes among autistics than among retarded and neurological controls. Tsai et al. (1983) also found a pattern of altered cerebral asymmetry. Campbell et al. (1982) have observed that some of their autistic patients have increased lateral ventricular size by linear measurement. The pattern is not an entirely clear one, in large part due to the relatively few studies in the literature.

Other Disorders

Several other childhood disorders have been studied to slight extent with computed tomography. In studies of children with attention deficit disorder a number of uncontrolled reports have been reviewed by Rapoport and Ismond (1982). In this review a surprisingly high incidence of abnormality seems to be present. Nasrallah et al. (1986) found that 66% of adults followed for a childhood history of attention deficit disorder or minimal brain dysfunction showed evidence of widened cortical sulci, compared to only 4% of matched controls. Hier et al. (1978) has also evaluated patients with developmental dyslexia and found that in this group 10 of 24 patients had reversed cerebral asymmetry as well as an association with lower IQ.

Clinical Applications

The foregoing portions of this chapter have discussed the technical principles of computed tomography and its application to clinical studies in psychiatry. The technique has proven to be a very powerful one for the detection of intracranial structural changes. The development of computing power and imaging software which led to the availability of computed tomography has provided the groundwork underlying all other major imaging techniques. The soft-tissue and bony structural information offered by computed tomography has been and continues to be the current major source of information regarding intracranial pathology for clinicians around the world. Due to its relatively low cost and resultant wide availability, the technique will probably remain on the scene for some time.

The practicing clinical psychiatrist will, at least for the foreseeable future, tend to apply computed tomography to circumstances not altogether different from those leading to its use by neurologists. Until further research provides greater understanding of the sensitivity, specificity, and overall utility of assessments of subtle structural changes in the brains of patients suffering from the various psychiatric disorders already discussed, the major use of computed tomography in general clinical settings will remain the detection of gross neuropathological conditions.

When computed tomography has been applied to populations of patients clinically diagnosed as suffering from chronic schizophrenia, in whom no previous evidence for neuropathology had been uncovered, a number of studies have found unsuspected diseases. Owens et al. (1980), in a randomly selected sample of 136 chronic schizophrenics, found previously unsuspected and undetected intracranial pathology in 12 individuals. The disorders uncovered included 7 cases of cerebral infarction, 2 subdural hematomas, one meningioma, a cystic enlargement of the pineal body, and porencephalic cyst. Reveley and Reveley (1983) identified previously unsuspected cases of hydrocephaly and aqueductal stenosis in 3 patients who had been diagnosed as schizophrenic by RDC criteria. Evans (1982), in examining 100 cases of psychiatric patients referred for clinical reasons for CT study, reported on the radiologist's evaluations and correlated these with clinical information. In this English study, Evans found that the elderly predominated in the group and that nearly half were felt to have some significant neuropathologic disorder, with 30 of the 100 patients diagnosed as suffering from dementia and an additional 17 having other "organic" diagnoses. Atrophy was read as present in 66 of the 100 patients, predominantly in the "organic" group; 24 of the patients had a scan read as normal; and specific lesions were detected in 8 of the 100, including 2 with tumors.

In only these few studies it becomes apparent that specific structural abnormalities are found relatively rarely in unscreened psychiatric patients but that the incidence is high enough that some rational approach to the selection of patients for scanning might be advisable. Such an impression is supported by two recent studies which discussed the use of computed tomography as a "screening" tool for unsuspected intracranial pathology. Rosenberg et al. (1982) studied all patients discharged from a neurology service in a year and examined CT and EEG results, where available, in patients who did not have any focal neurologic findings. They reported that only 6 (4.4%) of the 136 patients showed focal abnormalities on CT. They also noted that 4 of the 6 had EEGs indicative of focal pathology and concluded that EEG was sufficiently sensitive to be used as a screen for focal pathology. Larson et al. (1981) examined the use of CT in "ruling out" intracranial pathology. They examined the records of 123

consecutive patients suffering from psychiatric disorders who were referred for CT scans, and found that 85% of these scans were interpreted as
normal or "normal except for atrophy." They found 12 individuals with
positive findings on CT, 9 of whom had shown some evidence of focal
neurologic findings on examination. The authors concluded that computed tomography might be best used in psychiatric patients to confirm
findings from history and physical examination that suggest the possibility
of focal pathology, rather than applying the technique widely as a tool for
screening or "ruling out" focal pathology in the wider population of
psychiatric patients.

Weinberger (1984a) reviewed the brain disorders associated with
focal and diffuse pathology that lead secondarily to disorders commonly
seen by psychiatrists, such as psychosis and/or personality changes, depression, movement disorders, and dementia. Weinberger goes on to offer
a variety of reasonable suggestions as to when a CT scan might usefully be
applied. He suggests that for a patient with dementia of unknown etiology, a CT scan and neurologic consultation are mandatory. On the con-
trary, patients with well-established characterological diagnoses or long-
standing problems in living would not be likely to exhibit focal
neuropathology. In the middle ground are those patients with discrete
syndromes such as personality change, mood disorder, psychosis, and
disorders of movement. In order to deal with these issues, Weinberger
engages in a cost–benefit analysis. First of all he notes that the only
significant cost is the financial one. Radiation dose (2 to 3 rads) is low.
Weinberger summarizes the literature alluded to above as well as some
other studies which concur with the finding that 2% to 10% of preselected
psychiatric inpatients show diagnosable structural brain disease beyond
the atrophic processes previously discussed and that the yield increases
when neurologic exam findings are positive. However, he does note that
the study of Owens et al. (1980) is the only one which did not clinically
preselect patients for study and that preselection may contribute to the
high incidence of reported abnormalities. In order to provide some guid-
ance, Weinberger suggests special clinical cases which deserve greater
attention and in which a CT scan may yield significant information. He
suggests the following as indications: 1) confusion and/or dementia of
unknown cause, 2) first episode of a psychotic disorder of unknown
etiology, 3) movement disorder of uncertain etiology, 4) anorexia
nervosa, 5) prolonged catatonia, and 6) first episode of a major affective
disorder or personality change after age 50. Weinberger recommends
such studies in acute disorders where a CT scan may be advisable on
theoretical grounds and not unjustified on the basis of the benefit of
detecting previously unsuspected pathology at moderate cost ($200–
$400 per study).

Beyond the detection of focal pathology, the clinical utility of CT in psychiatry remains to be established. It may be that firm associations between structural abnormalities and clinical outcome or response parameters will be established. If this happens, one might, for instance, be able to use computed tomographic scans in the early phase of a schizophrenic disorder and determine that a patient has evidence of cerebral atrophy suggesting limited responsiveness to presently available antipsychotic medication. However, results are at this point extremely unclear in this regard.

Overall Assessment of the Technique

CT scanning remains a widely used and valuable tool for structural assessment of cranial and intracranial structures. Among its strengths are the long experience available and its relatively low cost. Its primary competitor is magnetic resonance imaging. Disadvantages of CT include its lesser degree of contrast between gray and white matter and the beam-hardening artifact effect on soft-tissue imaging adjacent to a bone. Primary advantages of CT are its lower cost, its wide availability, its ability to visualize bony structures, and its relative simplicity.

References

Allen JH, Martin JT, McLain LW. Computed tomography in cerebellar atrophic processes. Radiology 130:379, 1979

American Psychiatric Association, Committee on Nomenclature and Statistics. Diagnostic and Statistical Manual of Mental Disorders, 3rd Edition. Washington, D.C., American Psychiatric Association, 1980

Andreasen NC, Dennert JW, Olson SA, et al: Hemispheric asymmetries and schizophrenia. Am J Psychiatry 139:427-430, 1982a

Andreasen NC, Smith MR, Jacoby CG, et al: Ventricular enlargement in schizophrenia: definition and prevalence. Am J Psychiatry 139:292-296, 1982b

Andreasen NC, Olson SA, Dennert JW, et al: Ventricular enlargement in schizophrenia: relationship to positive and negative symptoms. Am J Psychiatry 139:297-302, 1982c

Barron SA, Jacobs L, Kunkel WR: Changes in size of normal lateral ventricles during aging determined by computed tomography. Neurology 26:1011-1013, 1976

Benes F, Sunderland P, Jones BD, et al: Normal ventricles in young schizophrenics. Br J Psychiatry 141:90-93, 1982

Bentson, JR, Reza M, Winter J, et al: Steroids and apparent cerebral atrophy on computed tomography scans. J Comput Assist Tomogr 2:16-19, 1978

Bird JM: Computerized tomography, atrophy, and dementia: a review. Prog Neurobiol 19:91-115, 1982

Boklage CE: Schizophrenia, brain asymmetry development, and twinning: cellular relationship with etiological and possible prognostic implications. Biol Psychiatry 12:19-35, 1977

Bondareff W, Baldy R, Levy R: Quantitative computed tomography in senile dementia. Arch Gen Psychiatry 38:1365-1368, 1981

Boronow J, Pickar D, Ninan RP, et al: Atrophy limited to third ventricle only in chronic schizophrenic patients: reports of a controlled series. Arch Gen Psychiatry 42:266-271, 1985

Bracewell RN: Strip integration in radio astronomy. Australian Journal of Physiology 9:198-217, 1956

Brewer C, Barrett L: Brain damage due to alcohol consumption: an airencephalographic psychometric and electroencephalographic study. Br J Addict 66:170-182, 1971

Brinkman SD, Sarwar M, Levin HS, et al: Quantitative indexes of computed tomography in dementia and normal aging. Radiology 138:89-92, 1981

Brooks, RA, DiChiro G: Beam hardening in x-ray reconstructive tomography. Phys Med Biol 21:390-398, 1976

Brooks RA, Glover AJ, Tolbert RL, et al: Aliasing, a source of streaks in computed tomograms. J Comput Assist Tomogr 3:511-518, 1979

Cala LA, Mastaglia FL: Computerized tomography in chronic alcoholics. Alcoholism 5:283-294, 1981

Calloway SP, Dolan R: ECT and cerebral damage. Br J Psychiatry 140:102-105, 1982

Campbell M, Rosenbloom S, Perry R, et al: Computerized axial tomography in young autistic children. Am J Psychiatry 139:510-512, 1982

Carlen PL, Wortzman G, Holgate RC, et al: Reversible cerebral atrophy in recently abstinent chronic alcoholics measured by computed tomography scans. Science 200:1076-1078, 1978

Carpenter WT, Bartko JJ, Strauss JS: A postscript on the 12-point flexible system for the diagnosis of schizophrenia: a report from the IPSS. Psychiatry Res 3:357-364, 1980

Carr EG, Wedding D: Neuropsychological assessment of cerebral ventricular size in chronic schizophrenics. Int J Neuropsychol 6:106, 1984

Coffman JA, Bloch S: Interhemispheric differences in regional density of the normal brain. J Psychiatr Res 18:269-275, 1984

Coffman JA, Nasrallah HA: Brain density patterns in schizophrenia and mania. J Affective Disord 6:307-315, 1984

Coffman JA, Mefferd J, Golden CJ, et al: Cerebellar atrophy in chronic schizophrenia. Lancet 1:666, 1981

Coffman JA, Andreasen NC, Nasrallah HA: Left hemispheric density deficits in chronic schizophrenia. Biol Psychiatry 19:1237-1247, 1984

Cormack AM: Representation of a function by its line integrals, with some radiological application. Journal of Applied Physics 34:2722-2727, 1963

Cormack AM: Representation of a function by its line integrals, with some radiological applications, II. Journal of Applied Physics 35:2908-2913, 1964

Courville CB: Effects of Alcohol on the Nervous System of Man. Los Angeles, CA, San Lucas Press, 1966

Dandy WE: Roentgenography of the brain after the injection of air into the spinal cord. Ann Surg 70:397, 1918

DeLeon MJ, Ferris SH, Blau I, et al: Correlations between computerized tomographic changes and behavioral deficits in senile dementia. Lancet 2:859, 1979

DeLisi LE, Schwartz CC, Targum SD, et al: Ventricular brain enlargement and outcome of acute schizophreniform disorder. Psychiatry Res 9:9-16, 1983

DeLisi LE, Goldin LR, Hamovit JR, et al: A family study of the association of increased ventricular size with schizophrenia. Arch Gen Psychiatry 43:148-153, 1986

DeMeyer MK, Gilmore R, DeMeyer WE, et al: Third ventricle size and ventricular brain ratio in treatment-resistant psychiatric patients. J Oper Psychiatry 14:2, 1984

DeRosier DJ, Klug A: Reconstruction of three-dimensional structures from electron micrographs. Nature 217:130-134, 1968

Dewan MJ, Pandurangi AK, Lee SH, et al: Central brain morphology in chronic schizophrenic patients: a controlled CT study. Biol Psychiatry 18:1133-1140, 1983a

Dewan MJ, Pandurangi AK, Lee SH, et al: Cerebellar morphology in chronic schizophrenic patients: a controlled computed tomographic study. Psychiatry Res 10:97, 1983b

DiChiro G, Brooks RA, Dubal L, et al: The apical artifact: elevated attenuation values toward the apex of the skull. J Comput Assist Tomogr 2:65-70, 1978

Dolan RJ, Calloway SP, Mann AH: Cerebral ventricular size in depressed subjects. Psychol Med 15:873-878

Donnelly EF, Weinberger DR, Waldman IN, et al: Cognitive impairment associated with morphological brain abnormalities on computed tomography in chronic schizophrenic patients. J Nerv Ment Dis 168:305-308, 1980

Duerinck AJ, Macovski A: Polychromatic streak artifacts in computed tomography images. J Comput Assist Tomogr 2:481-487, 1978

Earnest MP, Heaton RK, Wilkinson WE, et al: Cortical atrophy, ventricular enlargement and intellectual impairment in the aged. Neurology 29:1138, 1979

El-Tatawy S, Badrawi N, El-Bishlawy A: Cerebral atrophy in infants with protein energy malnutrition. AJNR 4:434-436, 1983

Enzmann DR, Lane B: Cranial computed tomography findings in anorexia nervosa. J Comput Assist Tomogr 1:410-414, 1977

Evans NJR: Cranial computerized tomography in clinical psychiatry: 100 consecutive cases. Compr Psychiatry 42:452-454, 1981

Feighner JP, Robins E, Guze SB, et al: Diagnostic criteria for use in psychiatric research. Arch Gen Psychiatry 26:57-63, 1972

Folstein MF, McHugh PR. Mini-mental state. J Psychiatry Res 12:189-198, 1975

Fox JH, Topel JL, Huckman MS: Use of computerized tomography in senile dementia. J Neurol Neurosurg Psychiatry 38:948-953, 1975

Frangos E, Athanassenas G: Differences in lateral brain ventricular size among various types of chronic schizophrenics, evidence basic on a CT study. Acta Psychiatr Scand 66:459-463, 1982

Gado M, Phelps M: Peripheral zone of increased density in computed tomography. Radiology 117:71-74, 1975

Gado M, Hughes CP, Danziger W, et al: Aging, dementia and brain atrophy: a longitudinal computed tomographic study. AJNR 4:699-702, 1983

Galaburda AM, LeMay M, Kemper TL, et al: Right–left asymmetries in the brain. Science 199:853-856, 1978

Gattaz WF, Kasper S, Kohlmeyer K, et al: Die kraniale computertomographie in der schizophrenieforschung. Fortschr Psychiatr Neurol 49:286-293, 1981

George AE, deLeon MJ, Ferris SH: Parenchymal CT correlates of senile dementia. AJNR 2:205, 1981

Glatt SL, Lantos G, Danziger A, et al: Efficacy of CT in the diagnosis of vascular dementia. AJNR 4:703-705, 1983

Gluck E, Radu EW, Gerhardt P: A computed tomographic prolective trohoc study of chronic schizophrenics. Neuroradiology 20:167-171, 1980

Golden CJ, Graber B, Coffman J, et al: Brain density deficits in chronic schizophrenia. Psychiatry Res 3:179-184, 1980a

Golden CJ, Moses JA, Zelazowski R, et al: Cerebral ventricular size and neuropsychological impairment in young chronic schizophrenics, measurement by the standardized Luria–Nebraska neurophysiological battery. Arch Gen Psychiatry 37:619-623, 1980b

Golden CJ, Graber B, Blose I, et al: Differences in brain densities between chronic alcoholics and normal control patients. Science 211:508-510, 1980c

Golden CJ, Graber B, Coffman J, et al: Structural deficits in schizophrenia, identification by computed tomographic scan density measurements. Arch Gen Psychiatry 38:1014-1017, 1981

Golden CJ, MacInnes WD, Ariel RN, et al: Cross-validation of the ability of the Luria–Nebraska Neuropsychological Battery to differentiate chronic schizophrenics with and without ventricular enlargement. J Consult Clin Psychol 50:87-95, 1982

Gyldensted C: Measurements of the normal ventricular system and hemispheric sulci of 100 adults with computed tomography. Neuroradiology 14:183-192, 1977

Handler LC, Stock MB, Smythe PM: CT brain scans: part of a 20-year development study following gross undernutrition during infancy. Br J Radiol 54:953-954, 1981

Hang JO: Pneumoencephalographic evidences of brain damage in chronic alcoholism. Acta Psychiatr Scand 203 (Suppl): 135-143, 1968

Haug G: Age and sex dependence of the size of normal ventricles on computed tomography. Neuroradiology 14:201-204, 1977

Heath RG, Franklin DE, Shraberg D: Gross pathology of the cerebellum in patients diagnosed and treated as functional psychiatric disorders. J Nerv Ment Dis 167:585-592, 1979

Heath RG, Franklin DE, Walker CF, et al: Cerebellar vermal atrophy in psychiatric patients. Biol Psychiatry 17:569-583, 1982

Heidrich R, Schmidt-Matthias H: Encephalographische befunde bei anorexia nervosa. Arch Psychiatr Nervenkr 101:183-201, 1961

Heinz ER, Martinex J, Haenggell A: Reversibility of cerebral atrophy in anorexia nervosa and Cushing's syndrome. J Comput Assist Tomogr 1:415-417, 1977

Hendee WR: The Physical Principles of Computed Tomography. Boston, Little Brown, 1983

Hier D, LeMay M, Rosenberger P, et al: Developmental dyslexia: evidence for a subgroup with reversed cerebral asymmetry. Arch Neurol 35:90-92, 1978

Hier D, Lemay M, Rosenberger P, et al: Autism and unfavorable left-right asymmetries of the brain. J Autism Dev Disord 9:153-159, 1979

Hounsfield GN: Computerized transverse axial scanning (tomography), part I: description of system. Br J Radiol 46:1016-1022, 1973a

Hounsfield GN: Computerized transverse axial scanning (tomography), part II:

clinical application. Br J Radiol 46:1023-1047, 1973b

Huckman M, Fox J, Topel J: The validity of criteria for the evaluation of cerebral atrophy by computed tomography. Radiology 116:85-92, 1975

Huckman MS, Fox JS, Ramsey RG: Computed tomography in the diagnosis of pseudotumor cerebri. Radiology 119:593, 1976

Jacobi W, Winkler H: Encephalographische studien an chronish schizophrenen. Arch Psychiat Nervenkr 81:299-332, 1927

Jacoby RJ, Levy R: Computerized tomography in the elderly, II: senile dementia, diagnosis and functional impairment. Br J Psychiatry 136:256-269, 1980a

Jacoby RJ, Levy R, Dawson JM: Computerized tomography in the elderly, I: the normal population. Br J Psychiatry 136:249-255, 1980b

Jacoby RJ, Levy R, Bird JM: Computed tomography and the outcome of affective disorder: a follow-up of elderly patients. Br J Psychiatry 139:288-292, 1981

Jaspers K: General Psychopathology. London, Manchester University Press, 1963

Jernigan TL, Zatz LM, Naeser MA: Semiautomated method for quantifying CSF volume on cranial computed tomography. Radiology 132:463-466, 1979

Jernigan TL, Zatz LM, Moses JA, et al: Computed tomography in schizophrenics and normal volunteers, I: fluid volume. Arch Gen Psychiatry 39:765-770, 1982a

Jernigan TL, Zatz LM, Moses JA, et al: Computed tomography in schizophrenics and normal volunteers, II: cranial asymmetry. Arch Gen Psychiatry 39:771-774, 1982b

Johnstone EC, Crow TJ, Frith CD, et al: Cerebral ventricular size and cognitive impairment in schizophrenia. Lancet 2:924-926, 1976

Johnstone EC, Crow TJ, Frith CD, et al: The dementia of dementia praecox. Acta Psychiatr Scand 57:305-324, 1978

Johnstone EC, Owens DGC, Crow TJ, et al: A CT study of 188 patients with schizophrenia, affective psychosis and neurotic illness, in Biological Psychiatry. Edited by Perris C, Struwe G, Jansson B. Amsterdam, Elsevier, 1982

Joseph PM: Image noise and smoothing in computed tomography (CT) scanners. Opt Engr 17:396-399, 1978

Joseph PM: Artifacts in computed tomography, in Radiology of the Skull and Brain: Technical Aspects of Computed Tomography vol. 5. St. Louis, Mosby, 1981

Kanba S, Shima S, Daizo T, et al: Brain CT density in chronic schizophrenia. Biol Psychiatry 19:273-274, 1984

Kellner CH, Rubinow DR, Gold PW, et al: Relationship of cortisol hypersecretion to brain CT scan alterations in depressed patients. Psychiatry Res 8:191-197, 1983

Kling AS, Kurtz N, Tachiki K, et al: CT scans in sub-groups of chronic schizophrenia. J Psychiatr Res 17:375-384, 1983

Kohlmeyer K, Lehmkuhl G, Poutska F: Computed tomography of anorexia nervosa. AJNR 4:437-438, 1983

Koller, WC, Glatt SL, Perlik S, et al: Cerebellar atrophy demonstrated by computed tomography. Neurology 31:405-412, 1981

Kraepelin E. Dementia Praecox and Paraphrenia (1919). New York, RM Krieger, 1971

Krawiecka M, Goldberg D, Vaughan M: A standardized psychiatric assessment scale for rating chronic psychotic patients. Acta Psychiatr Scand 55:299-303, 1977

Kuhl DE, Edwards RQ: Image separation isotope scanning. Radiology 80:653-661, 1963

Largen JW, Calderon M, Smith RC: Asymmetries in the density of white and gray matter in the brains of schizophrenic patients. Am J Psychiatry 140:1060-1063, 1983

Largen JW, Smith RC, Calderon M, et al: Abnormalities of brain structure and density in schizophrenia. Biol Psychiatry 19:991-1013, 1984

Larson EB, Mack LA, Watts B, et al: Computed tomography in patients with psychiatric illnesses: advantage of a "rule-in" approach. Ann Intern Med 95:360-364, 1981

LeMay M, Kido DK: Asymmetries of cerebral hemispheres on computed tomograms. J Comput Assist Tomogr 2:471-478, 1978

LeMay M: Morphological cerebral symmetries of modern man, fossil man, and nonhuman primate. Ann NY Acad Sci 280:349-366, 1976

LeMay M: Asymmetries of the skull and handedness. J Neurol Sci 32:243-253, 1977

Lippmann S, Manshadi M, Baldwin H, et al: Cerebellar vermis dimensions on computerized tomographic scans of schizophrenia and bipolar patients. Am J Psychiatry 139:667-668, 1982

Luchins DJ, Meltzer HY: A blind controlled study of occipital cerebral asymmetry in schizophrenia. Psychiatry Res 10:87-94, 1983

Luchins DJ, Weinberger DR, Wyatt RJ: Anomalous lateralization associated with a milder form of schizophrenia. Am J Psychiatry 136:1598-1599, 1979

Luchins DJ, Weinberger DR, Wyatt RJ: Schizophrenia and cerebral asymmetry detected by computed tomography. Am J Psychiatry 139:753-757, 1982

Luchins DJ, Jackman J, Meltzer HY: Lateral ventricular size and drug-induced parkinsonism. Psychiatry Res 9:9-16, 1983a

Luchins DJ, Lewine RJ, Meltzer HY: Lateral ventricular size in the psychoses: relation to psychopathology and therapeutic and adverse response to medication. Schizophr Bull 19:518-523, 1983b

Luchins DJ, Lewine RJ, Melzer HY: Lateral ventricular size, psychopathology, and mediention response in the psychoses. Biol Psychiatry 19:29-34, 1984

Lyon K, Wilson J, Golden CJ, et al: Effects of long-term neuroleptic use on brain density. Psychiatry Res 5:33-45, 1981

Martin F: Pathologie des aspects neurologiques et psychiatriques dans quelques manifestations carentielles avec troubles digestifs et neuroendocriniens, II: etudes des alterations du systeme nerveux central dans deux cas d-anorexie survenue chez la jeune fille (dite anorexie mentale). Helv Med Acta 22:522-529, 1955

Meese W, Lanksch W, Wende S: Cerebral atrophy and computerized tomography aspects of a qualitative and quantitative analysis from cranial computerized tomography, in Cranial Computerized Tomography. Edited by Lanksch W, Kasner E. Berlin, Springer-Verlag, 1976

Meese W, Kluge W, Grumme T, et al: CT evaluation of the CSF spaces of healthy persons. Neuroradiology 19:131-136, 1980

Mellanby AR, Reveley MA: Effects of acute dehydration on computerized tomographic assessment of cerebral density and ventricular volume. Lancet 2:874, 1982

Moriguchi I: A study of schizophrenic brains by computerized tomographic scans. Folia Psychiatr Neurol Jpn 35:54-63, 1981

Mundt C, Radu W, Gluck E. Computer tomographische Untersuchungen der Liquorraume an chronisch schizophrenen Patienten. Nervenarzt 51:743-748, 1980

Naber D, Albur M, Burke H, et al: Neuroleptic withdrawal in chronic schizophrenia, CT and endocrine variables relating to psychopathology. Psychiatry Res 16:207-219, 1985

Naeser MA, Gebhart C, Levin HL. Decreased computerized tomography numbers in patients with pre-senile dementia. Arch Neurol 37:401-409, 1980

Nasrallah HA, Kleinman JE, Weinberger DR, et al: Cerebral ventricular enlargement and dopamine synthesis inhibition in chronic schizophrenia. Arch Gen Psychiatry 34:1427, 1980

Nasrallah HA, Jacoby CG, McCalley-Whitters M: Cerebellar atrophy in schizophrenia and mania. Lancet 1:1102, 1981

Nasrallah HA, Jacoby CG, McCalley-Whitters M, et al: Cerebral ventricular enlargement in subtypes of chronic schizophrenia. Arch Gen Psychiatry 39:774-777, 1982a

Nasrallah HA, McCalley-Whitters M, Jacoby CG: Cortical atrophy in schizophrenia and mania: a comparative study. J Clin Psychiatry 43:439-441, 1982b

Nasrallah HA, Rizzo M, Damasio H, et al: Neurological differences between paranoid and non-paranoid schizophrenia, part II: computerized tomographic findings. J Clin Psychiatry 43:307-309, 1982c

Nasrallah HA, Kuperman S, Hamra BJ, et al: Clinical differences between schizophrenic patients with and without large cerebral ventricles. J Clin Psychiatry 44:407-409, 1983a

Nasrallah HA, Kuperman S, Jacoby CG, et al: Clinical correlates of sulcal widening in schizophrenia. Psychiatry Res 19:237-242, 1983b

Nasrallah HA, McCalley-Whitters M, Pfohl B: Clinical significance of large cerebral ventricles in manic males. Psychiatry Res 13:155-156, 1984

Nasrallah HA, Jacoby CG, Chapman S, et al: Third ventricular enlargement on CT scans in schizophrenia: an association with cerebellar atrophy. Biol Psychiatry 20:443-450, 1985

Nasrallah HA, Loney J, Jacoby CG, et al: Cerebral atrophy in young adults with history of hyperactivity in childhood. Psychiatry Res 17:241-246, 1986a

Nasrallah HA, Olson SC, McCalley-Whitters M, et al: Cerebral ventricular enlargement in schizophrenia: a preliminary follow-up study. Arch Gen Psychiatry 43:157-159, 1986b

Neito D, Escobar A: Major psychoses, in Pathology of the Nervous System. Edited by Minkler J. New York, McGraw-Hill, 1972

Nussbaum M, Shenker IR, Mar J, et al: Cerebral atrophy in anorexia nervosa. J Pediatr 96:867-869, 1980

Nyback H, Wiegel FA, Berggren BM, et al: Computed tomography of the brain in patients with acute psychosis and in healthy controls. Acta Psychiatr Scand 65:403-413, 1982

Obiols-Llandrich JE, Ruscallada J, Masferrer M: Ventricular enlargement in young chronic schizophrenics. Acta Psychiatr Scand 73:42-44, 1986

Oddy HC, Lobstein TJ: Hand and eye dominance in schizophrenia. Br J Psychiatry 120:331-332, 1972

Okasha A, Madkour O: Cortical and central atrophy in schizophrenia. Acta Psychiatr Scand 65:29-34, 1982

Okasha A, Madkour O, Madg FA: Cortical and central atrophy in chronic schizophrenia, a controlled study, in Biological Psychiatry. Edited by Perris C, Struwe G, Jansson B. Amsterdam, Elsevier, 1981

Okuno T, Ito M, Konishi Y, et al: Cerebral atrophy following ACTH therapy. J Comput Assist Tomogr 2:16-19, 1980

Oldendorf WH: Isolated flying spot detection of radiodensity discontinuities—displaying the internal structural pattern of a complex object. IRE Trans Bio-Med Elect BME-8:68-72, 1961

Owens DGC, Johnstone EC, Bydder GM, et al: Unsuspected organic disease in schizophrenia demonstrated by computed tomography. J Neurol Neurosurg Psychiatry 43:1065-1069, 1980

Owens DGC, Johnstone EC, Crow TJ, et al: Lateral ventricular size in schizophrenia: relationship to the disease process and its clinical manifestations. Psychol Med 14:27-41, 1985

Oxenstierna G, Bergstrand G, Bjerkenstedt L, et al: Evidence of disturbed CSF circulation and brain atrophy in cases in schizophrenic psychosis. Br J Psychiatry 144:654-661, 1984

Pandarangi AK, Dewan MJ, Lee SH, et al: The ventricular system in chronic schizophrenic patients, a controlled tomography study. Br J Psychiatry 144:172-176, 1984

Pearlson GD, Veroff AF: Computerized tomographic scan changes in manic depressive illness. Lancet 2:470, 1981

Pearlson GD, Garbacz DJ, Breakey WR, et al: Lateral ventricular enlargement associated with persistent unemployment and negative symptoms in both schizophrenia and bipolar disorder. Psychiatry Res 12:1-9, 1984

Pearlson GD, Garbacz DJ, Moberg PJ, et al: Symptomatic, familial perinatal, and social correlates of computerized axial tomography (CAT) changes in schizophrenics and bipolars. J Nerv Ment Dis 173:42-50, 1985

Penn RD, Belanger MG, Yasnoff WA: Ventricular volume in man computed from CAT scans. Ann Neurol 3:216-223, 1978

Radon J: Über die bestimmung von funktionen durch ihre integrelwerte längs gewisser mannigfaltigkeiten. Saechsische Akademie der Wissenschatten, Leipzig. Berichte über die ver handlungen 69:262-277, 1917. [Translation by Analogic Corp., 1976: On the determination of functions by their integral values along certain manifolds.]

Rapoport JL, Ismond DR: Biological research in child psychiatry. J Am Acad Child Psychiatry 21:543-548, 1982

Reveley AM, Reveley MA: Aqueduct stenosis and schizophrenia. Neurol Neurosurg Psychiatry 46:18-22, 1983

Reveley AM, Reveley MA, Clifford CA, et al: Cerebral ventricular size in twins discordant for schizophrenia. Lancet 1:540-541, 1982

Reveley MA, Reveley AM, Baldy R: Left cerebral hemisphere hypodensity in discordant schizophrenic twins: a controlled study. Arch Gen Psychiatry 44:625-632, 1987

Rieder RO, Donnelly EF, Herdt JR, et al: Sulcal prominence in young chronic schizophrenic patients: CT scan findings associated with impairment on neuropsychological tests. Psychiatr Res 1:1-12, 1979

Rieder RO, Mann LS, Weinberger DR, et al: Computed tomographic scans in patients with schizophrenia, schizoaffective, and bipolar affective disorder. Arch Gen Psychiatry 40:735-739, 1983

Rieder RO, Mann L, Weinberger DR, et al: CAT scans in schizophrenia and affective disorders. Paper presented at the 134th Annual Meeting of the American Psychiatric Association, New Orleans, LA, 1981

Riederer SJ, Pele NJ, Chesler DA: The noise power spectrum in computed x-ray tomography. Phys Med Biol 23:446-454, 1978

Roberts MA, Caird FI: Computerized tomography and intellectual impairment in the elderly. J Neurol Neurosurg Psychiatry 39:986-990, 1976

Ron MA, Acker W, Shaw GK, et al: Computerized tomography of the brain in chronic alcoholism: a survey and follow-up study. Brain 105:497-514, 1982

Rosenberg CE, Anderson DC, Mahowald MW, et al: Computed tomography and EEG in patients without focal neurologic findings. Arch Neurol 39:291-292, 1982

Schlegel S, Kretzschmar K: Computed tomography in affective disorders, Part I: ventricular and sulcal measurements. Biol Psychiatry 22:15-23, 1987a

Schlegel S, Kretzschmar K: Computed tomography in affective disorders, Part II: brain density. Biol Psychiatry 22:15-23, 1987b

Schulsinger F, Parnas J, Petersen ET, et al: Cerebral ventricular size in the offspring of schizophrenic mothers. Arch Gen Psychiatry 41:602-606, 1984

Schulz SC, Koller MM, Kishore PR, et al: Ventricular enlargement in teenage patients with schizophrenia spectrum disorder. Am J Psychiatry 140:1592-1595, 1983a

Schulz SC, Sinicrope P, Kishore P, et al: Treatment response and ventricular enlargement in young schizophrenic patients. Psychopharmacol Bull 19:510, 1983b

Scott ML, Golden CJ, Ruedrich SL, et al: Ventricular enlargement in major depression. Psychiatry Res 8:91-93, 1983

Shelton RC, Weinberger DR, Doran A, et al: Cerebral structural pathology in schizophrenia. Presented at the Fourth World Congress of Biological Psychiatry, Philadelphia, PA, 1984

Shepp LA, Stein JA: Simulated reconstruction artifacts in computerized x-ray tomography, in Reconstruction Tomography in Diagnostic Radiology and Nuclear Medicine. Edited by Ter-Pogossran M, Phelps M, Brownell GL, et al. Chicago, University Park Press, 1977

Shima S, Kanba S, Masuda Y, et al: Normal ventricles in chronic schizophrenia. Acta Psychiatr Scand 71:25-29, 1985

Smith RC, Largen J, Calderon M, et al: CT scans and neuropsychological tests as predictors of clinical response in schizophrenics. Schizophrenia Bull 19:505, 1983

Snyder SH: Schizophrenia. Lancet 2:970-973, 1982

Spitzer RL, Endicott J, Robins E: Research Diagnostic Criteria (RDC) for a Selected Group of Functional Disorders, 3rd ed. New York, Biometrics Research, 1977

Standish-Barry HMAS, Bouras M, Bridges PK, et al: Pneumoencephalographic and computerized axial tomography scan changes in affective disorder. Br J Psychiatry 141:614-617, 1982

Stevens JR: Neuropathology of schizophrenia. Arch Gen Psychiatry 39:1121, 1982

Synek V, Reuben J: The ventricular-brain ratio using planimetric measurement of EMI scans. Br J Radiol 49:233-237, 1976

Takahashi R, Inaba Y, Inanaga K, et al: CT scanning and the investigation of schizophrenia, in Biological Psychiatry. Edited by Perris C, Struwe G, Jansson B. Amsterdam, Elsevier, 1981

Tanaka Y, Hazama H, Kawahara R, et al: Computerized tomography of the brain in schizophrenic patients. Acta Psychiatr Scand 63:191-197, 1981

Tanaka Y, Hazama H, Fukuhara T, et al: Computerized tomography of the brain in manic depressive patients: a controlled study. Folia Psychiatr Neurol 36:137-144, 1982

Targum SD, Rosen LN, DeLisi LE, et al: Cerebral ventricular size in major depressive disorder: association with delusional symptoms. Biol Psychiatry 18:329-336, 1983a

Targum SD, Rosen LN, Citrin CM: Delusional symptoms associated with enlarged cerebral ventricles in depressed patients. South Med J 76:985-987, 1983b

Terrence CF, Delaney JF, Alberts MC: Computed tomography for Huntington's disease. Neuroradiology 13:173-175, 1977

Trimble M, Kingsley D: Cerebral ventricular size in chronic schizophrenia. Lancet 1:278-279, 1978

Tsai LY, Jacoby CG, Stewart MA: Morphological cerebral asymmetries in autistic children. Biol Psychiatry 18:317-327, 1983a

Tsai LY, Nasrallah HA, Jacoby CG: Hemispheric asymmetries on computed tomographic scans in schizophrenia and mania. Arch Gen Psychiatry 40:1286-1289, 1983b

Tsuang MT, Winokur G: Criteria for subtyping schizophrenia. Clinical differentiation of hebephrenic and paranoid schizophrenia. Arch Gen Psychiatry 31:43-47, 1974

Turner SW, Toone BK, Breet-Jones JR: Computerized tomographic scan changes in early chronic schizophrenia—their relationship to perinatal trauma, family history and alcohol intake: preliminary findings. Psychol Med 14:219-225, 1986

Victor M, Adams RD, Mancall EL: A restricted form of cerebellar cortical degeneration occurring in alcoholic patients. Arch Neurol 1:579, 1959

Villafana T: Physics and instrumentation, in Cranial Computed Tomography. Edited by Lee SH, Rao KCVG. New York, McGraw-Hill, 1983

Von Bonin G: Anatomical asymmetries of the cerebral hemispheres, in Interhemispheric Relations and Cerebral Dominance. Edited by Mountcastle VB. Baltimore, Johns Hopkins University Press, 1962

Weinberger DR: Brain disease and psychiatric illness: when should a psychiatrist order a CAT scan? Am J Psychiatry 141:1521-1527, 1984a

Weinberger DR: Brain disease and psychiatric illness: when should a psychiatrist order a CAT scan? Am J Psychiatry 141:1521-1527, 1984b

Weinberger DR: Computed tomography (CT) findings in schizophrenia: speculation on the meaning of it all. J Psychiatr Res 18:477-490, 1984c

Weinberger DR, Wyatt RJ: Brain morphology in schizophrenia: in vivo studies, in Schizophrenia as a Brain Disease. Edited by Henn FA, Nasrallah HA. New York, Oxford University Press, 1982

Weinberger DR, Torrey EF, Neophytides AN, et al: Lateral ventricular enlargement in chronic schizophrenia. Arch Gen Psychiatry 36:735-739, 1979a

Weinberger DR, Torrey EF, Neophytides AN, et al: Structural abnormalities in the cerebral cortex of chronic schizophrenic patients. Arch Gen Psychiatry 36:935-939, 1979b

Weinberger DR, Torrey EF, Wyatt RJ: Cerebellar atrophy in chronic schizophrenia. Lancet 1:718-719, 1979c

Weinberger DR, Cannon-Spoor E, Potkin SC, et al: Poor premorbid adjustment and CT abnormalities in chronic schizophrenia. Am J Psychiatry 137:1410-1413, 1980

Weinberger DR, DeLisi LE, Neophytides AN, et al: Familial aspects of CT abnormalities in chronic schizophrenic patients. Psychiatry Res 4:65-71, 1981

Weinberger DR, DeLisi LE, Perman GP, et al: CT scans in schizophreniform disorder and other acute psychiatric patients. Arch Gen Psychiatry 39:778-783, 1982a

Weinberger DR, Luchins DJ, Morihisa JM, et al: Asymmetrical volumes of the right and left frontal and occipital regions of the human brain. Ann Neurol 11:97-100, 1982b

Williams FJB, Walshe JM: Wilson's disease: an analysis of the cranial computerized tomographic appearances found in 60 patients and the changes in response to treatment with chelating agents. Brain 104: 735-752, 1981

Williams AO, Reveley MA, Kolakowska T, et al: Schizophrenia with good and poor outcome, II: cerebral ventricular size and its clinical significance. Br J Psychiatry 146:239-246, 1985

Withers E, Hinton J: Three forms of clinical tests of the sensorium and their reliability. Br J Psychiatry 119:1-8, 1971

Woods BT, Wolf J: A reconsideration of the relationship of ventricular enlargement to duration of illness in schizophrenia. Am J Psychiatry 140:1564-1570, 1983

Zatz LM: The effect of the kVp level on EMI values. Radiology 119: 683-688, 1976

Chapter 2

Nuclear Magnetic Resonance Imaging

Nancy C. Andreasen, M.D., Ph.D.

The basic principle of magnetic resonance, that the properties or structure of a tissue or substance can be observed through measuring changes that occur when atomic nuclei are placed in a magnetic field, was first discovered by Bloch at Stanford and by Purcell at Harvard in 1946 (Young 1984; Bloch 1946; Purcell et al. 1946). Both were awarded a Nobel Prize for this discovery in 1952. The principle of magnetic resonance was applied in basic science laboratories for many years, particularly to do chemical spectroscopic studies. The use of magnetic resonance for *imaging* was given its initial impetus by Lauterbur in 1973, when he pointed out that nuclear magnetic resonance could be used to code the properties of small units of tissue and then to use this information in order to create pictures (Pickett 1982; Lauterbur 1973). During the 1980s, magnetic resonance scanners have become increasingly available, and it appears likely that, in future years, magnetic resonance imaging will eventually replace CT scanning for many clinical purposes.

Like a CT scan, a magnetic resonance scan provides a clear picture of brain *structure*. As currently applied, magnetic resonance imaging is rarely used to examine dynamic function, as BEAM, SPECT, and PET do. In the future, however, magnetic resonance imaging may eventually be used

This research was supported in part by NIMH Grant MH31593; a Scottish Rite Schizophrenia Research Grant; the Nellie Ball Trust Research Fund, Iowa State Bank & Trust Company, Trustee; a Research Scientist Award; and Grant RR59 from the General Clinical Research Centers Program, Division of Research Resources, NIH.

to visualize both structure and function, as will be explained later in this chapter. Thus it is a particularly exciting new brain-imaging technique.

Magnetic resonance imaging has many strengths as a brain-imaging technique. Unlike CT, SPECT, and PET, it requires no ionizing radiation. There are only a few contraindications to the procedure (e.g., pacemakers, certain kinds of aneurysm clips), and it has no known physical hazards in human beings apart from these contraindications. Claustrophobia is a potential psychological hazard, since the patient must be inside a hollow tube while being imaged, but this problem arises very infrequently.

The pictures of the brain produced by magnetic resonance imaging are reminiscent of the postmortem brain slices seen in neuroanatomy laboratories and neuroanatomy atlases. This technique provides excellent resolution between gray matter and white matter, permitting visualization of relatively tiny structures, such as cranial nerves, nuclei of the basal ganglia, or limbic structures such as the hippocampus. While CT scanning is limited to a single plane, the magnetic resonance images can be obtained in three planes: sagittal, coronal, and transverse. As a consequence, magnetic resonance imaging provides a much greater potential for three-dimensional reconstruction of the brain.

Not only does magnetic resonance imaging permit visualization in new planes, such as in coronal sections, but it is also free of bony artifacts. Bone, in fact, cannot be visualized well with MRI (making MRI an inappropriate technique for studying bone abnormalities such as fractures). This limitation opens up new areas of the brain for study, however. With MRI it is possible to look into the posterior fossa, a region that is obscured by bone artifacts on CT scan. Further, with this technique fine shades of tissue abnormality can be identified very well. Although it is possible to see a hint of multiple sclerosis plaques with CT, they stand out clearly with MRI.

Basic Principles

Nuclear magnetic resonance imaging produces images using principles that are somewhat more complicated than those involved in computerized tomography. The images produced by CT depend on the degree to which radiation is attenuated as it passes through various tissues. Magnetic resonance imaging, on the other hand, manipulates the electromagnetic forces inherent in tissues and reconstructs images based on changes in these electromagnetic forces. The principles involved in producing the NMR signal are complex, but not incomprehensible. The average clinician ordering MRI scans does not need to understand these principles in detail, although a superficial knowledge is useful, particularly in interpreting the scans produced. For researchers, an understanding of the basic principles is mandatory.

Summary of Basic Principles

Magnetic resonance imaging draws on the physical principles of electricity and magnetism. The average psychiatrist needs to recall no more than the simple principles learned in an introductory physics class. The following description attempts to summarize the principles involved so that they can be understood by any physician who has no expertise in physics beyond that of an introductory course.

The fundamentals of NMR imaging are summarized in Table 1 and amplified in the following discussion (Fullerton 1982; Axel 1984, Ellis et al. 1985; DeMyer et al. 1985; Elster 1986; Brant-Zawadzki and Norman 1987).

Nuclear. This technique is referred to as *nuclear* magnetic resonance imaging because it exploits the inherent magnetic field produced by the nuclei of some atoms. By far the most common of these is hydrogen, which is composed of a single proton. Because hydrogen is so widely distributed throughout the body, it forms the basis for NMR imaging techniques currently in use, since its abundance produces a strong signal. Other nuclei that are likely to assume importance in the future are phosphorus-31, carbon-13, sodium-23, and potassium-39. All of these behave as spinning charged particles. As will be recalled from introductory physics, spinning charged particles induce a magnetic field. The strength and

TABLE 1.   Principles of NMR Imaging

Nuclear	Based on the inherent magnetic moment associated with the *nuclei of atoms* (e.g., the hydrogen proton in water)
Magnetic	Which is *concentrated* through the use of a *magnetic field* to align the nuclei in one plane, thereby creating a nonrandom magnetization that is strong enough to measure.
Resonance	These protons have their own specific spin and wobble (precession), which can be excited by a radio signal broadcast at their specific frequency (the Larmor frequency) by a radio-frequency transmitter; the gradual decay in this *resonance* can then be measured by a radio-frequency receiver.
Imaging	The radio-frequency signals can then be converted via computer to shades of gray, white, and black corresponding to the strength of the signal and used to make *images* or pictures.

orientation of this field is referred to as its magnetic moment. This basic principle is illustrated in Figure 1.

Before the principles of NMR were developed, the fact that our bodies are full of such spinning charged particles and magnetic fields was of no particular interest. The NMR concept, however, makes this fundamental fact useful by developing techniques by which the inherent magnetic moment can be measured. This is achieved by putting the body tissue inside a large static magnetic field. In the natural state, the tiny "bar magnets" inside our bodies are oriented in random directions and their moments cancel one another out, producing a net magnetic field of zero. When a sample of tissue (for our purposes, the brain) is placed inside a strong static magnetic field, these tiny bar magnets tend to line up with this external field. This produces a macroscopic net magnetization of the tissue so that it can yield a measurable signal. This principle is illustrated in Figure 2.

In actual clinical practice, this means that the patient's body (or head) is placed inside a magnet. Early in the history of NMR, these magnets were relatively weak, often in the range of .15 Tesla (1 Tesla = 10 kilogauss). More recently, medical imaging systems have enlarged to the range of .5 to 1.5 Tesla. In general, magnets of larger field strength reduce the signal:noise ratio, decrease scanning time, and improve the resolution of images.

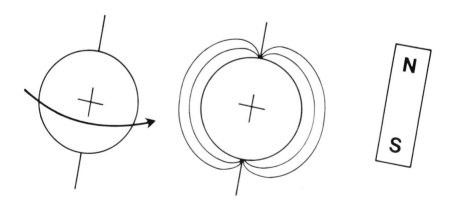

Spinning charged particles   induce a magentic moment   that acts like a
   in the nuclei of atoms   tiny bar magnet.

FIGURE 1.   How charged particles produce a magnetic field: the *Nuclear* in *N*MR.

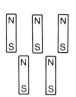

Without an external field the magnetic moments are random,	and therefore cancel one another and produce no net magnetization.	With an external magnetic field the protons are aligned and the magnetic moments concentrated,	producing a net positive magnetization.

WITHOUT AN EXTERNAL FIELD   WITH AN EXTERNAL FIELD

FIGURE 2. The effect of placing protons within an external magnetic field: the *Magnetic* in NMR.

Resonance. Placing the spinning hydrogen protons in a strong magnetic field has a second effect in addition to aligning them. When these protons are placed in a strong field their innate spin begins to wobble (or precess) around the longitudinal axis of the field. The simplest way to conceptualize this phenomenon is to think of a spinning top. When a top is set in motion, it does not remain totally upright as it spins, but rather tends to wobble; the wobbling is caused by the effects of the earth's gravitational field. In analogous fashion, the spinning protons also wobble or precess when placed within the magnetic field of an NMR system. This principle is illustrated in Figure 3.

This wobble, or precession, has a different rate for each nuclear species and is therefore characteristic of it. For example, the hydrogen proton differs from phosphorus-31, which differs from carbon-13, which differs from fluorine-19, and so on. This rate of wobble is called the Larmor frequency and is directly proportional to the strength of the magnetic field in which the nuclear species has been placed. This relationship is defined by the following equation:

$$\omega = \gamma B$$

where ω = Larmor frequency; γ = magnetogyric ratio (a constant); and B = strength of the magnetic field. The magnetogyric ratio, or gamma, is a constant that is specific for each particular nuclear species.

Our protons are now in a strong magnetic field, spinning and wobbling at a particular (resonant) frequency. Other forces must be applied

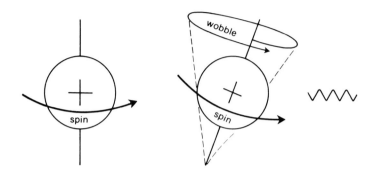

The spin is even.

The spin WOBBLES like a top, or precesses, with a resonant frequency specific to the nuclear species.

WITHOUT AN EXTERNAL FIELD   WITH AN EXTERNAL FIELD

FIGURE 3. How an external field produces resonance (precession): the *Resonance* in NMR.

to them, however, in order to permit this motion to be measured. In order to understand the next set of principles involved in NMR imaging, we must shift to a three-dimensional framework and see our spinning protons in x, y, and z axes. A set of pictures to illustrate these concepts appears in Figure 4.

The external magnetic field of the NMR system has aligned the protons so that they create a net magnetic moment that is aligned with the

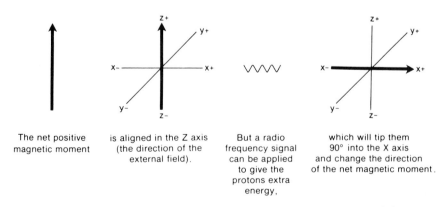

The net positive magnetic moment

is aligned in the Z axis (the direction of the external field).

But a radio frequency signal can be applied to give the protons extra energy,

which will tip them 90° into the X axis and change the direction of the net magnetic moment.

FIGURE 4. The use of radio-frequency signals to shift the direction of the magnetic moment.

direction of the external applied magnetic field, which is defined to be the z direction. They produce a net small magnetic moment pointing in the z direction, but it is unchanging and therefore cannot be measured. In order to permit the net magnetic moment to be measurable it has to be tipped into the $x-y$ axis by giving it extra energy and then measuring its gradual loss of this energy over time. The extra energy is given to it by taking advantage of the fact that the protons have their own inherent resonant frequency, or Larmor frequency, caused by their wobbling or precession.

In magnetic resonance imaging systems this extra energy is provided by transmitting a radio signal at the same frequency at which the protons are precessing. This principle is often explained by using the analogy of a tuning fork. If a tuning fork tuned to the note A is struck in the vicinity of another tuning fork tuned to that frequency, this second tuning fork will begin to hum. The first has produced energy which has been received by the second. Even if the first fork is stopped by having its vibration damped, the second will continue to vibrate for a period of time. It will gradually lose energy itself and reduce its signal. In NMR imaging a radio-frequency signal is transmitted to the receptive protons. This signal gives them additional energy and causes them to tip into the $x-y$ axis so that their net magnetic moment now points in a different direction. The strength of excitation or energy provided by the radio-frequency signal can vary depending on the strength of the signal itself.

The strength of the signal transmitted to the protons determines the angle at which the net magnetic moment is deflected in the $x-y$ axis. Thus the degree of deflection can be controlled. In actual practice, two signal strengths are commonly used. One tips the magnetic moment 90 degrees in the $x-y$ axis, and a second completely inverts the magnetic moment so that it points in the opposite direction. These are referred to as 90-degree and 180-degree pulses.

At this point NMR imaging now passes into its measurement phase. The actual process of measuring the NMR signal will be discussed in more detail below, but the basic principle involves the use of the resonance of the spinning protons. They have received extra energy during the radio-signal transmission phase. During the measurement phase, they are allowed to transmit back the signal produced by their resonant frequency. Following the analogy of the tuning fork, they have been given extra energy or activated, the initial tuning fork has been damped, and they are permitted to vibrate in isolation. Their signal gradually diminishes or decays over time (or relaxes, in NMR language), and the degree of relaxation over time is measured. Different tissues contain varying amounts of hydrogen protons, and thus the rate of decay varies. The difference in rate of decay produces radio-frequency signals of differing strengths, much as tissue attenuation differs in CT scanning and permits the development of pictures. (Further details about how the signal is used to differentiate tissues and produce images are described under the heading Production of Images.)

Thus the word *resonance* in magnetic resonance imaging refers to using the inherent resonant frequency, or Larmor frequency, produced by placing spinning charged particles (protons in this case) in an external magnetic field, adding extra energy to this resonance by exciting them with a radio signal broadcast at their specific frequency, and then measuring the gradual decay in this resonance by a radio-frequency receiver.

Imaging. Images, or pictures, are produced by assigning shades of gray, white, and black to the strength of the signal produced by the relaxing protons and received by a radio-frequency receiver. As in CT scanning, the signals are actually subdivided into tiny cubes or voxels (volume elements), which correspond to tiny chunks of brain tissue. Each of these has a different signal intensity and is therefore made a different shade of gray. The various shades of gray are put together to make the picture, composed of pixels (or picture elements) that correspond to the voxels.

NMR versus MRI. It should now be clear what the initials NMR or MRI stand for. This technology is referred to under both acronyms, although increasingly MRI or simply MR is preferred. NMR is an older term and was originally developed in the era when these principles were used largely for spectroscopic chemical studies. With the advent of NMR imaging, whereby the principles have been used to develop three-dimensional pictures, an "I" has been attached to the sequence of initials. Since the imaging procedures are now in use clinically, concern has arisen that some patients will misunderstand the use of the word "nuclear" and think that it refers to the use of ionizing radiation or the isotopes used in nuclear medicine. Thus, increasingly, radiologists have begun preferentially to use the term MRI, or simply MR.

Construction of Scanner

MRI suites look quite similar to other radiology suites. A picture of a typical MR unit appears in Figure 5. From the perspective of a patient, the major difference between an MR scanner and a CT scanner is that the patient's entire body must be moved inside the scanner. Subjectively, one has the experience of being moved inside a large hollow cave or tube. Further, the scanning procedure produces intermittent banging noises which are potentially distracting. However, when the procedure is ade-

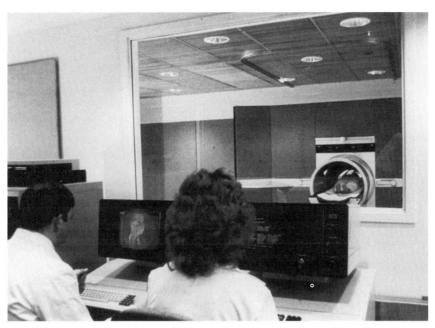

FIGURE 5.   A room in a typical NMR unit.

quately explained to the patient in advance, these minor psychological discomforts rarely produce any difficulty. Most psychiatric patients tolerate the procedure very well.

A summary of the components of an MR system appears in Table 2, while a schematic representation of a typical scanner appears in Figure 6.

The *static* magnet is used to apply a relatively large magnetic field in order to align the otherwise random magnetic moments generated by the spinning protons so that they produce a measurable magnetic moment. Two types of magnets are available for use: resistive magnets and superconducting magnets. Resistive magnets use wires wrapped around a coil to generate a field; they are less expensive and easier to maintain, but the fields that they generate are relatively small. In most modern scanning

TABLE 2.   Components of an NMR System

Static magnet	Radio-frequency receiver
Gradient magnets	Computer
Radio-frequency transmitter	Display system

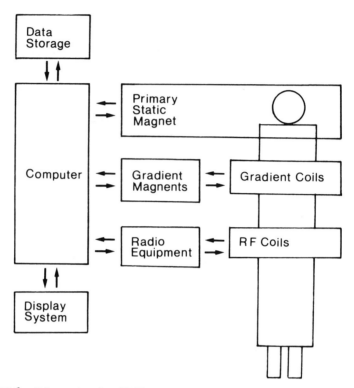

FIGURE 6.   Schematic of an NMR scanner.

equipment, superconducting magnets are used, instead. While they require more maintenance, they can also generate the large fields, in the range of .5 to 1.5 Tesla, that are needed to produce high-quality images.

The *gradient* magnets are necessary in order to permit localization of the signal so that it can be reconstructed as a series of slices. Without the use of gradient magnets, the MR signal generated by the process of excitation and measurement of resonance described above would lead to a generalized signal coming from the whole head. The signal would be coming from many different tissues with many different resonances, some of which would cancel one another out, and would produce an overall signal that would be unmeasurable or meaningless. Through the use of gradient magnets, the resonance can be activated selectively in adjacent slices of the brain independently, thereby producing the consecutive cuts that are seen in the sagittal, coronal, and transverse planes in the NMR images.

The *radio* equipment consists of *radio-frequency transmitters and receivers.* The transmitter is used to send the excitation signal at the

Larmor frequency that enhances the inherent resonance of the protons. After this radio signal is used to excite the protons, the transmitter is then turned off for a brief period of time and the enhanced resonance is allowed to relax or decay. As they resonate, however, these excited protons produce their own radio-frequency signal which is picked up on a radio-frequency receiver that collects data about the changing amplitude and frequency of this signal during the relaxation time period.

The *computer* is used to convert this complex mass of data into information that can be used to produce an image. The actual details about the techniques by which a set of phasic signals with changing amplitude and frequency can be converted into black, gray, and white dots is outside the range of this overview. A very rapid and efficient mathematical algorithm, known as fast fourier transformation, is applied to these complicated wave forms and turns them into an observable signal that is based on units of amplitude, frequency, and time. Because the gradient magnets permit the signal to be localized in slices of tissue, the signal can be measured simultaneously in tiny units of tissue or voxels. Signals of varying strength from each voxel are assigned varying shades of gray. Complex wave forms have now been digitalized, or turned into a series of dots, which can be used to produce a picture.

The *display system* is an interactive computer terminal that permits the radiologist or radiology technician to observe the quality of the scan as it is being obtained. Since modern MR systems are interactive, the technician sitting at the display system can request additional modifications in the scanning procedure, depending on what he or she sees, while the patient is still in the scanner. The scans can then be printed on film to provide a permanent visual record, while the signal intensity data used to reconstruct the images can be stored on tape or disc for a permanent data record.

Production of Images

MRI is a much more complex technology than CT scanning, with which it is similar in many respects. While images are produced in CT scanning simply through the attenuation of radiation as it passes through tissue, the image seen through magnetic resonance is produced by a number of different factors. Some of these are inherent in the tissue being studied (such as the density of protons in a particular voxel), and others are inherent in the particular imaging system being used (such as the field strength of the static magnet). But still other aspects of the scanning procedure are operator-controlled. As will become more apparent in the discussion below, the type of picture obtained can be manipulated by varying the timing and intensity of the excitation signal sent from the radio transmitter (*pulse sequence*). Further, the various gradient magnets can be manipulated in order to select particular imaging planes. With modern MR scanners, more options are available than can be used in a comfortable period of scanning time. The sequences that are best for seeing anatomic structures clearly may not be the best for seeing abnormal tissue or for measuring indices of tissue change (the relaxation times T1 and T2).

A psychiatrist–clinician who orders an MR scan for a patient will not, of course, be responsible for selecting a particular imaging sequence, but he or she should provide the radiologist with adequate detail about the questions to be asked so that the radiologist can select an appropriate group of scanning sequences. A clinical researcher must, however, be fully aware of the complexities involved in selecting scanning sequences, since he or she will want to select the ones most appropriate for the scientific question that he or she is asking.

Components of the MRI Signal

The MRI signal is produced by three different components, which are summarized in Table 3: proton density, T1 relaxation time, and T2 relaxation time. The relationship between them is defined by the Bloch equation:

$$\text{Intensity} = f(h)f(v) \, [1 - e^{-TR/T1}]e^{-TE/T2}$$

f(h) is a function of hydrogen proton concentrations, f(v) is a function of flow velocity and has a value of one for stationary tissue. TR and TE are repetition or echo times and under operator control; T1 and T2 are tissue-specific longitudinal and transverse relaxation times. These can be explained more specifically as follows:

Proton density is simply the number of protons present in a particular sample of tissue. Pulse sequences can be used that rely heavily on

TABLE 3.   Components of the NMR Signal

Proton Density—A measure of the number of hydrogen nuclei in the sample

T1—An exponential growth constant that reflects the return of magnetization within the nuclei to the resting state in the z axis (also called longitudinal relaxation time, or spin–lattice relaxation)

T2—An exponential decay constant that reflects loss of signal strength as dephasing of the spin occurs (also called transverse relaxation time, or spin–spin relaxation)

---

proton density (e.g., a pulse sequence referred to as saturation recovery), but these sequences give very poor contrast and consequently are now infrequently used. The imaging sequences currently most widely used are more heavily influenced either by T1 or T2 relaxation times.

T1 relaxation time is an exponential growth constant that reflects the return of magnetization of the protons to their equilibrium state in the z axis. (Since the z axis is longitudinal, T1 is also sometimes called longitudinal relaxation time; since the energy released during relaxation passes into the "lattice," T1 is also sometimes referred to as spin–lattice relaxation.)

The processes that underlie T1 relaxation and that make it useful for imaging are summarized in Figures 7 through 9. In order to understand both T1 and T2, we must return to the concept of manipulating the magnetic moment in three-dimensional space, as was portrayed earlier, in Figure 4. When a portion of the human body, such as a head, is placed within the magnetic field of an MR scanner, the protons in its tissue are aligned along the direction of the magnetic field (or the z axis). This produces a small magnetic moment in the tissue pointing in the z direction. Since this is in equilibrium with the external magnetic field, it produces no measurable time-dependent phenomenon. In order to permit measurement, it has to be manipulated in some way. One technique is to administer a radio-frequency signal that will deflect the magnetic moment 90 degrees, which tips it into the x–y plane. This type of radio-frequency signal is referred to as a 90-degree pulse. The time when the pulse is administered is referred to as the excitation phase. After the 90-degree pulse is administered, the excited protons gradually relax. As they relax, the longitudinal component of the net magnetization returns back to its equilibrium value while the transverse component of the magnetization decays to zero in a T2 relaxation process, described below. Thus, through the process of relaxation, the net magnetization in the z axis gradually increases, until it is again back to its original level.

As indicated in Figure 8, T1 is defined as the time required for the net magnetization in the z axis to return to 63 percent of its original value. Since the relaxation process leads to an increase in the magnetic moment in the z axis, T1, when portrayed graphically, has the appearance of an exponential growth constant, as shown in Figure 8.

Various tissues within the body differ in their proton composition and therefore in the rate at which relaxation occurs. Thus T1 varies in different tissues. As illustrated in Figure 9, relaxation occurs more quickly in normal brain tissue than in abnormal brain tissue, while both return more quickly than cerebrospinal fluid (CSF) or water (except early in the relaxation process). In general, pathological processes lead to an increase in fluid within brain tissue and therefore lengthen or increase T1 relax-

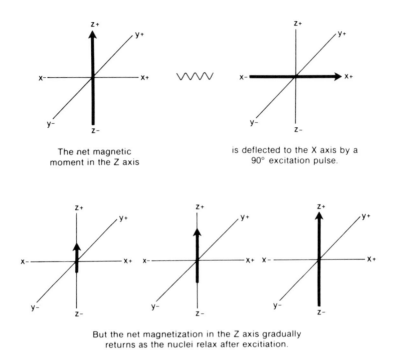

The net magnetic
moment in the Z axis

is deflected to the X axis by a
90° excitation pulse.

But the net magnetization in the Z axis gradually
returns as the nuclei relax after excitiation.

FIGURE 7.   Measurement of T1 relaxation: basic principles.

ation time. These differences in T1 among tissues therefore permit them to be visualized differently in the image or picture that is ultimately produced by the MR scanning process.

T2 relaxation time is an exponential decay constant that reflects loss of signal strength as dephasing of spin occurs after excitation. Since this relaxation process occurs in a *x–y* plane, it is sometimes referred to as transverse relaxation. Since the dephasing of spin occurs because of interaction with other spinning nuclei, it is also sometimes called spin–spin relaxation time.

The processes underlying T2 relaxation are illustrated in Figures 10 through 12. While T1 and T2 relaxation have been separated for purposes of discussion, it is important to realize that they are occurring simultaneously during any given imaging procedure, and both are contributing some relative amount to the imaging process. As Figure 10 illustrates, measurement of T2 also begins with an excitation pulse that moves the alignment of net magnetization out of the *z* axis. As was described for T1, a 90-degree pulse will tip the net magnetic moment into the *x–y* axis. When the hydrogen nuclei are tipped, initially the spinning of this group of

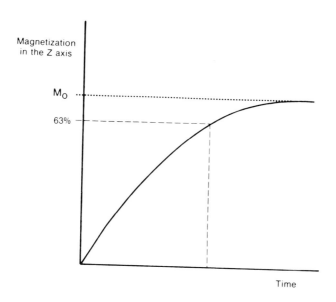

T1 is the time required for net magnetization in
the Z axis to return to 63% of equlibrium value, M_O.

FIGURE 8.   Measurement of T1 relaxation: definition of T1.

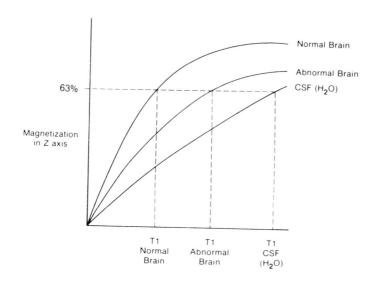

Different tissues have different rates of relaxation.
Therefore measurement of T1 can potentially be used
as a measureable index of tissue variation, tissue
function, and tissue pathology.

FIGURE 9.   Measurement of T1 relaxation: differentiation among tissues.

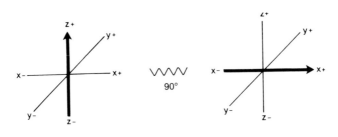

T2 is a relaxation process occurring in the X axis
after a 90° pulse has been applied.

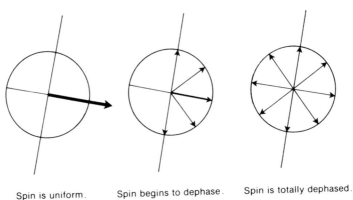

Spin is uniform.   Spin begins to dephase.   Spin is totally dephased.

It reflects dephasing of the spin of the nuclei until
the net magnetic moment relaxes to zero.

FIGURE 10.   Measurement of T2 relaxation: basic principles.

nuclei is "in phase" because of the relatively uniform alignment induced by the static magnetic field. (For those who like to think visually, it may help to imagine the aligned hydrogen protons as a group of spinning tops that are precessing in unison.) As the nuclei relax, the uniformity of spin gradually decreases among them, and they no longer precess in unison. Gradually some spin faster, while some spin more slowly. As this dephasing of spin occurs, the net magnetic moment in the x–y plane is gradually reduced until the nuclei are randomly oriented in the x–y plane and the net magnetic moment is reduced to zero.

As Figures 11 and 12 indicate, T2 is portrayed visually as an exponential decay constant. T2 is defined as the time required for net magnetization to decay to 37 percent (i.e., 100 minus 63 percent) of its original value in the x–y plane. Because magnetization is steadily decreasing in this plane, a graphic plot of its appearance appears as an exponential

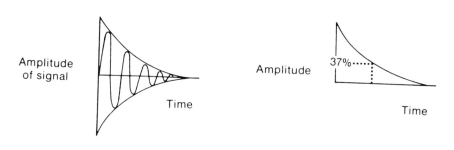

The signal decays over
time as dephasing of spin occurs.

T2 is defined as the time
required for the signal to
return to 37% of its original value.

FIGURE 11.   Measurement of T2 relaxation: definition of T2.

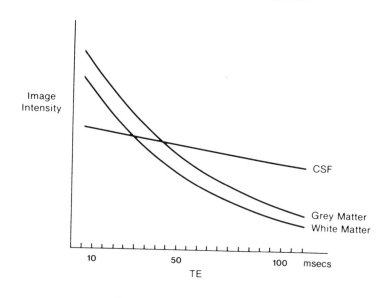

Different tissues also have different
rates of T2 relaxation:

CSF > Grey Matter > White Matter

Source: Pfefferbaum A, Zatz LM, Jernigan TL, et al:
Quantitative approach to the analysis of CT and NMR scans.
*Abstracts of Panels and Posters Presented at the Annual
Meeting of the American College of Neuropsychopharmacology,*
December 1985.

FIGURE 12.   Measurement of T2 relaxation: differentiation among tissues.
Image intensity at various TE for spin-echo sequence with
TR = 2000 msec.

decay. As in the case of T1, the rate of decrease in T2 also varies in tissues. For example, T2 is longer in white matter than in gray matter tissue, and it is longest in CSF or water.

T1 and T2 are specific tissue characteristics. Their size will vary depending on other factors such as magnetic field strength. Nevertheless, at a given field strength and radio-frequency strength, different tissues will have different characteristic T1s and T2s. This fact is summarized in Table 4. Table 4 indicates that when one compares the T1 and T2 for water and muscle at 4 MHz, the T1 and T2 for water are essentially identical (2,700 milliseconds); but T1 for muscle is 600 milliseconds while T2 for muscle is 30 milliseconds.

Common Pulse Sequences. While a variety of pulse sequences were used in the early days of magnetic resonance imaging (e.g., saturation recovery), scanners in current clinical use rely primarily on two types of pulse sequences: inversion recovery and spin-echo. The characteristics of these two pulse sequences are summarized in Table 5. Inversion-recovery pulse sequences are best for visualizing anatomical structures, since they produce pictures with excellent gray–white resolution. This pulse sequence relies more heavily on the T1 component of the NMR signal and therefore is said to produce "T1-weighted" images. Spin-echo sequences produce pictures that are less anatomically clear, but this technique is far more sensitive for detecting subtle abnormalities of tissue such as tumors or multiple sclerosis plaques. Because detection of lesions not otherwise readily visualized is a major clinical goal of MR imaging, spin-echo sequences are more often chosen for clinical evaluations. Spin-echo images often draw heavily on the T2 component of the MR signal and therefore are sometimes said to produce "T2-weighted" images. (Spin-echo images

TABLE 4. Tissue Differentiation: T1 and T2 for Water versus Muscle at 4 MHz

	Water	Muscle
T1	2,700 msec	600 msec
T2	2,700 msec	30 msec

TABLE 5. Common Imaging Sequences

Inversion Recovery:	Good gray–white resolution, T1-weighted images
Spin-Echo:	Good detection of small focal lesions
	T2-weighted images with long TE and long TR
	T1-weighted images with short TE and short TR

can also be obtained in such a manner so as to yield T1-weighted images, however, if shorter pulse sequences are used; and due to continuing improvements in software, these T1-weighted spin-echo images now often have very impressive anatomic definition.)

The mechanisms and principles involved in selection and application of pulse sequences are relatively complicated. The clinician interested in a broad general grasp of magnetic resonance may wish to skip the remainder of this section, armed with the knowledge that there are two basic types of pulse sequences in common clinical use, and move ahead to the next section, on interpreting MR images. Readers interested in the research applications of magnetic resonance need to have a fundamental understanding of these pulse sequences, however, and so this material is included in order to assist them.

Inversion-recovery sequences involve the application of two radio-frequency signals. The basic principles involved are summarized in Figures 13 and 14. The first pulse is a 180-degree pulse and serves as the excitation pulse. This pulse tips the alignment of the magnetic moment 180 degrees in the z axis so that it is *inverted*. After this inversion the magnetic moment steadily relaxes and realigns itself to its former level, following the principles discussed in the previous section. Since this relaxation is occurring in the z axis, however, it cannot be measured. Only when there is a transverse component of the magnetization precessing in the x–y plane will radio-frequency waves be emitted. Consequently, for

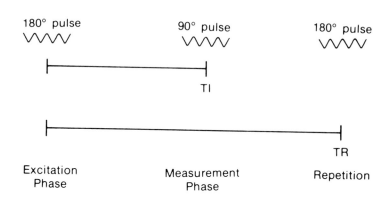

TI = Time to inversion

TR = Repetition time

FIGURE 13.   Principles of inversion-recovery imaging: timing of pulse sequences.

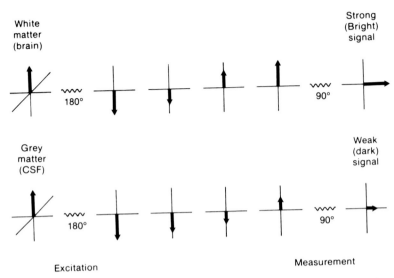

FIGURE 14.   Principles of inversion-recovery imaging: tissue differentiation.

measurement to occur, it is necessary to apply a second 90-degree pulse that tips the magnetization into the x–y plane. The time between the 180-degree excitation pulse and the 90-degree pulse that permits measurement is referred to as the inversion time (TI). After measurement has occurred, the relaxation process is allowed to complete itself, and the pulse sequence is then begun again with another 180-degree pulse. The time interval from the initial excitation pulse of the first sequence until the initial excitation pulse of the next sequence is called repetition time.

Since relaxation times are fixed tissue characteristics, it is important to time the pulses in a way that will maximize resolution. While T1 and T2 are fixed, pulse sequence parameters such as TI and TR are under operator control. Figure 14 illustrates how the relative differences in rate of relaxation between white and gray matter (or between brain and CSF) produce relatively different signals. Since white matter returns to its original net magnetization more quickly, it produces a stronger, brighter signal than do the slower gray matter or CSF. If, however, TI were too short, the differences might be slight and therefore produce very little difference in signal size. On the other hand, if TI is left too long so that all tissues have reached nearly complete relaxation, discrimination between tissues will also be poor. Specific rules for selection of the timing parameters TI and TR cannot be provided in this book, since they will vary from scanner to scanner depending on magnetic field strength, available software, and so forth.

Spin-echo pulse sequences are somewhat more difficult to understand than are inversion recovery sequences. The basic principles underlying this pulse sequence are summarized in Figures 15 and 16. Spin-echo pulse sequences derive much of their signal strength from the T2 component and largely reflect relaxation in the x–y plane. This relaxation occurs as the precession of nuclei, originally occurring more or less in unison, gradually dephases. The speed of this dephasing is caused by two factors: lack of homogeneity in the external static magnetic field, and intrinsic properties of the spinning nuclei themselves. The spin-echo sequence has been designed in order to eliminate the effect of lack of homogeneity in the external magnetic field (since this is an artifact or "nuisance variable") and to provide a relatively pure measure of T2 relaxation.

In the spin-echo sequence, a 90-degree pulse is administered in order to tip the magnetic moment into the x–y plane where it can be measured. Dephasing of spin begins to occur immediately, but after a specific time (referred to as tau) a 180-degree pulse is administered that tips the magnetic moment 180 degrees in the opposite direction. At a time that is twice tau (2τ), a measurement is obtained. For reasons explained in the next paragraph, this measurement provides a relatively pure reflection of T2 without any contribution from nonhomogeneity of the magnetic field. The time between the original 90-degree excitation pulse and measure-

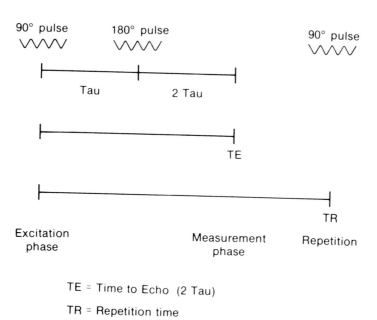

FIGURE 15. Principles of spin-echo imaging: timing of pulse sequences.

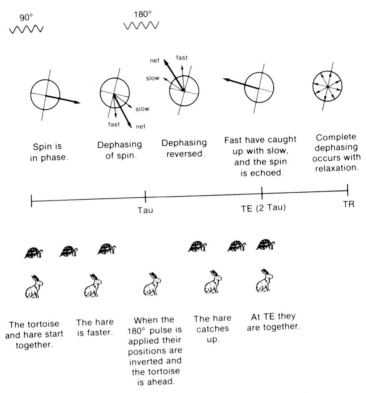

FIGURE 16.   Principles of spin-echo imaging: how the spin echoes.

ment is referred to as time-to-echo (TE) and is always equivalent to 2τ. After a period of time to permit complete relaxation, the sequence is initiated again with another 90-degree pulse. The time between pulse sequences is referred to as the repetition time (TR).

As Figure 16 illustrates, this pulse sequence capitalizes on the fact that different nuclei dephase at different rates. After excitation, the magnetic moment is concentrated in the x–y plane. As dephasing occurs, however, some nuclei get ahead of others, just as if a tortoise were racing a hare. When the 180-degree pulse is administered, however, the position of the two racers is reversed, and the tortoise is suddenly ahead of the hare. (Or, the position of the nuclei dephasing relatively slowly is ahead of those that were dephasing more quickly.) As time elapses in this race, the tortoise and hare are finally side by side again, just as they were at the start of the race. (Or, the faster nuclei have now caught up again with the slower nuclei, and the net magnetic moment is concentrated again.) From the point of view of signal measurement, the signal emitted by the nuclei has nearly returned to the strength that it had at excitation; in other words, it has produced an echo of its original intensity. That is why this sequence is called spin-echo: the signal that is measured is produced when the dephasing nuclei, tipped into their mirror position as racers, have met one another again and produced a signal that echoes their original signal. As more time is permitted to elapse, complete dephasing occurs, and then the process is begun again. Through the use of the spin-echo technique, it is possible to remove the component of spin dephasing that is due to magnetic field nonhomogeneity and to obtain a relatively pure signal based primarily on the T2 component of spin dephasing.

This discussion, while relatively complicated, is still over-simplified. Inversion recovery has been presented as if signal intensity is due simply to T1 relaxation, while spin-echo has been described as if it produces only a T2-weighted signal. In fact, however, in MR imaging, the signal emitted has three components as mentioned above (proton density, T1, and T2). Different pulse sequences maximize the relative contribution of these components, but all pulse sequences still produce a mixed signal.

In spin-echo in particular, the relative contributions of T1 and T2 can vary markedly, depending on the time-to-repetition (TR). If TR is relatively long, then relaxation in the z axis (the T1 component) will be nearly complete, and the T1 will provide a relatively small contribution to the signal. On the other hand, when TR is relatively short, T1 may provide a large contribution.

Interpretation of Images

The signal emitted in response to the various manipulations described above is turned into images by assigning various shades of gray, white, and black to tiny blocks of tissue according to their difference in signal intensity. The stronger the signal, the brighter the image. The factors that increase signal intensity are summarized in Table 6. In general, signal intensity increases with increased proton density, decreased T1, and increased T2. Tissues with a short T1 relax and return to equilibrium more quickly and therefore give off a brighter signal. Tissues with a long T2 stay in phase longer and give out a brighter signal.

TABLE 6.   Reading NMR Images: Why Are Parts Bright or Dark?

Increased signal intensity causes brightness in the image. Factors that increase signal intensity and therefore brightness are:
Increased proton density (free H_2O, CSF)
Decreased T1
Increased T2

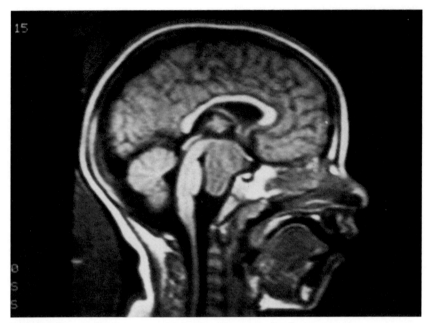

FIGURE 17.   Inversion-recovery image of a posterior fossa tumor.

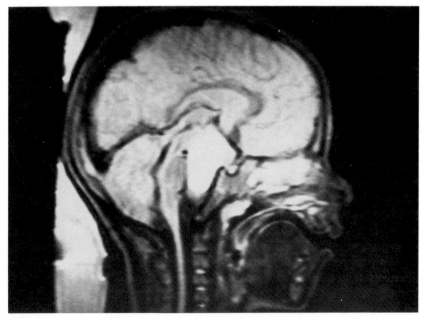

FIGURE 18.   Spin-echo image of a posterior fossa tumor.

MR images may appear quite different depending on the imaging sequence being used. Figures 17 and 18 illustrate this quite clearly. These depict identical midsagittal cuts showing the head of a child with a posterior fossa brain tumor. Figure 17 is an inversion recovery image which is T1-weighted, while Figure 18 is a spin-echo image that is T2-weighted. These figures demonstrate many of the differences between these two types of imaging sequences. Both images show the tumor well, since it is quite large, although it may be somewhat more obvious in Figure 18. The inversion-recovery image has clear gray–white resolution, while the gray–white resolution is somewhat less distinct in the spin-echo image.

Some aspects of the image remain more or less the same no matter which imaging sequence is used. Relatively consistently, fat is bright (short T1, long T2). Air, calcification, and cortical bone are dark (low proton density). Rapid flow (i.e., in blood vessels) produces no signal and is black. However, most other structures may appear either light or dark, depending on the type of imaging sequence. One must know whether the image is T1- or T2-weighted in order to interpret it.

Most pathological processes lengthen T1 and T2. As has been emphasized in Figures 9 and 12, the relative range of relaxation time varies, with normal tissue relaxing more quickly than abnormal, and abnormal more quickly than water or CSF. The relaxation time in abnormal tissue is probably increased because of increased water content. Figure 19 shows a transverse cut of a patient suffering from multiple sclerosis, in which the MS plaques are clearly highlighted by a spin-echo sequence.

As Figures 17 and 18 illustrate, many tissues have a different degree of brightness on T1- versus T2-weighted images. On T1-weighted images abnormal tissues are relatively dark, while on T2-weighted images they are relatively bright. The posterior fossa tumor in these scans is dark in Figure 17 and bright in Figure 18. White and gray matter have different appearances as well. The inversion-recovery scan of Figure 17 shades white and gray matter much as they are shaded in the brain. The corpus callosum, for example, appears as a clear white strip because it is a densely packed bundle of white-matter tracts, while the callosum is relatively dark in Figure 18. CSF is relatively dark with both imaging sequences. The cortical bone of the skull cannot be seen because it is too dark, but the area of the skull is clearly demarcated by the bright white fat of the bone marrow which lies inside it.

As the sample scan also indicates, MR scanning (like nearly all brain scanning) involves a *partial volume effect*. This term refers to the fact that the brain slices that are imaged are not clean slices of the sort seen in anatomy laboratories, but rather represent an average through a section of tissue of specified thickness (often around 1 cm). Thus this midsagittal cut depicts not only midline structures, but also structures that appear

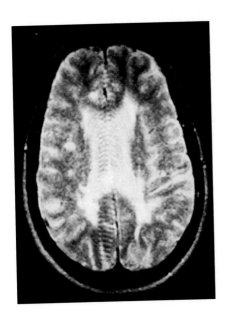

FIGURE 19.   Transverse spin echo scan showing multiple sclerosis plaques.

slightly on either side of the midline. For example, one can clearly see the thalamus and the columns of the fornix, which stand out against the darker background of CSF in the lateral ventricles that lie on either side of the midline septum pellucidum.

Scanning sequences can be manipulated to produce different kinds of images. For example, the relative contributions of T1 and T2 can be changed within spin-echo sequences by varying TE and TR. When TE and TR are relatively short, the T1-weighting of the images is increased. These *fast spin-echo sequences* produce images similar to those obtained through inversion recovery. When TE and TR are relatively long, the contribution of T2 to the signal increases. These T2-weighted images produce the greatest contrast between normal and abnormal tissues. Unfortunately, they also have less impressive anatomic definitions and a poorer signal:noise ratio because of the decay in signal intensity with longer time delay.

All these factors make MR imaging more difficult to use and to interpret than the more familiar CT-scanning technique. The sequences that are best for seeing structure are not the best for seeing abnormal tissue. It is important to decide on the purpose of the MR scan in advance so that an appropriate pulse sequence and an appropriate plane can be selected in order to evaluate the presence or absence of a particular pathological process. Every possible option cannot be explored, because more are available than can be used in a comfortable period of scanning time.

Types of Equipment Available

Commercial imaging systems have been available since the early 1980s, and their quality has improved exponentially in a very rapid time period. Although the early systems used resistive magnets, superconducting magnets are now standard. Most newer commercial systems are operating at a field strength of 1.5 Tesla, and the upper limit of field strength for clinical imaging has not yet been established. Larger field strengths permit shorter imaging time and improved resolution.

The various commercial imaging systems available are probably all of high quality, but they vary in their capacities according to the software available. All provide imaging in at least three planes, but some permit the operator to shift the angle at will, while others require that the three planes be perpendicular to one another. Some software packages provide a balanced blend of inversion-recovery and spin-echo sequences, while others emphasize spin-echo primarily. The thickness of the cut also may or may not be fixed at some specified interval such as 1 cm. The comparability of CT scans obtained through different imaging systems has always been questioned, but with MR imaging it is even more likely that it will be difficult to compare scans obtained in different centers using different equipment, at least for the purpose of research investigations.

Applications in Psychiatry

Magnetic resonance imaging has a broad range of applications in medicine. It can be used to examine for disc disease in the spine, to conduct cardiovascular imaging, and to explore for mediastinal masses. Many of the most promising applications of MRI are, however, in brain imaging. Exploration of the relevance of MRI to psychiatry is just beginning.

Background

Studies using magnetic resonance imaging are currently applied from two different vantage points. One vantage point involves the use of MRI to search for anatomical or structural abnormalities that may characterize various types of mental illness. Following the lead of research using CT, which has found evidence of ventricular enlargement and sulcal enlargement which may indicate cortical or subcortical atrophy in some patients with serious mental illnesses such as schizophrenia, magnetic resonance research is also exploring the possibility of structural abnormalities. If such anatomical abnormalities exist in schizophrenia, magnetic resonance imaging offers a superior capacity to detect them, since it has markedly improved gray–white resolution and permits imaging in multiple planes. A second line of research involves searching for indications of regional tissue pathology by determining whether specific regions of interest (e.g., limbic tissue, basal ganglia, etc.) display any abnormalities in T1 and T2 relaxation times.

Structural Studies: Methodological Aspects. The possibilities for using magnetic resonance imaging to conduct structural studies of the brain in mental illness are very exciting. Prior to MRI, such structural studies could only be done on postmortem brains. While eminently worthwhile, postmortem studies have certain intrinsic limitations. Patients studied at postmortem are typically relatively old, and it is therefore difficult to separate aging effects from effects due to the illness. Further, some patients whose brains come to postmortem have had long-term institutionalization, which might provide at least a partial alternate explanation for any findings obtained. It is frequently difficult to obtain adequate clinical description of the patient's symptoms of mental illness prior to death. Finally, preservation artifacts may distort brain size or shape. These various problems can be bypassed using a technology such as MRI, which permits study of brain structure in young patients while they are living and while they can be evaluated systematically relatively early in their illness.

Studies that focus on examining for possible structural abnormalities must deal with a number of different methodological issues. These include selection of the appropriate scanning sequence, selection of appropriate cuts, and developing techniques for measurement.

The *scanning sequence* most appropriate for conducting structural studies is either inversion-recovery or a fast spin-echo (i.e., T1-weighted) sequence. As is by now apparent from the above section on generation and interpretation of MR images, this technology involves a series of trade-offs. The sequences best for detailed structural definition differ from those best for picking up regions of tissue abnormality.

Inversion-recovery sequences probably give the most impressive anatomical definition, but good inversion-recovery sequences are not available on all scanners that are currently manufactured. If a good inversion-recovery sequence is lacking, spin-echo sequences with a short TE and TR offer relatively good gray–white resolution as well.

Selection of cuts will depend in large part on the hypotheses to be investigated. Figures 20, 21, and 22 illustrate some of the structures that are seen using midsagittal, coronal, and axial or transverse cuts. They indicate that perhaps the largest amount of anatomical information is provided by coronal cuts. This method for sectioning the brain was of course the choice of neuroanatomists for the past century, at least prior to the invention of CT scanning. Once CT scanning was developed,

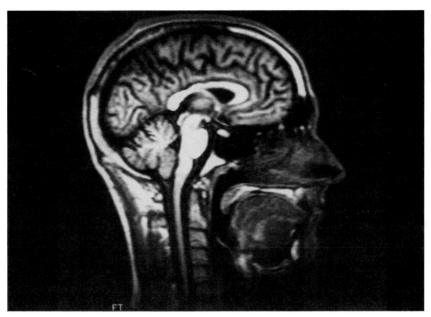

FIGURE 20. Structures seen on midsagittal cuts (inversion recovery).

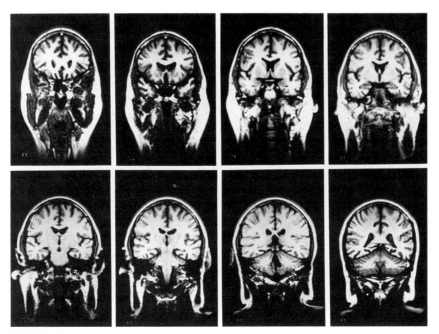

FIGURE 21. Structures seen on coronal cuts (inversion recovery).

neuroanatomists and neuropathologists began to switch to transverse cuts in order to provide sections comparable to those seen through CT. Now that MRI is available, many more options are also available. An obvious advantage of MRI over neuroanatomical sectioning is that the neuroanatomists can only cut through the brain once in one set of planes, while MRI permits multiple cuts, at least in theory. (Time limitations may preclude achieving this in actuality for many patients.)

The midline sagittal cut is anatomically quite interesting (Figure 20), but more lateral sagittal cuts primarily provide sections through white-matter tracts and are not particularly useful for visualizing subcortical nuclei or structural asymmetry. The coronal cuts yield a large amount of information, since they permit comparison of left versus right differences, good visualization of the basal ganglia and limbic structures such as the hippocampus and amygdala, and clear differentiation of frontal and temporal lobes (Figure 21). The transverse cuts provide clear sections through the basal ganglia, the ventricular system, the thalamus, and other regions of interest but are less useful for observing asymmetry (Figure 22).

Techniques for measuring structures (i.e., morphometric techniques) are still in a "growth phase." The natural inclination of most investigators is simply to extrapolate from previous CT studies and to measure things that have been observed on CT scans. This represents an unimaginative use of a flexible and interesting technology, however, and over the long run methods for measuring MRI scans are likely to develop independently of those used for CT scans.

Measurement techniques range from visual inspection, to linear measurements, to area and volume measurements.

The simplest method for evaluating MR scans involves direct visual inspection. While this may not seem very "scientific" because it is not quantitative, it is clearly foolish not to look at what one measures before one measures it. Further, visual inspection is necessary in order to determine whether head position is standardized, whether the scan is of adequate quality, whether movement or other artifacts are present, whether it indeed passes through the appropriate structures, whether there are any clear pathological abnormalities, and whether there are overall indications of cerebral atrophy as indicated in sulcal and/or ventricular enlargement. Visual inspection can be used to apply rating scales for designating atrophy (of regions such as the cortex or cerebellum) as mild, moderate, or severe, since no quantitative measurements are readily available for evaluating these structures anyway.

Subjective visual inspection suffers from the deficiencies inherent in any subjective system of measurement, such as potentially poor reliability and lack of quantification. On the other hand, subjective visual inspection

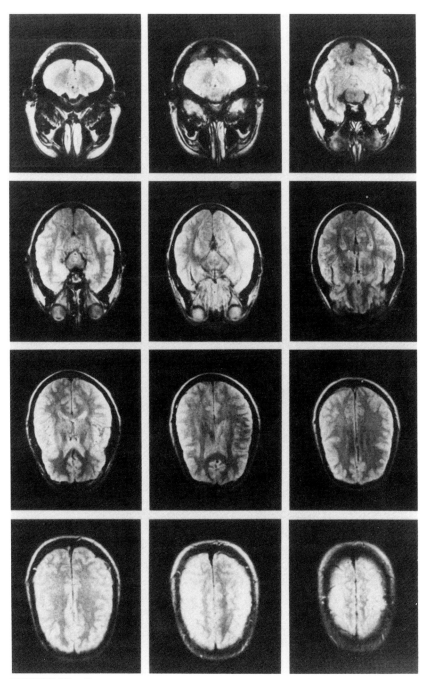

FIGURE 22. Structures seen on transverse cuts (spin-echo).

is the only method available for evaluating some aspects of the scan. It also serves as a useful check on more complex methods of measurement, is the method most commonly used by neuroradiologists, and therefore has considerable face validity.

Linear measurements were originally developed for pneumo-encephalography and later for CT scanning. A large body of literature exists for the evaluation of atrophic processes and ventricular enlargement by making linear measurements on CT scans. Linear measurements have a number of drawbacks, however. First, they permit only a one-dimensional representation of the brain and therefore can only roughly approximate measures of structures that have intricate or complex shapes, such as the ventricular system. Further, they tend to be relatively insensitive and skewed by a variety of other factors. For example, it has been shown that increases in the linear dimensions of the ventricular system do not vary directly with the volume of the system as the ventricles enlarge. Linear measurements may nevertheless be useful for evaluating some aspects of brain anatomy. For example, linear measurements may be the best way to obtain indices of cerebral asymmetry, such as left versus right sylvian fissure height and angle as seen on coronal cuts.

Area measurements have been the mainstay for measuring structures using CT scanning, and they are likely to have a similar role in MR studies. Most imaging programs include a calibration ruler on each scan, permitting area measurements to be calculated in order to reflect actual brain size in square centimeters. Alternatively, investigators have used ratios, such as the ventricular:brain ratio. Ratios have the advantage of inherently controlling for "nuisance variables" such as difference in head and brain size due to differences in body size. Their major disadvantage is that they treat the numerator as a structure of interest and assume that no characteristic pathology will be observed in the structure used as a denominator. Some evidence suggests, however, that patients with schizophrenia may have reduced brain size. This makes the interpretation of ratios much more difficult and suggests that absolute measures may be appropriate if statistical techniques such as regression are used to correct for nuisance effects such as sex differences or body size.

Using MR, investigators can determine the area of many more structures than was possible on CT scans. Figure 23 indicates a large number of structures that can be clearly visualized and measured on midsagittal cuts alone. Using MR one can specifically determine the size of regions such as the frontal lobes, the cingulate gyrus, the corpus callosum, and so forth.

The coronal cuts offer even greater opportunities to visualize and measure structural features. Coronal cuts also present many practical and theoretical measurement problems, however. If a standard series of 8–16 cuts is used in order to obtain images, for example, differences in head

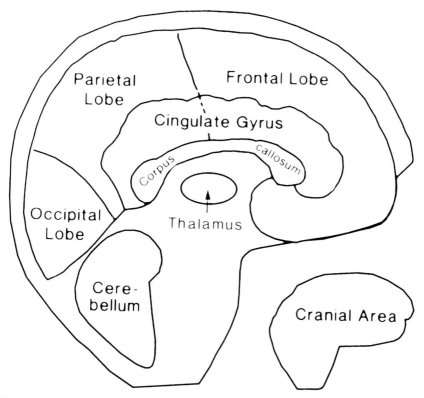

FIGURE 23.   Measurement of midsagittal cuts.

size may cause structures to appear in different cuts in different individuals. Therefore, it is necessary to develop a way to standardize measurement procedures in order to reduce this effect to a minimum. Perhaps the simplest is to designate a central cut as the reference cut in all individuals and to make comparisons of structures seen anterior or posterior to this reference cut. The cut that passes through the optic chiasm provides a very good central reference point.

Volumetric measurements provide an alternative to area measurements. In theory, volumetric measurements may be more meaningful than area measurements, in that they provide detailed information about the true size of a particular structure, such as the ventricles, frontal lobes, and so forth. In practice, however, there are some difficulties with volumetric measurements, since all volumetric measurements involve an extrapolation between points located at some distance apart that may involve structures that are quite small (e.g., thalamus, basal ganglia, etc.) or structures that have a very complicated shape (e.g., the ventricular system).

Even if volumetric measurements can be conducted in a valid and reliable manner, one cannot assume that they are necessarily "the best" (i.e., the most meaningful) thing to measure. While they may give some indication of the overall size of a structure, such as the lateral ventricular system, they may not be useful in assessing focal atrophy or focal ventricular enlargement due to a pathological process occurring in a relatively specific brain region. For example, if an illness such as schizophrenia principally affects a particular brain region, such as the frontal lobes, then volumetric measurements of the ventricular system would not be as sensitive as area measurements of the frontal horns of the ventricles or the frontal lobes. Alternatively, one could measure frontal lobe volume, however.

Measurements can be done using either manual or computerized methods. Each of these has its inherent advantages and disadvantages. Manual methods usually involve enlarging scans via an overhead projector, tracing around regions of interest, and using a planimeter to measure area. The strength of manual methods is that they provide a paper record of all work completed and facilitate later rechecking. The principal objection to manual methods is that they are relatively time-consuming and are potentially less reliable than computerized methods.

Computerized methods are, at least in theory, highly objective. In practice, however, computers cannot make refined judgments such as distinguishing between the ventricular system and cisterns filled with CSF. Likewise, the human brain processing a scan is able to distinguish the amygdala from the hippocampus based on shape and to some extent location, while computers are in general unable to make such distinctions. One useful compromise is to identify and measure structures at the viewing console in a radiology suite by outlining regions of interest with a joystick or an edge detection program and letting the MR computer calculate areas or volumes.

Whatever method is used, and whatever structures are measured, it is imperative to document that the measurements are reliable. Two types of reliability are pertinent: interrater reliability and test–retest reliability. Interrater reliability usually involves having two different clinician-tracers outline regions of interest on the same scan and then compare their degree of agreement using some appropriate statistic, such as the intraclass R or the Pearson R. Table 7 shows reliability data collected in our center for midsagittal structures using a manual method. They indicate that, when appropriate care is used, good interater reliability can be achieved with manual methods. Test–retest reliability involves determining whether measurements are reproducible from one occasion to the next. In order to conduct test–retest studies, an individual must be scanned two times. Because scans are relatively costly, very few test–retest

TABLE 7. Interrater Reliability of NMR Measurements: Structures Seen on a Coronal Cut Passing Through the Optic Chiasm

Region		Intraclass R*	Pearson R*
Cranial area		.8143	.9865
Frontal area	Left	.8824	.9875
	Right	.8739	.9876
Medial frontal area	Left	.7278	.9719
	Right	.9045	.9742
Dorsolateral frontal area	Left	.7235	.7058
	Right	.7498	.7102
Orbital frontal area	Left	.6374	.6543
	Right	.5652	.7834
Temporal area	Left	.8531	.9175
	Right	.7856	.9172
Ventricular area	Left	.9621	.9749
	Right	.9412	.9712
Caudate area	Left	.7857	.8747
	Right	.3153	.8551
Putamen + globus pallidus	left	.6901	.8901
	Right	.6480	.8800
Amygdala	Left	.8637	
	Right	.8385	
Cingulate height	Left	.6775	.8650
	Right	.7160	.8186
Corpus callosum thickness		.6448	.7272
Cranial breadth		.4687	.9062

*Based on measurements done of 20 subjects by 4 different individuals.

reliability studies have been conducted in brain-imaging centers to date. Nevertheless, test–retest studies are very important as an index of the reproducibility of findings.

A number of methodological problems are inherent in brain imaging. Some of them are inevitable, and they are mentioned in order to indicate that results should be interpreted relatively conservatively. Other problems can be minimized or eliminated through careful technique. These problems include variations in head position, variations in head size, and partial volume effects.

Head position: Obtaining standardized positioning of the head in the scanner is a recurrent problem in brain-imaging research. This problem can be particularly serious in the measurement of some areas such as frontal lobes since a variation in the angle of the coronal cut can markedly increase or decrease an area in any given site. If possible, a fixed head-holder should be provided. Clinicians evaluating scans must also do a preliminary visual check in order to insure that the sagittal scan is midline, since this provides an index of head position. After visual review, it may be necessary to exclude from study some scans in which the head is not appropriately positioned.

Head size: There is considerable variation in human head size both within sexes and across sexes. This makes it difficult to standardize measurement of structures in a series of cuts. One solution for this problem is to select a central midline reference point, as discussed above. A stereotactic method has also been proposed in order to correct for variations in brain and structure size (Fox et al. 1985). These investigators suggest the use of the proportional grid system developed by Talairach, which uses the anterior and posterior commissures as reference points. When absolute measures of structure size are determined, it may be necessary to use statistical corrections for variations in body size.

Partial volume effect: Because most brain-imaging techniques provide a two-dimensional representation of three-dimensional structures, some portions of structures overlap with others, and the boundaries are difficult to visualize or are inaccurately visualized. This problem is reduced, at least to some extent, however, in MR scanning, since the gray–white resolution is much superior to CT scanning. In addition, because MR scanning can be done in a number of different planes, it is possible to select cuts in which partial volume effect is relatively minimal. For example, partial volume effect is a serious problem in measuring lateral ventricular size in transverse cuts, since the ventricles are relatively small and most cuts in the transverse area include some ventricle and some brain tissue. On the other hand, the coronal cuts pass directly perpendicular to the ventricular system and provide a relatively clean separation of CSF and brain tissue.

Medication Effects: Medications have no known effect on observation of brain structure with magnetic resonance imaging. On the other hand, however, they could potentially affect T1 and T2 relaxation times, since these parameters reflect specific tissue characteristics that could be influenced by factors such as fluid or water balance. Some common pharmaceuticals have been shown to produce significant changes in T1 and T2 relaxation times in animals, but most of these effects were on the lung, uterus, liver, and spleen. Only two drugs were shown to affect T1 and T2 relaxation times in the brain: digoxin and heparin. Drugs that could theoretically affect the central nervous system, such as cimetidine, flurazepam, lorazepam, or triazolam, had no effect. Neuroleptics and antidepressants were not studied (Karlik 1986). Among the most commonly used psychoactive drugs, lithium seems most likely to have some effect on T1 and T2, but rigorous studies have not as yet been done to examine the effects of lithium on T1 and T2 in the normal brain in either humans or animals.

Clinical Applications

Because it allows visualization of specific brain regions, magnetic resonance can be used to determine whether specific differences in brain anatomy occur in the major mental illnesses. While a search for regional brain differences might have been scoffed at 50 years ago as a foolish elaboration of phrenology, the striking demonstration by Geschwind and Levitsky (1968) concerning the asymmetry of the planum temporale in the human brain has made such hypothesizing intellectually respectable. Geschwind's discovery that the planum temporale was significantly larger on the left side, where the regions governing human speech reside, has demonstrated clearly that functional differences may be due to structural organization.

Studies exploring structural abnormalities in the major mental illnesses have focused to date on patients suffering from schizophrenia, autism, affective disorder, and dementia. They have examined a number of different brain regions. These include the frontal system, the corpus callosum, the cerebellum, and the temporolimbic system.

Schizophrenia. Research in schizophrenia has emphasized the study of the frontal lobes, the corpus callosum, and overall brain size. The frontal lobes comprise the single largest cortical region in the human brain. As is demonstrated in other chapters in this book, a substantial amount of evidence suggests that frontal system abnormalities may occur in schizophrenia. The frontal system is the brain region that mediates a large number of volitional, intellectual, and social functions that are sometimes impaired in mental illness. Studies of experimental lesions in animals and traumatic or disease-induced lesions in human beings have indicated that injury to the prefrontal cortex leads to disorders of cognitive function (concreteness, impaired attention, difficulty abstracting or categorizing), diminished spontaneity of speech, decrease in voluntary motor behavior, decreased will and energy, a tendency to engage in repetitious or perseverative behavior, difficulty in shifting response set, and abnormalities of affect and emotion (particularly apathy, indifference, shallowness, and *witzelsucht*) (Fuster 1980; Damasio 1979; Luria 1980; Nauta 1971; Dabrowska 1971; Hebb 1945; Jacobsen 1935; Milner 1964).

The symptoms of schizophrenia are strikingly similar to the symptoms observed in such lesion studies, particularly the negative or deficit symptoms of schizophrenia.

Recognition that some type of frontal dysfunction could account for the symptoms of schizophrenia has led to substantial research in this area, and recent work by a number of investigators has provided support for the hypofrontality hypothesis. This support includes studies using brain electrical activity mapping, regional cerebral blood flow, and positron emission tomography (Ingvar 1974; Mathew 1982; Andreasen 1986a; Weinberger 1986; Berman 1986; Morihisa 1986; Buchsbaum 1985; Morihisa 1985). Evidence for hypofrontality in schizophrenia using each of these techniques is summarized in their respective chapters in this book.

Given the substantial amount of evidence from other brain-imaging modalities, it is logical to attempt to determine whether *structural* abnormalities might occur in the frontal system in patients suffering from schizophrenia. To explore this possibility, several MRI studies have been done. Initial work focused on examination of the midsagittal cut, in which the central sulcus can be clearly seen and frontal lobe size can be clearly delimited (Andreasen 1986b). In this particular study, an inversion-recovery pulse sequence was used (TI = 600 milliseconds), and 38 schizophrenic patients were compared with 45 normal controls. Figure 20 indicates the appearance of a midsagittal cut using this type of inversion-recovery pulse sequence.

In this morphometric study, cerebral size and frontal lobe size were measured using the central sulcus as the posterior boundary of the frontal lobe. Schizophrenic patients were observed to have a statistically significant decrease in both frontal and cerebral size. This could not be accounted for by possible confounding variables such as height, weight, or sex, although there was some suggestion that the abnormality was more prominent in the male patients. In addition, in post hoc analyses, decreased cranial size was observed in the schizophrenic patients.

The results of this preliminary study suggest that some patients suffering from schizophrenia may have had some kind of cerebral insult early in life which has partially inhibited brain growth (and therefore cranial growth) and that this inhibition has had relatively specific effects on the frontal lobes. Since most skull growth is completed by age two, the factor producing this effect must have occurred during a relatively early developmental phase. Possible factors that might be implicated in producing this result include prenatal factors such as maternal nutrition, maternal smoking, and maternal substance abuse; perinatal factors such as birth complications; and postnatal factors such as head trauma, infections, psychological and intellectual simulation, and nutrition.

This study also examined the relationship between clinical

phenomenology and brain abnormalities. Negative symptoms (alogia, affective blunting, avolition, anhedonia, and attentional impairment) were noted to have some relationship to decreased cranial and cerebral size, but not to decreased frontal lobe size (Andreasen 1983; Andreasen 1984). Cognitive tests designed to test frontal function were also administered (i.e., Wisconsin Card Sorting, Stroop, and fluency tests) (Stroop 1935; Milner 1963; Benton 1968; Jones-Gotman and Millner 1977). A relationship was found between poor performance on these tests and decreased cranial and cerebral size, but not frontal size.

This initial study had a number of limitations. It examined only a single midsagittal cut. Further, the normals were recruited from hospital employees, including house staff, faculty, physicians, and x-ray technologists, a socially and educationally advantaged group that was not sociodemographically matched to the schizophrenic sample. The sample size, although not small, was not large enough to address questions such as whether a sex effect was present.

For these reasons, a second MRI study was done in the same center in order to correct some of the limitations of the earlier study. Although this second study is not as yet complete, preliminary results are in conflict with the previous study and indicate some of the methodological problems that arise in conducting morphometric studies.

The results of both studies for male patients are shown in Table 8. As this table indicates, in the second MRI study no significant differences were found between schizophrenics and controls in any of the areas previously examined; both groups appear to have regressed to the mean. The schizophrenic subjects in Study 2 continue to have smaller brain

TABLE 8. Midsagittal Measure (in square centimeters) for Male Subjects

| | MRI Study 1: | | | | | |
| | Schizophrenics (N = 26) | | Controls (N = 27) | | | |
	x	SD	x	SD	t	p
Frontal area	50.57	3.00	54.92	5.37	3.36	.0015
Cerebral area	86.72	8.08	95.22	9.05	3.61	.0007
Cranial area	152.58	9.78	164.33	11.52	4.01	.0002

| | MRI Study 2: | | | | | |
| | Schizophrenics (N = 26) | | Controls (N = 27) | | | |
	x	SD	x	SD	t	p
Frontal area	51.95	5.59	51.14	4.56	.544	NS
Cerebral area	91.55	9.49	88.86	7.80	1.052	NS
Cranial area	163.04	14.27	160.02	9.46	.847	NS

measures than the controls in Study 1, but are similar and even larger when compared to the more closely matched controls of Study 2.

The two groups of schizophrenic patients do not differ in any relevant characteristics, such as age, educational level, severity or duration of illness, number of hospitalizations, or types of symptoms present. The major differences are between the control groups: nearly all controls in Study 1 were college graduates and many had doctoral and postdoctoral training, while the controls in Study 2 had only a high school education. These results highlight the importance of selecting appropriate control groups. The schizophrenic patients differ from the socially and educationally advantaged controls of Study 1 in cerebral and frontal lobe size (at the < .08 and .03 levels, respectively), but not from the matched controls. This may suggest that their socioeconomic peers suffer from similar disadvantages that produce a similar limitation in cerebral development. In the patients who developed schizophrenia, some additional predisposing factor may have occurred that led to the illness. Several other investigators have found supportive evidence for cranial and cerebral abnormalities in schizophrenia (Pearlson 1987; McNeil T, personal communication, 1987).

Coronal MRI cuts provide an interesting opportunity to examine temporolimbic regions in order to determine whether specific abnormalities can be observed in patients suffering from schizophrenia. Several studies have reported abnormalities in these regions in schizophrenia (Bogerts et al. 1985; Kovelman and Schiebel 1984). Using inversion-recovery or T1-weighted spin-echo images in the coronal plane, these structures can be clearly seen with magnetic resonance imaging (Naidich et al. 1987). To date, however, these findings have not been confirmed with magnetic resonance imaging. In Iowa MRI Study II, the sizes of the hippocampus, amygdala, and parahippocampal gyrus were compared in schizophrenic patients and controls, and no significant differences in size were observed using area measurements. The slice thickness in these studies was 1 cm, however; smaller slice thicknesses would permit volumetric measures of these structures and might permit greater sensitivity for detecting differences in these relatively small structures.

Abnormalities of the Corpus Callosum.   The corpus callosum is a large bundle of white-matter tracts that connects the right and left cerebral hemispheres. The frontal lobes are connected through the anterior callosum (i.e., the rostrum and genu), the temporal and parietal lobes through the body of the callosum, and the occipital lobes through the posterior portion (i.e., the splenium). Embryologically, the callosum is related to limbic structures such as the hippocampus and septal nuclei (Rakic et al. 1968).

A number of studies of hemispheric specialization in schizophrenia have suggested the possibility of impaired transfer of information between the two hemispheres via the callosum among patients suffering from schizophrenia (Rosenthal 1972; Nasrallah 1986; Beaumont 1973; Bigelow 1983; Gruzelier 1979; Gur et al. 1982; Diamond 1980). These have used a variety of experimental techniques, such as dichotic listening. In addition, some reports of structural anatomical abnormalities in the callosum in schizophrenia have been reported (particularly, increased "thickness"), but the number of such studies has been relatively small (Beaumont et al. 1973; Rosenthal et al. 1972; Bigelow et al. 1983). Further, some reports of callosal dimensions in normal individuals have suggested that there may be differences in gender and handedness in the normal population, with left-handers and ambidextrous individuals having larger corpora callosa and with females showing some differences in callosal shape (i.e., a more bulbous configuration in the anterior regions) (De Lacoste-Utamsing 1982; Witelson 1985).

Using the sample described for Iowa MRI Study 1, differences in callosal size and shape were also studied (Nasrallah et al. 1986). The method for measuring the callosum is portrayed in Figure 24. The schizophrenics were found to have a larger callosal area than the controls. When specific regions of the callosum were compared, the schizophrenics as a whole appeared to have an increase in mean callosal thickness in the middle and anterior portions, but not in the posterior region. These find-

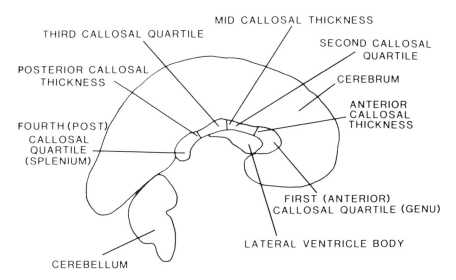

FIGURE 24.   Measurement of the corpus callosum.

ings confirm previous postmortem studies that found a larger callosal size in schizophrenia. However, when the patients and controls were compared by gender and handedness, schizophrenic males were found not to differ from control males in callosal thickness, regardless of handedness, while schizophrenic females were found to have a highly significant increase in the thickness of the callosum in anterior and middle regions as compared to control females.

These data suggest several possible interpretations. If one assumes that thickness of the callosum means an increase in interhemispheric connections and that an increase in connections leads to less hemispheric specialization or differentiation, then one might conclude that schizophrenic females have a lesser degree of hemispheric specialization than do normal females. The schizophrenic males do not, however, display this functional abnormality.

Studies of callosal size and shape have a number of problems. Investigators have not consistently replicated one another's findings in normals. Mathew et al. (1985) observed the corpus callosum to be longer in schizophrenic patients than in normals, but did not observe a larger area. Nasrallah et al. (1986) did note the sexual dimorphism in normals observed by De Lacoste-Utamsing et al. (1982), but were not able to confirm differences in right- versus left-handers. Holloway et al. (1986) and De Lacoste-Utamsing et al. (1986) report confirmation of gender-related differences in the callosum, but Weber et al. (1986) and Oppenheim et al. (1987) have failed to confirm gender-related differences. These various studies differ methodologically, with some using postmortem brains and some using magnetic resonance; further, no single, standard, agreed-upon method is in use for measuring callosal size and shape. Further, the functional significance of differences in size and shape is unclear. While some investigators have tended to assume that a larger size indicates a larger density of axons, this assumption has not been confirmed through postmortem human studies that actually count the number of axons, and animal studies suggest that this assumption could be questionable (Rakic et al. 1968; Musiek 1986; Foxman et al. 1986).

Since the corpus callosum is related embryologically to the limbic system, developmental abnormalities are of potential interest as well. Lewis and Mezey (1985) have reported an increased incidence of cavum septum pellucidum in patients suffering from schizophrenia. This developmental abnormality is a *form fruste* of callosal agenesis and suggests that patients with schizophrenia may have a higher rate of developmental brain abnormalities. In the Iowa MRI series, we have observed one patient with cavum septum pellucidum and a second with nearly complete agenesis of the corpus callosum. A coronal scan of this latter patient appears in Figure 25. The clinical picture of both these patients was characterized by severe, treatment-refractory positive symptoms. The base rate of developmental callosal abnormality in the general population is unknown, but certainly infrequent; common clinical correlates observed in other MRI studies include mental retardation, the Dandy–Walker syndrome, seizures, visual and auditory impairment, cranial and facial abnormalities, and a variety of other findings (Atlas et al. 1986; Curnes et al. 1985; Davidson et al. 1985; Parrish et al. 1979; McLeod et al. 1987; Lynn et al. 1980; Sauerwein et al. 1981; Kendall 1983; Lassonde 1981). MRI is clearly a powerful technique for studying midline abnormalities in major mental illnesses and can potentially teach us a great deal about underlying anatomic substrates of clinical phenomena.

Cerebellar Size. Two studies have examined cerebellar size in schizophrenia, following reports in the earlier CT literature suggesting that cerebellar atrophy may occur in some patients suffering from schizophrenia. MR work has not confirmed this finding, however. Absence of cerebellar atrophy has been demonstrated both by the work of Mathew et al. (1985) and by the work of Coffman et al. (1984).

Affective Disorders. Very little work has been done, to date, in order to determine whether morphometric abnormalities can be observed in patients suffering from affective disorders. The emphasis on schizophrenia is not surprising, given the preponderance of CT studies indicating structural abnormalities in schizophrenia, and the relative paucity in affective illness. Nevertheless, one group has observed some abnormalities in bipolar patients. Specifically, they have reported a significantly increased number of small areas of increased signal intensity, which appear as bright dots on the MRI scan and are referred to colloquially as "UBOs" (unidentified bright objects) (Dupont et al., personal communication). Areas of increased signal intensity are apparently seen in normal individuals with no evidence of psychopathology or neuropathology, but larger and more extensive areas probably do reflect some type of intracerebral pathology (Zimmerman et al. 1985). The significance of these findings in bipolar illness is at present unclear.

Dementias. Magnetic resonance imaging is potentially useful for evaluating dementia syndromes, in that its high resolution permits clear visualization of atrophic changes. MRI is particularly preferable to CT for observing the morphological changes of Huntington's disease (Simmons et al. 1986), in that caudate atrophy can be clearly observed. More generalized atrophy is observed in Alzheimer's disease. This finding is of course not diagnostic, since generalized atrophy occurs in many other disorders as well (McGeer et al. 1986). PET and SPECT undoubtedly

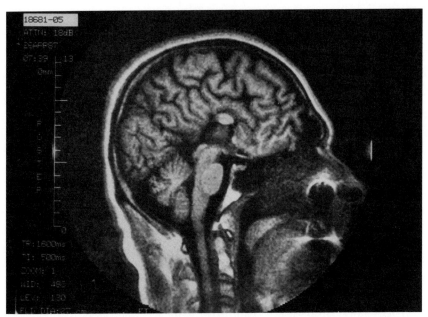

FIGURE 25.   Sagittal (above) and coronal (opposite, top and bottom) scans showing nearly complete agenesis of the corpus callosum.

surpass MRI in sensitivity and specificity for detecting Alzheimer's disease.

An interesting new application of MRI with high field strength magnets involves the imaging of endogenous paramagnetic substances, principally iron, that are present in the caudate, putamen, globus pallidus, red nucleus, substantia nigra, and dentate nucleus (Rutledge et al. 1987; Drayer et al. 1986a; 1986b; Pastakia et al. 1986). Iron is not present in the brain at birth, but accumulates rapidly between ages eight and 25, thereafter continuing to accumulate more gradually. Characteristic patterns of signal increase and decrease, based on changes in iron concentration in the extrapyramidal motor system, are currently being mapped. They will permit improved differential diagnosis of various types of movement disorders, including primary and secondary Parkinson's disease, dystonias, chorea and hemiballismus, Wilson's disease, and the Shy–Drager syndrome.

Autism.   Clinically, autism manifests as an early developmental abnormality reflected by impaired language development, impaired social attachment, and impaired intellectual functioning. A recent report indicates that the early developmental abnormality may have a neural ana-

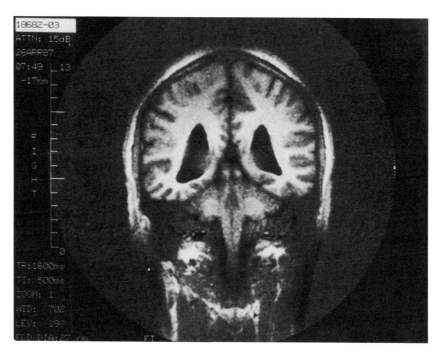

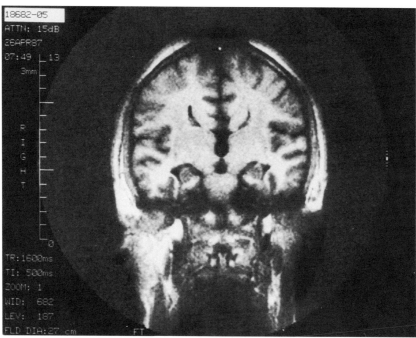

tomical substrate. Courchesne et al. (1987 and in press) describe a characteristic abnormality involving hypoplasia of vermal lobules VI and VII in the cerebellum in 14 out of 18 patients with classic autism. The other vermal lobules were normal in size. These lobules are phylogenetically and ontologically distinct from the other parts of the vermis, in that they are neocerebellar as opposed to paleocerebellar and are linked via a distinct set of circuits to the brain stem and thalamus and to the cerebral cortex. The relationship between this area of hypoplasia and the clinical picture of autism is unclear, but may reflect the modulatory activities of the fastigial nucleus and its links to the hippocampus.

Measurement of T1 and T2.   Since T1 and T2 represent specific tissue parameters and in some sense reflect *tissue behavior*, they are potentially a sensitive index of brain dysfunction, particularly regional brain dysfunction. Nevertheless, T1 and T2 are difficult to measure. T1 and T2, as characterized in the chemical experiments conducted with NMR prior to the advent of magnetic resonance imaging, are the relaxation characteristics of pure substances. As evaluated through MRI, T1 and T2 are averages of a mixture of chemical substances that are combined in the tiny blocks of tissue present in the MR voxel. Thus, properly speaking, the T1 and T2 that are measured through MRI are "T1-*like*" and "T2-*like*" rather than T1 and T2, per se. Nevertheless, the linguistic conventions of MRI tend to refer to these measures as T1 and T2, and this convention is also followed herein.

Estimates of T1 and T2 using MRI have a number of problems. Several studies have evaluated measurement of T1 and T2 using phantoms containing pure substances with known T1 and T2 values. In general, estimates of T1 and T2 based on MRI show substantial inaccuracies (Rosen et al. 1984; Majumdar et al. 1987). This is due to a variety of problems, including distortion produced by radio-frequency pulse imperfections and by inhomogeneity of the magnetic field (Majumdar et al. 1986a, 1986b). Several techniques to correct for the imperfections are currently being developed (Majumdar et al. 1986b, Rosen et al. 1984).

In addition to the problems produced by field inhomogeneity and variation in pulses, measurement of T1 and T2 is technically difficult and relatively time-consuming. As Figures 8 and 11 have shown, both T1 and T2 represent exponential curves, with repetition time (TR) forming the *x*-axis for T1 and echo time (TE) forming the *x*-axis for T2. In order to define these curves accurately, multiple echo and repetition times are required. Software programs provided by MRI manufacturers typically provide only two-point curves and are therefore likely to be highly unreliable. To develop true measurements of T1 and T2, multiple TR and TE values must be collected. A suggested matrix, currently in use in Iowa MRI studies,

TABLE 9.   Matrix of Reconstructions

TR = 400	800	1200	2000
TE = 26	26	26	26
52	52	52	52
78	78	78	78
104	104	104	104
130	130	130	130
154	154	154	154

appears in Table 9. The varying echo and repetition times must be obtained for a single slice that is collected because it is likely to be informative; obtaining a multiple matrix of TEs and TRs for a single slice required 20 to 25 minutes of scanning time in this particular study. (Newer software may make such studies simpler in the future.)

These varying TEs and TRs can then be used to create a series of simultaneous equations based on the original Bloch equation, as follows:

$$
\text{Signal Intensity} = \left(M_0 \cdot e^{\frac{-TE}{T2}} \right) \cdot \left[\left(1 \cdot e^{\frac{-TR}{T1}} \right) + \left(2 \cdot e^{\frac{-TR + \frac{1}{2}TE_1}{T1}} \right) - \left(2 \cdot e^{\frac{-TR + \frac{3}{2}TE_1}{T1}} \right) \right.
$$
$$
\left. + \left(2 \cdot e^{\frac{-TR + \frac{5}{2}TE_1}{T1}} \right) - \left(2 \cdot e^{\frac{-TR + \frac{7}{2}TE_1}{T1}} \right) + \left(2 \cdot e^{\frac{-TR + \frac{9}{2}TE_1}{T1}} \right) - \left(2 \cdot e^{\frac{-TR + \frac{11}{2}TE_1}{T1}} \right) \right]
$$

In these equations there are three unknowns (M, T1, and T2). Because of the large number of equations, however, T1 and T2 are easily calculated.

Investigators have attempted to determine whether T1 and T2 can be used diagnostically. Many of these attempts have focused on the diagnosis of malignancies (Komiyama et al. 1987; Mills et al. 1984). In general, investigators have found differences in T1 and T2 between normal and abnormal tissue. On the other hand, however, it is difficult to differentiate tumor tissue types using T1 and T2, so that malignant tumors cannot be consistently distinguished from nonmalignant tumors.

Several investigators have also attempted to examine T1 and T2 in patients suffering from schizophrenia. Besson et al. (1987) have examined T1 in a series of 23 patients suffering from schizophrenia, 15 of whom showed evidence of tardive dyskinesia. They measured T1 in the basal ganglia and in frontal and parietal white matter. They also subdivided their patients into those with high- and low-negative symptoms. They observed the patients with prominent negative symptoms to have increased T1 in the left frontal region. Patients with tardive dyskinesia also tended to have increased T1 in the basal ganglia.

Fujimoto et al. (1984) have also examined T1 relaxation time in patients suffering from schizophrenia. They have studied 46 patients with schizophrenia compared to 20 normal controls. They also observe a decreased T1 in frontal white matter, and the findings are particularly strong on the left side. T1 was increased in the putamen as well, but no correlation with tardive dyskinesia was done, nor was there any attempt to relate observed abnormalities to positive and negative symptoms. Thus this work appears to conform to some of the findings reported by the Besson group.

Rangel-Guerra et al. (1982) also examined T1 relaxation time in patients suffering from affective disorder. They studied 20 bipolar patients before and after treatment with lithium carbonate and compared their T1 values to 18 normal controls. They observed that 17 out of 20 patients had pre-lithium values higher than the controls, but the T1 values dropped to normal levels after lithium treatment. This study may suggest some abnormality in hydrogen proton behavior in patients suffering from bipolar affective disorder that is normalized through lithium therapy.

Although it is outside the range of brain imaging per se, a study conducted by Rosenthal et al. (1986) has extended the work of Rangel-Guerra by examining the behavior of blood cells of patients suffering from affective disorder before and after lithium treatment using NMR spectroscopy. Their findings are in a similar direction to those reported by Rangel-Guerra, with T1 elevation prior to treatment and normalization after treatment.

Clinical Applications.   Clinical applications are still in their preliminary phase. Research studies suggest that schizophrenics as a group may have some type of structural abnormality that can be measured and visualized on MRI scan and that patients with tardive dyskinesia may have evidence of subtle tissue abnormality in the basal ganglia. Further, it is possible that magnetic resonance may be used to monitor response to lithium.

Nevertheless, none of these studies is definitive. Consequently, MRI must be considered an appropriate laboratory test in psychiatry at approximately the same degree that CT scans are appropriate and useful. That is, there are no indications as yet that MRI offers any findings that are diagnostically specific. Psychiatrists will order this brain-imaging technique for many of the same reasons that they have ordered CT scans. It is likely to be useful in any patients in whom there is a difficult differential diagnosis (e.g., depression versus dementia, schizophrenia versus dementia, etc.). Just as a CT scan is not definitive in helping to determine the final diagnosis, but does provide some assistance, so too MRI may help sway evidence in one direction or another if findings suggestive of atrophy abnormal for the age of the patient are observed.

MRI will also be appropriate for patients whose clinical picture is atypical and arouses suspicion of some nonpsychiatric pathological process. For example, an MRI scan may be appropriate for a patient with a late onset of a schizophrenia-like syndrome, a late onset of mania, or a severity of cognitive impairment inconsistent with the degree of psychosis. In such patients, one is seeking evidence in order to assist in a differential diagnosis between schizophrenia or affective disorder and a brain tumor, unobserved head injury, exposure to a toxin, or possibly some infectious process. An MRI scan may also be appropriate for patients with a long-standing history of substance abuse. In many of these cases, an EEG and neuropsychological testing are also indicated as useful adjuncts.

Overall Assessment of the Technique

In its present form, MR imaging is a *structural* technique. Although it may eventually have dynamic capacities, the most relevant comparisons of its strengths and weaknesses at this moment are with CT scanning, the other major structural imaging technique.

In most respects, MRI is superior to CT and likely to supplant it eventually. One major asset is the strikingly improved tissue resolution. Gray- and white-matter structures are precisely imaged and differentiated. This capacity makes MRI particularly preferable for studies of brain anatomy (e.g., VBR, cerebral asymmetry). Its capacity to image in various planes (i.e., coronal and sagittal in addition to transverse) also makes MRI superior to CT for anatomical studies.

A second superiority of MRI is the fact that the MRI signal contains more information than does the CT signal. Instead of simply indicating attenuation of x-rays through tissue, MRI provides information about proton density, the interaction of protons with their environment (T1), and the interaction of protons with other protons (T2). In actual clinical practice, this aspect of the MRI signal makes it much more useful in imaging pathological lesions. MRI is clearly superior for studying demyelinating diseases such as multiple sclerosis. It can be used to trace the progressive myelinization of the brain in infants and young children. Some of the studies described earlier in this chapter indicate that MRI may also be useful for identifying tissue abnormalities in regions such as the basal ganglia or the periventricular area in psychiatric patients, although these studies do await further confirmation.

The final strength of MRI is the range of brain structures that can be observed. Partly because of problems with bony artifacts, CT has not been able to look into the posterior fossa well. This region of the brain can be well imaged with MRI. As mentioned, the capacity to look in multiple planes also permits more complete imaging of various brain regions.

In comparison with MRI, the major strength of CT is its ability to image bone, which is not at all well observed with MRI. This limitation is of minor relevance for psychiatry, however. At the present time CT scanners are still more widely available, and CT scans somewhat cheaper than MRI scans. Prices for both of these scanning techniques usually range from $400–800, with CT scans usually being several hundred dollars cheaper. As MRI scanners become more widely available, however, costs may become more comparable.

When MRI is compared with RCBF, SPECT, and PET, its major limitation is its inability to measure dynamic functions. Measuring of metabolic processes or neurotransmitter communication is outside its present range. As discussed below, however, at least some of these applications may become available for MRI research and clinical studies during the coming years.

Future Directions

In order to have applications in magnetic resonance, the nuclei being studied should have two major properties. They must have a reasonably high prevalence within the body, and they must have a net charge that makes them magnetic. Hydrogen has a single proton and is widely abundant throughout the body. The nucleus of the widely abundant carbon-12 is not magnetic, but C-13 (an isotope of carbon) has six protons and seven neutrons. Other isotopes of potential interest for magnetic resonance are phosphorus-31, sodium-23, chlorine-19, oxygen-17, and nitrogen-15.

One possibility for enlarging the information available through magnetic resonance imaging is the use of various types of exogenously administered paramagnetic isotopes. Paramagnetic substances are characterized by the presence of at least one unpaired electron. This characteristic causes them to align with an external magnetic field and to create local fields that affect the relaxation of protons. Manganese and gadolinium have these characteristics and are potentially available to make compounds that can be used as contrast agents. Some of these are experimentally available at present. Of greater interest to psychiatry, however, would be the possibility of labeling compounds that can be used to study either metabolism or neurotransmission, but no such compounds are available at present.

Another application of future interest is the use of magnetic resonance spectroscopy. Spectroscopy moves magnetic resonance into the functional arena and allows study of metabolic processes in order to assess both normal and abnormal tissue function. For example, techniques have recently been proposed, using high field strength magnets, for measuring N-acetyl aspartate, GABA, lactate, and phosphocholine (Luyten et al. 1987). Sodium imaging has been used to explore vasogenic edema and stroke (Perman et al. 1986; Turski et al. 1986). Phosphorus-31, although less abundant than sodium or hydrogen, is a potentially informative nucleus in human biology because of its importance in energy metabolism. High field strength magnets can also be used to examine concentrations of various phosphorus-containing metabolities such as adenosine triphosphate, phosphocreatinine, or inorganic phosphate (Bottomley et al. 1984; Cohen et al. 1984).

It is not yet clear whether these applications will be useful in psychiatry. Spectroscopic techniques at present measure activity from the whole brain and are used as an index of general brain metabolism. It seems likely that if spectroscopic techniques are to be useful as a means for studying metabolic activity in mental illness, refinements must be developed in order to permit the study of small subregions, since whole-brain abnormalities are not likely to be useful. Likewise, the use of paramagnetic tracers will require further refinement before they find a use in psychiatry. Ideally, one would like to observe energy metabolism and neurotransmitter function with magnetic resonance. This hope may be realized during future years.

References

Andreasen NC: The Scale for the Assessment of Negative Symptoms (SANS). Iowa City, Iowa, The University of Iowa, 1983

Andreasen NC: The Scale for the Assessment of Positive Symptoms (SAPS). Iowa City, Iowa, The University of Iowa, 1984

Andreasen NC (Ed): Can Schizophrenia Be Localized in the Brain? Washington, DC, American Psychiatric Press, Inc., 1986

Andreasen NC, Nasrallah HA, Dunn V, et al: Structural abnormalities in the frontal system in schizophrenia: a magnetic resonance imaging study. Arch Gen Psychiatry 43:136-144, 1986

Atlas SW, Zimmerman RA, Bilaniuk LT, et al: Corpus callosum and limbic system: neuroanatomic MR evaluation of developmental anomalies. Radiology 160:355-362, 1986

Axel L, Margulis AR, Meaney TF: Glossary of NMR terms. Magnetic Resonance in Medicine 1:414-433, 1984

Beaumont JG, Diamond SJ: Brain disconnection in schizophrenia. Br J Psychiatry 123:661-662, 1973

Benton AL, Hancher ADS: Multilingual Aphasia Examination. Iowa City, Iowa, The University of Iowa, 1968

Berman KF, Zec RF, Weinberger DR: Physiologic dysfunction of dorsolateral prefrontal cortex in schizophrenia, II: role of neuroleptic treatment, attention, and mental effort. Arch Gen Psychiatry 43:126-135, 1986

Besson JAO, Corrigan FM, Cherryman GR, et al: Nuclear magnetic resonance brain imaging in chronic schizophrenia. Br J Psychiatry 150:161-163, 1987

Bigelow LB, Nasrallah HA, Rauscher FP: Corpus callosum thickness in chronic schizophrenia. Br J Psychiatry 142:284-287, 1983

Bloch F: Nuclear induction. Physics Review 70, No. 7:8, 1946

Bogerts B, Meertz E, Schonfeldt-Bausch R: Basal ganglia and limbic system pathology in schizophrenia. Arch Gen Psychiatry 42:784-791, 1985

Bottomley PA, Hart HR Jr, Edelstein WA, et al: Anatomy and metabolism of the normal human brain studied at 1.5 Tesla. Radiology 150:441-446, 1984

Brant-Zawadzki M, Norman D (Eds): Magnetic Resonance Imaging of the Central Nervous System. New York, Raven Press, 1987

Buchsbaum MS, DeLisi LE, Holcomb HH, et al: Anteroposterior gradients in cerebral glucose use in schizophrenia and affective disorders. Arch Gen Psychiatry 41:1159-1166, 1983

Coffman JA, Andreasen NC, Nasrallah HA: Left hemisphere density deficits in chronic schizophrenia. Biol Psychiatry 19:1237-1247, 1984

Cohen MM, Pettegrew JW, Kopp SJ, et al: P–31 nuclear magnetic resonance analysis of brain: normoxic and anoxic brain slices. Neurochem Res 9:785-801, 1984

Courchesne E, Hesselink JE, Jernigan TL, et al: Abnormal neuroanatomy in a nonretarded person with autism. Arch Neurol 44:335-341, 1987

Courchesne E, Yeung-Courchesne R, Press G, et al: Hypoplasia of cerebellar vermal lobules VI and VII in infantile autism. Science (in press)

Curnes JT, Laster DW, Koubek TD, et al: MRI of corpus callosal syndromes. Am J Neurol 7:617-622, 1986

Dabrowska J: Association of impairment after lateral and medial prefrontal lesions in dogs. Science 171:1037-1038, 1971

Damasio A: The frontal lobes, in Clinical Neurology. Edited by Hellman KM, Valenstein E. New York, Oxford University Press, 1979

Davidson HD, Abraham R, Steiner RE: Agenesis of the corpus callosum: magnetic resonance imaging. Radiology 155:371-373, 1985

De Lacoste-Utamsing C, Holloway RL: Sexual dimorphism in the human corpus callosum. Science 216:1431, 1982

De Lacoste MD, Holloway RL, Woodward DJ: Sex differences in the fetal human corpus callosum. Hum Neurobiol 5:93-96, 1986

DeMyer MK, Hendrie HC, Gilmor RL, et al: Magnetic resonance imaging in psychiatry. Psychiatric Annals 15:262-267, 1985

Diamond SJ, Scammell R, Pryce IL, et al: Some failures of intermanual and cross-lateral transfer in chronic schizophrenia. J Abnorm Psychol 89:505-509, 1980

Drayer BP, Burger P, Darwin R, et al: Magnetic resonance imaging of brain iron. AJNR 7:373-380, 1986a

Drayer BP, Olanow W, Burger P, et al: Parkinson plus syndrome: diagnosis using high field MR imaging of brain iron. Radiology 159:493-498, 1986b

Drewe EA: An experimental investigation of Luria's theory of the effects of frontal lobe lesions in man. Neuropsychologia 13:421-429, 1975

Ellis JH, Meiere FT: NMR physics for physicians. Indiana Medicine 78:20-28, 1985

Elster AD: Magnetic Resonance Imaging: A Reference Guide and Atlas. Philadelphia, J.B. Lippincott, 1986

Fox PT, Perlmutter JS, Raichle ME: A stereotactic method of anatomical localization for positron emission tomography. J Comput Assist Tomogr 9:141-153, 1985

Foxman BT, Oppenheim J, Petitio CKK, et al: Proportional anterior commissure area in humans and monkeys. Neurology 36:1513-1517, 1986

Fujimoto T, Yokoyama Y, Fujimoto A, et al: Spin-lattice relaxation time measurement in schizophrenic disorders. Abstracts, Society for Magnetic Resonance Imaging, 1984

Fullerton GD: Basic concepts for nuclear magnetic resonance imaging. Magnetic Resonance Imaging 1:39-55, 1982

Fuster JM: The Prefrontal Cortex. New York, Raven Press, 1980

Geschwind N, Levitsky W: Human brain: left-right asymmetries in temporal speech region. Science 151:186-187, 1968

Gruzelier J, Flor-Henry P (Eds): Hemisphere Asymmetries of Function in Schizophrenia. New York, Elsevier Biomedical Press, 1979

Gur RC, Gur RE, Obrist WD, et al: Sex and handedness differences in cerebral blood flow during rest and cognitive activity. Science 217:659-661, 1982

Hebb DO: Man's frontal lobes: a critical review. Archives of Neurology and Psychiatry 54:431-438, 1945

Holloway RL, De Lacoste MD: Sexual dimorphism in the human corpus callosum: an extension and replication study. Hum Neurobiol 5:87-91, 1986

Ingvar DG, Franzen G: Abnormalities of cerebral blood flow distribution in patients with chronic schizophrenia. Acta Psychiatr Scand 15:425-462, 1974

Jacobsen CS: Functions of the frontal association area in primates. Archives of Neurology and Psychiatry 33:558-569, 1935

Jones-Gotman M, Milner B: Design fluency: the invention of nonsense drawings after frontal cortical lesions. Neuropsychologia 15:653-675, 1977

Karlik SJ: Common pharmaceuticals alter tissue protein NMR relaxation properties. Magnetic Resonance in Medicine 3:181-193, 1986

Kendall BE: Dysgenesis of the corpus callosum. Neuroradiology 25:239-256, 1983

Komiyama M, Yagura H, Baba M, et al: MR imaging: possibility of tissue characterization of brain tumors uing T1 and T2 values. AJNR 8:65-70, 1987

Kovelman JA, Scheibel AB: A neurohistological correlate of schizophrenia. Biol Psychiatry 19:1601-1621, 1984

Lassonde MC, Lortie J, Ptito M, et al: Hemispheric asymmetry in callosal agenesis as revealed by dichotic listening performance. Neurophysiologia 19:455-458, 1981

Lauterbur PC: Image formation by induced local interactions: examples employing nuclear magnetic resonance. Nature 242:190, 1973

Lewis SW, Mezey GC: Clinical correlates of septum pellucidum cavities: an unusual association with psychosis. Psychol Med 15:43-54, 1985

Luria AR: Higher Cortical Functions in Man. New York, Basic Books, 1980

Luytens PR, den Hollander JA: Observation of metabolites in the human brain by MR spectroscopy. Radiology 161:795-798, 1986

Lynn RB, Buchanan DC, Fenichel GM, et al: Agenesis of the corpus callosum. Arch Neurol 37:444-445, 1980

Majumdar S, Gore JC: Effects of selective pulses on the measurement of T2 and apparent diffusion in multiecho MRI. Magnetic Resonance in Medicine 4:120-128, 1987

Majumdar S, Orphanodakis SC, Gmitro A, et al: Errors in the measurement of T2 using multiple-echo MRI techniques, I: effects of radiofrequency pulse imperfections. Magnetic Resonance in Medicine 3:397-417, 1986

Mathew RJ, Partain CL: Midsagittal sections of the cerebellar vermis and fourth ventricle obtained with magnetic resonance imaging of schizophrenic patients. Am J Psychiatry 142:970-971, 1985

Mathew RJ, Meyer HS, Francis DJ, et al: Regional cerebral blood flow in schizophrenia: a preliminary report. Am J Psychiatry 138:112-113, 1981

Mathew RJ, Duncan GC, Weinman ML, et al: Regional cerebral blood flow in schizophrenia. Arch Gen Psychiatry 39:1121-1124, 1982

Mathew RJ, Partain CL, Prakash R, et al: A study of the septum pellucidum and corpus callosum in schizophrenia with MR imaging. Acta Psychiatr Scand 72:414-421, 1985

McGeer PL, Kamo H, Harrop R, et al: Comparison of PET, MRI, and CT with pathology in a proven case of Alzheimer's disease. Neurology 36:1569-1574, 1986

McLeod NA, Williams JP, Machen B, et al: Normal and abnormal morphology of the corpus callosum. Neurology 37:1240-1242, 1987

Mills CM, Crooks LE, Kaufman L, et al: Cerebral abnormalities: use of calculated T1 and T2 magnetic resonance images for diagnosis. Radiology 150:87-94, 1984

Milner B: Effects of different brain lesions in card sorting. Arch Neurol 9:90-100, 1963

Milner B: Some effects of frontal lobectomy in man, in The Frontal Granular Cortex and Behavior. Edited by Warren JM, Ackert K. New York, McGraw-Hill, 1964

Morihisa JM, McAnulty GE: Structure and function: brain electrical activity mapping and computed tomography in schizophrenia. Biol Psychiatry 20:3-19, 1985

Morihisa JM, Weinberger DR: Is schizophrenia a frontal lobe disease?, in Can Schizophrenia Be Localized in the Brain? Edited by Andreasen NC. Washington, DC, American Psychiatric Press, Inc., 1986

Musiek FE: Neuroanatomy, neurophysiology, and central auditory assessment, part III: corpus callosum and efferent pathways. Ear and Hearing 7:349-358, 1986

Naidich TP, Daniels DL, Haughton VM, et al: Hippocampal formation and related structures of the limbic lobe: anatomic-MR correlation, part I: surface features and coronal sections. Radiology 162:747-754, 1987

Nasrallah HA, Andreasen NC, Coffman JA: A controlled magnetic resonance imaging study of corpus callosum thickness in schizophrenia. Biol Psychiatry 21:274-282, 1986

Nauta WJH: The problem of the frontal lobes: a reinterpretation. J Psychiatr Res 8:167-187, 1971

Oppenheim JS, Benjamin CP, Lee RN, et al: No sex-related differences in human corpus callosum based on magnetic resonance imagery. Ann Neurol 21:604-606, 1987

Parrish ML, Roessmann U, Levinsohn MW: Agenesis of the corpus callosum: a study of the frequency of associated malformations. Ann Neurol 6:349-354, 1979

Pastakia B, Polinsky R, Di Chiro G, et al: Multiple system atrophy (Shy-Drager syndrome): MR imaging. Radiology 159:499-502, 1986

Perman WH, Turski PA, Houston LW, et al: Methodology of in vivo human sodium MR imaging at 1.5 T. Radiology 160:811-820, 1986

Pickett IL: NMR imaging in medicine. Sci Am 46:78-88, 1982

Purcell EM, Taurry HCC, Pound RV: Resonance absorptions by nuclear magnetic components in a solid. Physics Review 59:37, 1946

Ra JB, Hilal SK, Cho ZH: A method for in vivo MR imaging of the short T2 component of sodium-23. Magnetic Resonance in Medicine 3:296-302, 1986

Rakic P, Yakovlev PI: Development of the corpus callosum and cavum septi in man. J Comp Neurol 132:45-72, 1968

Rangel-Guerra RA, Perez-Payan M, Todd LE, et al: Nuclear magnetic resonance in bipolar affective disorders. Magnetic Resonance Imaging 1:229-239, 1982

Rosen BR, Pykett IL, Brady TJ: Spin lattice relaxation time measurements in two-dimensional nuclear magnetic resonance imaging: corrections for plane selection and pulse sequence. J Comput Assist Tomographr 8:195-199, 1984

Rosenthal R, Bigelow LB: Quantitative brain measures in chronic schizophrenia. Br J Psychiatry 121:259-264, 1972

Rosenthal J, Strauss A, Minkoff L, et al: Identifying lithium-responsive bipolar depressed patients using nuclear magnetic resonance imaging. Am J Psychiatry 143:779-780, 1986

Rutledge JN, Hilal SK, Silver AJ, et al: Study of movement disorders and brain iron by MR. AJNR 8:397-411, 1987

Sauerwein HC, Lassonde MC, Cardu B, et al: Interhemispheric integration of sensory and motor functions in agenesis of the corpus callosum. Neurophysiologia 3:445-454, 1981

Simmons JT, Pastakia B, Chase TN, et al: Magnetic resonance imaging in Huntington's disease. AJNR 7:25-28, 1986

Stroop JR: Studies of interference in serial verbal reaction. J Exp Psychol 18:643-662, 1935

Turski PA, Perman WH, Hald JK, et al: Clinical and experimental vasogenic edema: in vivo sodium MR imaging. Radiology 160:821-825, 1986

Vaghi M, Visciani A, Testa D, et al: Cerebral MR findings in tuberous sclerosis. J Comput Assist Tomogr 11:403-406, 1987

Vanier M, Ethier R, Clark J, et al: Anatomical interpretation of MR scans of the brain. Magnetic Resonance in Medicine 4:185-188, 1987

Weber G, Weis S: Morphometric analysis of the human corpus callosum fails to reveal sex-related differences. J Hirnforsch (Berlin) 27:237-240, 1986

Weinberger DR, Berman KF, Zec RF: Physiological dysfunction of the dorsolateral prefrontal cortex in schizophrenia, I: regional cerebral blood flow evidence. Arch Gen Psychiatry 43:114-124, 1986

Witelson SF: The brain connection: the corpus callosum is larger in left-handers. Science 229:665-668, 1985

Young SW: Nuclear Magnetic Resonance Imaging: Basic Principles. New York, Raven Press, 1984

Zimmerman RD, Fleming CA, Lee BCP, et al: Periventricular hyperintensity as seen by magnetic resonance: prevalence and significance. AJNR 7:13-20, 1985

Chapter 3

Computerized EEG and Evoked Potential Mapping

John M. Morihisa, M.D.

Among the relatively new techniques for imaging the brain, computerized mapping of electrophysiologic data from the human central nervous system is among the first to have been attempted. Indeed, the use of topographic techniques to display data derived from electroencephalograph (EEG) or evoked potential recordings has been under development for over three decades. However, recent advances in solid state electronics and computer software development have revolutionized this approach. In this chapter we will review the history of this approach, describe its application, and discuss some of the findings that it has elaborated.

History of Technology

In 1929, Hans Berger, a psychiatrist, first reported recording electrical activity from the human brain. Almost from his first measurement he was beset with methodological issues and technical difficulties in his assessment of these data. Interestingly, two important concerns basic to Berger's investigation remain pivotal issues in electrophysiological research today. The first was the level of technology that could be applied to the problem of recording electrical activity from the brain. The second was the question of the ultimate source of these electrical pertubations that could be detected across the human scalp. In the first case, advances in electrophysiological research have been closely tied to technological developments ranging from refinements in EEG amplifiers to the introduction of digital computers. In the second case, the exact nature of the neural generators that are responsible for the brain electrical phenomena being measured remains a highly controversial yet crucial issue. In many respects far more progress has been achieved in the evolution of technology to record this brain electrical activity than in our understanding of its nature. It is a central goal of this evolving process that sufficient advances in the ability to detect, analyze, and interpret brain electrical activity may eventually allow us to better understand the character of these neural generators.

Since 1929, the measurement of brain electrical activity has been refined and developed into the field of electroencephalography and has extended into sleep studies (Gillin et al. 1972; Kupfer et al. 1973), telemetry (Stevens and Livermore 1982), spectral analysis (Itil et al. 1972), as well as evoked potentials (Roth 1977; Buchsbaum 1977; Shagass et al. 1979, 1980). What began as a research tool has been integrated into medicine, for the assessment of clinical situations that range from a multitude of neuropsychiatric disorders to the determination of brain death. Throughout its development this field has held out the promise of far more than its present applications. As early as its first introduction by Berger, it was hoped that it would uncover the underlying pathophysiology of the mental disorders. To some degree, this resulted from the unrealistic expectations that often greet any new research approach. However, a number of researchers suspected that the inability to deal effectively with the massive amount of data generated by electrophysiological recordings greatly hampered its clinical utility. This assumption led several generations of researchers to attempt to unlock this potential information from the EEG through the development of new approaches to the measurement of brain electrical activity.

One of the first research teams to map the human EEG were Adrian and Yamagiwa (1935) who investigated the topographic distribution of the alpha rhythm. Of particular importance was their discovery that the alpha rhythm had the dynamic characteristics of a traveling wave form. In an insightful review of the evolutionary process to develop topographic EEG approaches, Petsche (1976) emphasizes the significance of the work of Adrian and Yamagiwa as the first indication that the electrical fields of the EEG were constantly changing their shape and location across the scalp.

It became the work of other research teams to elaborate this novel concept into one of the fundamental characteristics of brain electrical activity. Evidence of the wavelike propagation of brain electrical activity was also reported by Kornmuller and Janzen (1939) and Jasper and Hawke (1938). In 1944 Motokawa and Tuziguti reported that the electrical activity of the frontal and parietal areas were out of phase, suggesting a wave propagation. These scientists as well as an independent group led by Petsche pioneered the graphic depiction of these data by using vector diagrams to represent spatio-temporal discontinuities. The wavelike nature of brain electrical activity was most specifically conceptualized by Walter in 1947, when he concluded from his study of spike-and-wave patterns that the spike was a traveling wave moving over the cortex. These findings about the basic nature of the electrical activity of the brain contributed fundamental concepts that laid the groundwork for the entire field of topographic investigations of EEG.

From this point of evolutionary significance, the next period of development in the topographic analysis of EEG occurs at the beginning of the next decade with the introduction of the toposcope, a device for the visualization of brain electrical activity. One of the first of these devices was described in 1951 by Walter and Shipton. This toposcope used multiple cathode ray tubes to present EEG data. Toposcopic systems were then introduced by the seminal research groups of Petsche (Petsche and Marko 1954) and Remond (1955).

However, a fundamental problem with these approaches was the great difficulty in developing satisfactory quantitative analysis of information generated visually by these techniques. The enormity of this problem limited this avenue of investigation until the effective application of digital computers. This addition to the research armamentarium had far-reaching ramifications in influencing not only the basic direction of research but also in shaping the very manner in which data could be presented.

Overview

One might state that one of the greatest strengths of the computer is not that it can accomplish mathematical calculations beyond human conception, but rather that it can compress the time that is required for the computation of an extraordinary amount of information. Inherent in this ability is the heart of computerized data presentation. The human brain, although without question the most versatile computer known, has certain basic limitations. Of particular importance to this field of study is the brain's limit concerning how many different pieces of novel mathematical data may be recorded, manipulated, and compared at any given time. The mind cannot remember thousands of pieces of mathematical data and compare them to thousand more. A computer, however, is ideally suited for the acquisition, analysis, and presentation of massive amounts of data in relatively short time periods. This ability allows two fundamental processes: first, the data can be acquired from the physiological experiment, then categorized and compared in the mathematical fashion desired; second, the data may then be condensed and summarized in the manner most amenable for human assimilation. This process takes advantage of the basic strengths of the computer and allows the human brain to apply to advantage its own particular strengths. The brain can analyze and interpret novel pictorial representations, such as photographs, with a speed and flexibility far beyond the capability of most computers presently available. Although computers with sophisticated pattern-recognition software can detect subtle differences or similarities between separate events, they cannot begin to approach the human mind's ability to interpret along multiple divergent lines of inquiry and derive meaning from these similar or disparate patterns. The utility of brain electrical mapping techniques derives from the successful marriage of these two sets of formidable strengths. Unfortunately, this approach has the inherent danger of wedding the combined weaknesses of these two analytic systems. This concern will be addressed further in the section on Overall Assessment.

Over the next two decades a series of research groups applied topographic techniques in the investigation of brain electrical activity. This important period of investigation was highlighted by the work of Estrin and Uzgalis (1969), Lehman (1971), Bickford et al. (1972), Gotman and Gloor (1975), and Petsche (1976).

In 1979, Duffy introduced a topographic system called brain electrical activity mapping (BEAM) which has subsequently been applied to the study of electrophysiological abnormalities in patients with brain tumors, dyslexia, Alzheimer's disease, or covert epilepsy (Duffy et al. 1979, 1980, 1982; Lombroso 1980). This technique of brain electrical activity mapping was used in a psychiatric population in a case study (Morihisa et al. 1982), and was first applied systematically to the study of a psychiatric population in 1983, in a study of schizophrenia (Morihisa, Duffy, and Wyatt 1983).

In 1982, Coppola introduced a topographic system for the computer generation of surface-distribution maps of measures of brain activity that has been applied to psychiatric research (Buchsbaum et al. 1982a, 1982b; Weinberger et al. 1986; Karson et al. 1987).

Construction of Systems and Production and Analysis of Images

The computerized topographic systems developed by Duffy and Coppola have some differences in their technical approach to the investigation of electrophysiological phenomena in the human brain. However, these two systems are prototypical of the most widely used EEG and evoked potential computerized topographic systems presently used in psychiatric research.

Both systems build upon basic techniques of electroencephalography and evoked potential studies. For EEG studies the electrophysiological data are classically broken down into the following separate frequency bands: delta (f < 4 Hz), theta (4 Hz sf < 8 Hz), alpha (8 Hz ≤ f < 13 Hz), and varying bands of beta (f ≥ 13 Hz). Different techniques use some variations in the frequency cut-off between these bands but most are relatively similar. For evoked potentials, the subject perceives multiple (sometimes several hundred) presentations of the same stimulus. In some cases the stimulus can be a flash of light, auditory tones or clicks, or any number of more complex stimuli or patterns. In all cases electrophysio-logical data must be recorded for multiple trials so that they may be averaged together to detect the brain's specific response to each stimulus. This averaging process is necessary because the evoked response is a relatively subtle pattern buried within the background electrical activity of the entire brain.

These two computerized topographic systems are based upon a stan-dard system of placing electrodes on the cortical surface of the skull. This technique is called the International 10–20 System and uses percentages of anatomic measurements to place electrodes in the same relative posi-tion on skulls of varying size. These electrodes are referenced to linked ears. Although this type of reference is commonly used in clinical electro-encephalography it has been pointed out that it introduces some distor-tion into the recording. For this reason techniques are being developed in a number of laboratories to eliminate or diminish this distortion.

The system developed by Duffy in 1979, called brain electrical activ-ity mapping or BEAM, uses 20 sites of the 10–20 International System of electrode placement, as shown in Figure 1. EEG and evoked potential data are amplified by standard clinical EEG amplifiers (Grass 7P511) and can then be recorded on magnetic tape (Honeywell 5600E FM analog tape recorder) for off-line computer processing. The computer used for the findings reported here was a DEC PDP 11-60. The data are carefully examined to remove artifacts from eye movements, eye blinks, muscle artifact, movement artifacts, and 60 Hz interference. The EEG data are analyzed with a fast Fourier transform algorithm (Cooley and Tukey 1976) and displayed in a map format that uses a projection looking down at the top of the head.

Evoked potentials are averaged and any 4-msec epoch can be viewed (Figure 2). For either evoked potentials or EEG the electrophysiologic data provide numerical values reflecting brain electrical activity at each of the 20 scalp electrode sites. A 64 × 64 grid matrix is overlaid over these data points to define 4096 picture elements or pixels of the brain map. These picture elements are given values by linear interpolation between the three nearest electrodes. The map can be defined by assigning differ-ent colors or shades of gray to specific voltage ranges of brain electrical activity. Finally, statistical relationships between a single subject and a normative group or between groups can also be displayed in a color map

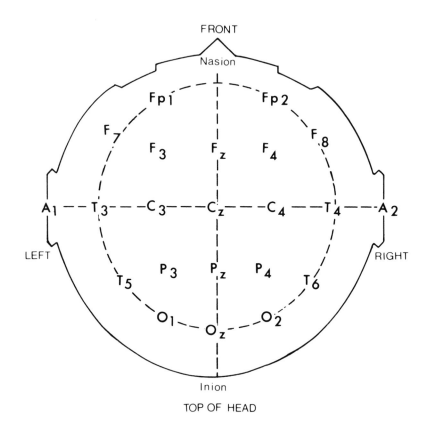

FIGURE 1.   Brain electrical activity mapping bases electrode placement upon the 10–20 International System. Data are displayed within this graphic representation of the top of the head with ears to the right and left, and the nose at the top of the picture. Provided by John M. Morihisa, M.D., Georgetown University School of Medicine, and Veterans' Administration Medical Center, Washington, D.C.

format (Figure 3). Multivariate discriminant analysis can be developed using the numerical indices underlying the topographic maps. In this manner, statistical computations can be performed that allow us to compare individuals to a control group or a group of subjects to a control group. Furthermore, this technique can assist us in investigating topographic differences between the test group and the control group.

The second prototypical topographic system in use was developed by Coppola et al. (1982) and Buchsbaum (1982b) and presents data as surface distribution maps of brain activity. This system also is based upon the International 10–20 System of electrode placement, but adds four additional placements per hemisphere that provide greater resolution of

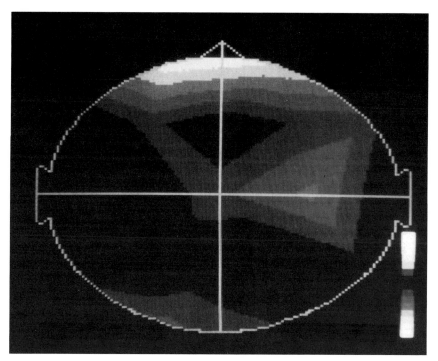

FIGURE 2.   This is a brain electrical activity map of a portion of a visual evoked potential of a patient with schizophrenia. Greatest brain electrical activity is depicted in white. Provided by John M. Morihisa, M.D., Georgetown University School of Medicine, and Veterans' Administration Medical Center, Washington, D.C.; and Frank H. Duffy, M.D., Boston Children's Hospital and Harvard Medical School.

posterior regions. This system has been most commonly used with 16 leads on the left hemisphere alone or with 32 leads over both hemispheres (duplication of midline leads), although it has the potential for a multitude of electrode montages (arrangements). Figure 4 demonstrates the left-hemispheric placements in this system (Coppola 1982). EEG or evoked potential data are amplified by standard clinical EEG amplifiers (Grass 7P511) and can be recorded on magnetic tape or floppy disk for subsequent analysis. In this system a 128 × 128 rectilinear grid of picture elements is overlaid over the data values. Each picture element is assigned a value employing a "four nearest neighbor" interpolation algorithm in which data from the four nearest electrodes are used and weighted in inverse linear proportion to their distance from each picture element (Buchsbaum 1982b). This system uses a mapping technique that is an approximate equal areas projection, which means the projection of the

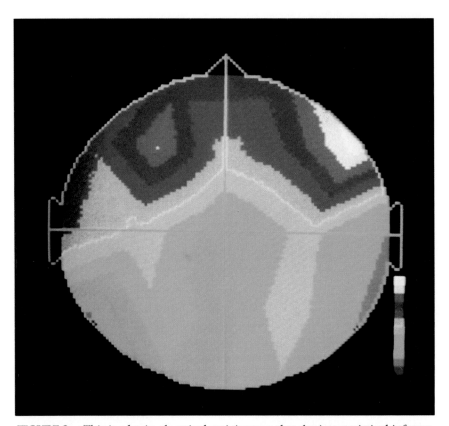

FIGURE 3.   This is a brain electrical activity map that depicts statistical information comparing two groups. In this case a group of schizophrenic patients with frontal atrophy is compared to a group of patients without atrophy, defining regional electrophysiologic differences in an auditorily evoked potential. Provided by John M. Morihisa, M.D., Georgetown University School of Medicine, and Veterans' Administration Medical Center, Washington, D.C.; and Gloria B. McAnulty, Ph.D., Boston Children's Hospital and Harvard Medical School (Morihisa and McAnulty 1985).

area from the three-dimensional scalp is represented by an equal area on the two-dimensional map (Coppola 1982) displayed within a left or right profile of the head (Figure 5). This approach limits gradient distortion and therefore allows gradient comparisons (Figure 6). Along these lines the same mapping program has been used by groups using positron emission tomography and regional cerebral blood flow (Weinberger et al. 1986), thereby facilitating topographic comparisons.

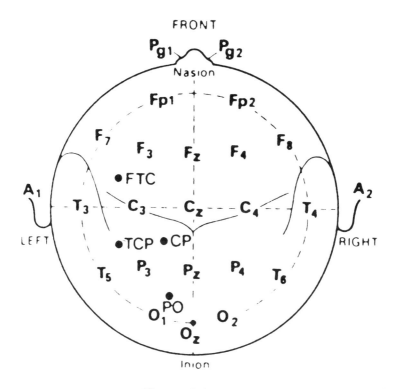

Top of Head

FIGURE 4. Depiction of the left-hemispheric electrode placements of the Coppola system. Twelve of the positions are standard 10–20 positions and four additional ones are labeled FTC, TCP, CP, and PO. Provided by Richard Coppola, Ph.D., National Institute of Mental Health, Bethesda, Maryland (Coppola 1982).

Overall Assessment: Strengths and Limitations

Strengths

In one important respect, computerized topographic mapping of electrophysiological data is distinct from the other techniques for imaging brain function. In all other functional brain imaging approaches, such as regional cerebral blood flow (rCBF) and positron emission tomography (PET), the subject is exposed to radiation of varying intensities. The absence of radiation exposure allows this technique to be repeated as frequently as desired and for extended periods of study.

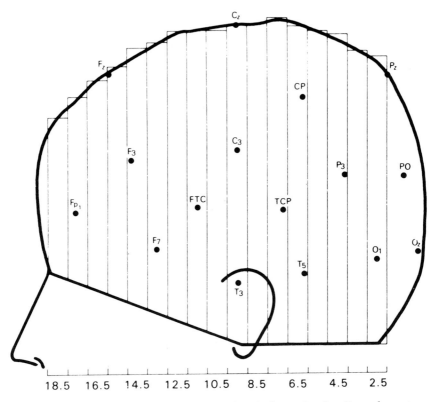

FIGURE 5. A lateral projection of one hemisphere, in the Coppola system, within a graphic outline of a profile of the head. Provided by Richard Coppola, Ph.D., National Institute of Mental Health, Bethesda, Maryland (Coppola 1982).

In addition, the chronologic resolution of this approach is several orders of magnitude greater than the PET scan or rCBF. While imaging techniques using radioactive isotopes require several minutes, computerized topographic mapping of evoked potentials can explore phenomena that are measured in milliseconds.

It should be noted that one of the most promising new brain-imaging approaches is magnetic resonance imaging (MRI) which presently provides new structural insights into the brain. This technique of MRI also has the potential to image functional aspects of the human brain with further technical development. When this is realized a new, very powerful technique for functional imaging will become available that does not expose the subject to radiation.

The cost of computerized EEG mapping equipment varies consider-

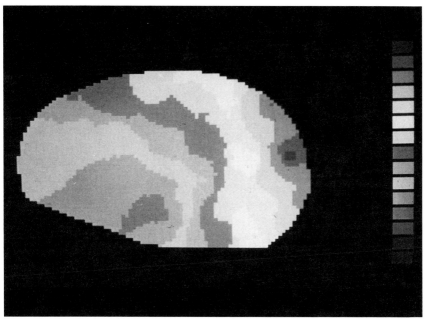

FIGURE 6.   A surface distribution map using the Coppola system to depict the left-hemispheric topographic distribution of alpha activity recorded from a normal volunteer resting with eyes closed. Note the normal peak of alpha activity at the back of the head (occipital area). Provided by Richard Coppola, Ph.D., National Institute of Mental Health, Bethesda, Maryland.

ably (approximately 30,000 to up to several hundred thousand dollars) depending upon the capability desired and the use of standard computers as opposed to packaged systems. This is much less than the present cost for CT, PET, rCBF, or MRI. This lower cost is related in part to the fact that EEG mapping requires no radioactive isotopes and can be used in conjunction with equipment that is routinely found in many clinical EEG laboratories. Indeed, some of the systems which use standard computers (i.e., computers that are not dedicated only to EEG studies, as part of a commercially packaged system) can use hardware that is readily available in most medical centers. Conversely, some of the commercially available packaged systems provide convenience and technical features that would be difficult to develop and maintain without sophisticated software and hardware systems-engineering support staff. However, the most significant point that should be emphasized is that, unlike CT scanning, this technique of computerized EEG mapping has not been scientifically proven to provide clear clinical superiority over more conventional EEG laboratory techniques.

Limitations

A major limitation of this EEG topographic method is that we are record-ing electrical activity from the surface of the human scalp. We would like to assume that there is a clear relationship between what can be detected from scalp electrodes and what is occurring intracranially. Unfortunately, although some research (Cooper et al. 1965) suggests that electrical activity recorded from the scalp usually reflects the activity of a relatively large, electrophysiologically synchronized cortical area directly underly-ing the electrode, there is also evidence that volume conduction can significantly affect the signals detected (Vaughan and Ritter 1970). Be-yond the fact that there is considerable question as to the exact nature of the neural generators of this electrical activity, one must also be chastened by the varying conductive properties of human skull anatomy as well as the peculiar structure of the brain which contains numerous complex folds. Finally, this somewhat obscured view is then compressed into two dimensions as the average of all detectable electrical activity in the region of the electrode. It is from this narrow window with glass of varying thicknesses that we must attempt to discern electrophysiological patterns of function.

A perpetual hazard of electrophysiological research that has plagued researchers from the moment brain electrical activity was first detected is artifactual contamination. Three major sources of artifact are eye move-ment, muscle activity, and 60 Hz interference. In a recent study (Karson et al. 1987) the importance of eliminating eye-movement artifact from EEG recordings was emphasized and its contamination of the delta band of EEG was demonstrated. Attempts to develop strengths and technology to limit the contribution made by artifacts represents an entire area of investiga-tion. Indeed, both of the approaches described here use elaborate proto-cols to limit contamination of the data by artifact. This study (Karson et al. 1987) utilized an on-line, time-locked electro-oculogram to delineate electrical activity attributable to eye movement. These data were sub-jected to the same spectral analysis (i.e., measurement of delta, theta, alpha, and beta activity) as the EEG data. This allowed us to determine the relative contribution by eye-movement artifact to our measurement of delta activity from the cortical surface. Despite the efforts of many re-searchers, contamination by movement artifact remains a significant chal-lenge to investigations utilizing computerized EEG mapping.

Another important source of artifact is the effect of medications on the EEG. This factor is particularly difficult to control in psychiatric patients, in whom certain medications have sometimes been used for extended periods. The EEG has been shown to be exquisitely sensitive to some drugs and, even in drug-free patients, the possible long-term effects of psychoactive drugs cannot be excluded as a possible source of error.

Perhaps the greatest concern over the use of computerized topographic analysis of EEG is paradoxically related to its great utility at communicating large quantities of condensed and summarized information about brain function. In part this is related to the fact that the process of data analysis and data summarization is performed by computers whose software or instructions have been defined in some predetermined fashion by a programmer. The software that is the basis for computer operations is built upon a series of assumptions and a necessarily refined focus of investigation. In some cases these assumptions are simplifications that do not consider all aspects of the information about the brain. In other cases these assumptions may be controversial or even known compromises containing mathematical sources of inaccuracies. These powerful effects are difficult to assess or even detect in the final form in which the data are presented. Thus, it is of vital importance in this field for clinicians to work closely with computer scientists and statisticians in the development of these approaches as well as in the interpretation of the data they produce. In other words, the very ability of computers to summarize and condense information into easily assimilated packages carries the danger that valuable information has not been presented or that certain assumptions or methods of simplification have introduced inaccuracies or misleading implications.

Finally, there is a special subset of danger inherent in the power of the computerized imaging of brain function. This danger lies in the seductive beauty of the images themselves. The images, especially those fitted to color scales, have a certain unfortunate esthetic beauty that in no way is correlated with the inherent validity or importance of the data used to generate them. The most compelling and "meaning-filled" picture may be created with the entry of random numbers as data points into a color mapping computer program. In a more subtle fashion, even pictures generated from carefully collected data and analyzed with classically accepted statistics may provide temptation for overinterpretation far beyond what can be justified by the data. The use of these approaches requires careful explanation of how they are generated and a healthy reluctance to interpret past what the data can clearly support.

Applications in Psychiatry

Both of the techniques described here have been applied to the study of several psychiatric populations with the primary focus thus far being in the area of schizophrenia research. Indeed, although EEG and evoked potentials have an important place in clinical psychiatry, the clinical role of computerized mapping of EEG and evoked potentials is yet to be delineated and it therefore remains a research tool at this time.

The first systematic application of the brain electrical activity mapping technique in a psychiatric population was reported in 1983 in a study of drug-free and medicated schizophrenic patients who fulfilled *Diagnostic and Statistical Manual of Mental Disorders, Third Edition* criteria and Research Diagnostic Criteria, compared to controls who were not significantly different for age, gender, or handedness (Morihisa, Duffy, and Wyatt 1983). Drug-free patients were unmedicated for at least four weeks and medicated patients were on a standard dose of haloperidol (0.4 mg/kg) for at least four weeks. The major finding of this study was that schizophrenic patients demonstrated more delta activity than normal controls over the entire cortical surface.

This finding of increased delta was consistent with the work of Itil et al. (1972) who reported more delta activity in schizophrenic patients in one of the first applications of analog computer power spectral analysis to determine delta, theta, alpha, and beta activity.

A recent study (Karson et al. 1987) has replicated, in a new patient population, the major finding of generally increased delta activity over the entire cortical surface in drug-free schizophrenic patients compared to normal controls. However, this study also emphasizes that artifactual contamination from eye movement can falsely indicate a frontal focus of this increased delta. It is prudent to avoid interpretations of topographic localization unless one can be assured, by an on-line, time-locked spectral analysis of the data from artifact-generating regions, that regional localizations are not artifact induced. Thus, these computerized EEG findings of generally increased delta, from our laboratory, should be conservatively interpreted as evidence for abnormalities of brain function in schizophrenic patients without specific topographic localization.

The significant physiological and artifactual limitations of computerized EEG to make regional distinctions demonstrate the importance of interpreting these findings with the assistance of complementary brain-imaging techniques which can measure metabolic and structural parameters that can complement our electrophysiological findings.

One of the earliest applications of a brain-imaging system capable of delineating regional differences did focus attention on the frontal lobes in schizophrenia. This was the work of Ingvar and Franzen (1974) who used regional cerebral blood flow to demonstrate that schizophrenic patients exhibited a relative decrease in frontal blood flow compared to alcoholic controls. Although significant limitations to this early application of rCBF have been shown, it remains one of the earliest attempts to distinguish regionally specific pathophysiology (Berman et al. 1984).

Both regional cerebral blood flow and computerized EEG mapping are functional brain-imaging techniques, as they attempt to measure and topographically map the activity of the brain. Recently a measure of brain function has been introduced with which we may complement our EEG findings, positron emission tomography (PET scan) that can provide investigations of brain activity in three dimensions.

In one of the first systematic applications of positron emission tomography to a psychiatric population, Buchsbaum and colleagues (1982a) reported an abnormality of the anterior–posterior gradient of brain glucose metabolism in schizophrenic patients, compared to controls. This particular finding would be consistent with Ingvar's regional cerebral blood flow findings. However, differences in both how the data are derived, as well as in the manner they are presented, make direct comparisons of these studies problematic. Indeed, the abnormalities of anteroposterior gradient reported by Buchsbaum and colleagues may not specifically demonstrate localized dysfunction of the frontal lobes.

However, in a more recent study, Wolkin and colleagues (1985) reported an actual decrease in absolute frontal brain metabolism in schizophrenic patients compared to controls. Using magnetic resonance imaging (MRI), Andreasen and colleagues (1986) have reported frontal structural abnormalities which provides anatomic evidence for frontal lobe pathology in schizophrenia. These findings appear to support the notion of abnormalities of brain function in schizophrenia. Both rCBF, PET, and MRI complement the attempt to localize functional abnormalities that was begun using electrophysiological approaches. In each approach there is a suggestion of abnormal function that might be associated with the frontal lobes.

One way in which we may refine the focus of our investigation of schizophrenia is to use these brain-imaging techniques in combination with cognitive-activation paradigms that place a demand on functionally specific anatomic regions. Weinberger and colleagues (Weinberger et al. 1986; Berman et al. 1984) have utilized just such a strategy coupled with the Xenon-133 regional cerebral blood flow technique. This group found when a specific cognitive demand is placed upon the dorsolateral prefrontal cortex (Milner 1963) using the Wisconsin Card-Sort Test, normal controls activate this region and schizophrenic patients fail to do so. Thus, further evidence is added that supports frontal lobe dysfunction in schizophrenia and the electrophysiological finding of increased delta is perhaps extended and localized to a specific portion of the frontal lobes.

This use of information from multiple brain-imaging approaches in an attempt to localize functional abnormalities of the brain enhances our chances to detect meaningful patterns amidst the complex and sometimes contradictory reports of computerized EEG research. Further, the specific use of cognitive-activation tests may provide a strategy by which we may more finely focus our electrophysiological measures. Thus, we (Morihisa 1986a) would suggest that the use of the Wisconsin Card-Sort paradigm in computerized topographic EEG research may allow us to increase the utility of this approach and specifically test a theoretical localization of abnormality in brain function in schizophrenia. In addition, the use of cognitive-activation tasks in computerized topographic EEG studies is a superior strategy over the study of the resting state because the resting state has a greater potential for variation between individuals.

Despite the apparent convergence of information from several different approaches that support the EEG topographic findings of increased delta in schizophrenia, caution and skepticism should be applied, in both the interpretation of these findings as well as how we conceptualize this general body of findings about the brain. Specifically, data which appear to coalesce into relatively coherent theories of abnormal function should be used as tools and not as assumptions upon which we rush to build further speculation. For example, these findings should not in any way discourage the pursuit of alternative or conflicting theories. This avenue of investigation is in its infancy and to take a gnomic stance at this point and develop maxims of interpretation would be premature and dangerous. It is possible that these early findings may be ultimately most useful in helping us to develop a set of effective strategies and to identify limitations of the system, rather than to provide basic laws of brain function.

Indeed, several studies have been reported that contradict each of the findings that we have presented and that use each of the brain-imaging approaches considered. Furthermore, frontal abnormalities have also been reported in other diagnostic categories than schizophrenia (Buchsbaum et al. 1984). The divergent wealth of findings is perhaps most evident in computerized topographic studies of EEG in psychiatric populations.

Most recently, using the computerized topographic technique developed by Coppola et al. (1982) and Buchsbaum et al. (1982b), Buchsbaum and colleagues (1987) have extended the investigation of left-hemispheric abnormalities in schizophrenia, in a study employing somatosensory evoked potentials. This group found that schizophrenic patients demonstrated more diffuse evoked potential activity which did not exhibit the stimulus intensity-linked variation shown by normal controls. These findings build upon the pioneering work of Shagass (1979, 1980) and Buchsbaum (1979) and others in the delineation of abnormalities in evoked potentials in schizophrenia.

Future Directions

Potential correlations between CT scans, PET scans, regional cerebral blood flow, and computerized topographic studies of EEG and evoked potentials have supported the strategy of combining multiple brain-imaging techniques in concert in an attempt to extend the utility of our investigations of mental illness. Future brain-imaging studies may utilize multiple approaches that measure several parameters of the brain in an attempt to enhance our ability to discern patterns of both normal and pathologic brain function.

One of the first combined applications of computerized topographic electrophysiologic techniques and computed tomography (CT scan) was reported in 1985 (Morihisa and McAnulty) in an investigation of structural abnormalities in schizophrenia related to evoked potentials. In this pilot study, two small groups of schizophrenic patients were electrophysiologically compared: those with evidence of frontal lobe atrophy versus those without evidence of frontal lobe atrophy. Only four correlations were detected, and in each case the regional differences delineated involved areas that overlay the frontal lobes (Figure 3). This preliminary study suggests that structural differences in anatomy might be reflected in electrophysiological differences between two groups of schizophrenic patients. This direction represents an attempt to achieve one of the basic goals of topographic electrophysiological research which is to relate electrophysiological manifestations to their structurally specific underlying neural generators. This goal is presently beyond our capability, and it is possible that inherent limitations in this approach may prohibit clinically useful localization of functional brain activity with computerized topography of EEG and evoked potentials. However, it is most likely through strategies that employ complementary brain-imaging techniques that we will have our best chance of overcoming the limitations of any single approach.

Neuroscience Issues in Computerized EEG Topography

All of this research most certainly is derived from basic neuroscience efforts that continue to provide the foundation of innovations in the strategic approach to imaging the function of the brain. Indeed, the central assumption in the search for topographic localizations of EEG events, that they reflect the functional activity of the underlying neural generators, is based upon knowledge about the central nervous system contributed by neuroscience investigations.

More specifically, recent neuroscience findings provide support for the potential value of further elaboration of the two examples (Morihisa, in press a) of computerized topographic findings discussed here. For example, in the case of evidence implicating frontal lobe dysfunction in schizophrenia, research in the neurosciences has demonstrated several suggestive characteristics of the prefrontal cortex (Weinberger 1987; Morihisa and Weinberger 1986b). This region has been shown to connect with almost every lobe of the brain and with all types of association cortex

(Fuster 1980; Nauta 1971) and receives and sends projections to limbic, diencephalic, and mesencephalic nuclei relevant to the regulation of behavior. Recent studies in the neurosciences indicate that integrity of the prefrontal cortex is necessary for functions as basic as the ability to develop and implement strategies to achieve future goals as the relevant rules undergo continuing change (Fuster 1980).

Interestingly, in an animal model of this functional system in the nonhuman primate, an experimental lesion may not become behaviorally manifested until sexual maturity (Alexander and Goldman 1978). Thus, the work of Weinberger and colleagues (1986) in highlighting possible dysfunction of the dorsolateral prefrontal cortex in schizophrenia is not only consistent with the neuroscience findings, but could be extended to suggest a certain theoretical convergence of findings (Weinberger 1987). Specifically, if it is true that some schizophrenic patients have a dorsolateral prefrontal deficit, and that deficits in this region only become fully relevant in the human upon sexual maturity as in the case in an experimental animal model, an explanation might be hypothesized for what has been a well-known but unexplained clinical observation in schizophrenia. Schizophrenia seldom occurs before adolescence, and if schizophrenia were indeed linked to a dorsolateral prefrontal deficit, then based upon these neuroscience findings one might speculate that, in humans, the disease schizophrenia only becomes manifest upon sexual maturity. This is a tempting explanation to what has long been observed about the classical age of onset of schizophrenia. However, this theory (Weinberger 1987) about the pathophysiology of schizophrenia makes basic assumptions about the relevance of nonhuman primate models to human disease processes. Further, the great heterogeneity of this disorder emphasizes that this theory is but one of many viable and useful conceptual alternatives. What is certainly required is an extensive exploration of this possible pathophysiological model of schizophrenia, and tests of its utility.

In the case of Buchsbaum's work (Buchsbaum et al. 1987) showing an apparent deficit in pain sensitivity in schizophrenic patients who fail to exhibit evoked-potential (EP) activity variation across intensities, it has been suggested that the parietal region is involved in deficits of pain perception and attention in schizophrenia. This proposal is supported by the neuroscience work of Mesulam and Geschwind (1978) who reported that in the rhesus monkey parietal ablations produce unilateral inattention and significant sensory deficits (Buchsbaum et al. 1987).

Although faster computers with more sophisticated software will be developed, as well as new technologies which may use the magnetic fields generated by brain electrical activity to create three-dimensional pictures of brain function, it is most likely that the future of this field will be most closely linked to developments in the neurosciences. It is the basic principle of brain function being elucidated in the neurosciences that will help us to develop useful research strategies in the use of computerized EEG and evoked potential mapping.

Conclusion

Finally, there is an additional price to be paid that must be added to the inherent dangers and limitations to which we have already alluded. Indeed, the computer creates a host of new problems and difficulties, sometimes derived from its very strengths. However, it would be difficult, if not impossible, to avoid grappling with these fundamental technical issues and we shall surely require the efforts of such innovative scientists as Duffy (1979) and Coppola (1982) who have brought to their clinical research an extensive grasp of basic engineering and technical issues. Nevertheless, we agree with Petsche (1976) that the greatest hope for this field, and an important guiding strategy, will be to steadfastly focus upon the "clinically and physiologically relevant" issues in our attempt to apply computerized topography of EEG and EP to the study of the brain.

At present the interpretation of this computer-generated deluge of information will require significant refinement and testing in both larger and more diverse subject populations, before we may even hope that this flood can evolve into a wellspring of knowledge. For example, careful evaluation of the test–retest reliability of these techniques must be investigated, as well as the possible long-term effects of medication. Furthermore, an order-of-magnitude larger (100 versus 10) number of subjects must be tested using these computerized techniques before even the research findings of these approaches can be effectively evaluated. In addition, different clinical populations must be extensively studied and compared before any assessment of the diagnostic capability of such techniques can have any clear clinical applications.

Present studies merely suggest that computer programs can sort schizophrenic patients from normal controls. This could be true even if differences were related to medication effects of undetected abnormal movements in the patients rather than to any electrophysiological trait characteristic of pathologic brain function in schizophrenia. It is of course our hope that this approach may eventually delineate pathophysiologic traits in psychiatric disorders that may define basic neuroscience principles of brain function.

For now it would appear prudent to observe that these computerized EEG/EP techniques remain promising research tools but that their general superiority over competent standard EEG/EP techniques remains to be scientifically proven. Thus, it is premature to assign any clear indication for the application of these techniques in clinical practice. Certainly, there is yet no clear and compelling basis for standard EEG/EP laboratories to convert to the new computerized technology until further research and development of these approaches has been achieved.

Despite the formidable obstacles to our attempt to understand brain function in psychiatry, we are fortunate to also have powerful allies. Perhaps the most promising source of support in our quest to understand the mind will be realized in a growing collaboration with the neurosciences (Morihisa 1987). As we have seen in the brain-imaging work presented here, research in the neurosciences can provide crucial insights and vital guidelines in our attempt to interpret our massive and sometimes conflicting data.

Finally, it is essential to realize that, in the search for meaning in the central nervous system, we must not seek unitary strategies to embrace as true but, instead, marshal a multitude of basic science and clinical science approaches. Only by following each of the clues provided by clinical psychiatry, neurosciences, and new fields such as molecular biology can we hope to address the complex and frustrating mysteries of mental illness.

References

Adrian ED, Yamagiwa K: The origin of the Berger rhythm. Brain 58:323-351, 1935

Alexander GE, Goldman PS: Functional development of the dorsolateral prefrontal cortex: an analysis utilizing reversible cryogenic depression. Brain Research 143:233-249, 1978

American Psychiatric Association: Diagnostic and Statistical Manual of Mental Disorders, 3rd edition. Washington, DC, American Psychiatric Association, 1980

Andreasen N, Nasrallah HA, Dunn V, et al: Structural abnormalities in the frontal system in schizophrenia. Arch Gen Psychiatry 43:136-144, 1986

Berger H: Uber das elektrenkephalogram des Menschen I. Arch Psychiatr Nervenkr 87:527-571, 1929

Berman KF, Weinberger DR, Morihisa JM, et al: Regional cerebral blood flow in psychiatry: application to clinical research, in Brain Imaging in Psychiatry. Edited by Morihisa JM. Washington, DC, American Psychiatric Press, 1984

Bickford RG, Billinger TW, Fleming NII, et al: The compressed spectral array (CSA): a pictorial EEG. Proceedings of the San Diego Biochemical Symposium 11:365-470, 1972

Bickford RG, Brimm J, Berger L, et al: Application of compressed spectral array in clinical EEG, in Automation of Clinical Electroencephalography. Edited by Kellaway P, Petersen J. New York, Raven Press, 1973

Buchsbaum MS: The middle evoked response components and schizophrenia. Schizophrenia Bull 3:93-104, 1977

Buchsbaum MS: Neurophysiological aspects of the schizophrenic syndrome, in Disorders of the Schizophrenic Syndrome. Edited by Belak L. New York, Basic Books, 1979

Buchsbaum MS, Coppola R, Gershon ES, et al: Evoked potential measures of attention and psychopathology. Advances in Biological Psychiatry 6:186-194, 1981

Buchsbaum MS, Ingvar DH, Kessler R, et al: Cerebral glucography with positron tomography: use in normal subjects and in patients with schizophrenia. Arch Gen Psychiatry 39:251-259, 1982a

Buchsbaum MS, Rigal F, Coppola A, et al: A new system for gray-level surface distribution maps of electrical activity. Electroencephalogr Clin Neurophysiol 53:237-242, 1982b

Buchsbaum MS, DeLisi LE, Holcomb HH, et al: Anteroposterior gradients in cerebral glucose use in schizophrenia and affective disorders. Arch Gen Psychiatry 41:1159-1166, 1984

Buchsbaum MS, Awsare SV, Holcomb HH, et al: Topographic differences between normals and schizophrenics: the N120 evoked potential component. Neuropsychobiology 15:1-6, 1986

Cooley JW, Tukey JW: An algorithm for the machine calculation of complex Fourier series. Math Comput 19:297-301, 1976

Cooper AL, Winter HJ, Crow TJ, et al: Comparison of subcortical, cortical, and scalp activity using chronically indwelling electrodes in man. Electroencephalogr Clin Neurophysiol 18:217-228, 1965

Coppola R: Topographic methods of functional cerebral analysis, in Frontiers of Engineering in Health Care. Edited by Potvin AR, Potvin JH. New York, IEEE Press, 1982

Coppola R: Issues in topographic analysis of EEG activity, in Topographic Mapping of the Brain. Edited by Duffy FH. Stoneham, MA, Butterworth (in press)

Coppola R, Buschbaum MS, Rigal F: Computer generation of surface distribution maps of measures of brain activity. Comput Biol Med 12:191-199, 1982

Duffy FH, Burchfiel JL, Lombroso CT: Brain electrical activity mapping (BEAM): a method for extending the clinical utility of EEG and evoked potential data. Ann Neurol 5:309-332, 1979

Duffy FH, Denckla MD, Bartels PH, et al: Dyslexia: regional differences in brain electrical activity by topographic mapping. Ann Neurol 7:412-420, 1980

Estrin T, Uzgalis R: Computer display of spatio-temporal EEG patterns. IEEE Trans Biomed Eng 16:192-196, 1969

Fuster J: The Prefrontal Cortex. New York, Raven Press, 1980

Gillin J, Post R, Wyatt RJ, et al: Infusion of threodihydroxyphenylserine (DOPS) and 5-hydroxytryptophan (5HTP) during human sleep. Sleep Research 1:45, 1972

Gotman J, Gloor R, Ray WG: A quantitative comparison of traditional reading of the EEG and interpretation of computer extracted features in patients with supratentorial brain lesions. Electroencephalogr Clin Neurophysiol 38:623-639, 1975

Gur RE: Regional cerebral blood flow in psychiatry: the resting and activated brains of schizophrenic patients, in Brain Imaging in Psychiatry. Edited by Morihisa JM. Washington, DC, American Psychiatric Press, 1984

Ingvar DH, Franzen G: Abnormalities of cerebral blood flow distribution in patients with chronic schizophrenia. Acta Psychiatr Scand 50:425-462, 1974

Ingvar DH, Sjolund B, Ardo A: Correlation between dominant EEG frequency, cerebral oxygen uptake and blood flow. Electroencephalogr Clin Neurophysiol 41:268-276, 1976

Itil TM, Saletu B, Davis S: EEG findings in chronic schizophrenics based on digital computer period analysis and analog power spectra. Biol Psychiatry 5:1-13, 1972

Jasper HH, Hawke WA: Electroencephalography IV: localization of seizure waves in epilepsy. Archives of Neurology and Psychiatry 39:885-901, 1938

Karson CN, Coppola R, Morihisa JM, et al: Computed electroencephalographic activity mapping in schizophrenia. Arch Gen Psychiatry 44:514-517, 1987

Kornmuller AE, Janzen R: Uber die normalen bioelektrischen Erscheinungen des menschlichen Gehirns. Arch f Psychiat 110:224-252, 1939

Kupfer DH, Foster FG, Detre TP: Sleep continuity changes in depression. Diseases of the Nervous System 34:192-195, 1973

Lehman D: Multichannel topography of human alpha EEG fields. Electroencephalogr Clin Neurophysiol 31:439-449, 1971

Lombroso CT, Duffy FH: Brain electrical activity mapping as a adjunct to CT scanning, in Advances in Epileptology: 11th International Epilepsy Symposium. Edited by Canger R, Angeleri F, Penry JK. New York, Raven Press, 1980

Mesulaum M, Geschwind N: On the possible role of neocortex and its limbic connection in attention in schizophrenia, in The Nature of Schizophrenia. Edited by Wynee, Cromwell, Matthysee. New York, John Wiley and Sons, 1978

Milner B. Effects of different brain lesions on card sorting. Arch Neurol 9:100-110, 1963

Morihisa JM: Electrophysiological evidence implicating frontal lobe dysfunction in schizophrenia. Psychopharmacol Bull 22(3):885-889, 1986a

Morihisa JM, McAnulty GB: Structure and function: brain electrical activity mapping and computed tomography in schizophrenia. Biol Psychiatry 20:3-19, 1985

Morihisa JM, Weinberger DR: Is schizophrenia a frontal lobe disease? An organizing theory of relevant anatomy and physiology, in Can Schizophrenia Be Localized in the Brain? Edited by Andreasen N. Washington, DC, American Psychiatric Press, 1986b

Morihisa JM, Duffy F, Wyatt RJ: Topographic analysis of computer processed electroencephalography in schizophrenia, in Biological Markers in Psychiatry and Neurology. Edited by Usdin E, Hanin J. New York, Pergamon Press, 1982

Morihisa JM, Duffy FH, Wyatt RJ: Brain electrical activity mapping (BEAM) in schizophrenic patients. Arch Gen Psychiatry 40:719-728, 1983

Morihisa JM: Functional brain imaging techniques, in American Psychiatric Association Annual Review, vol 6. Edited by Hales RE, Frances AJ. Washington, D.C., American Psychiatric Press, 1987

Motokawa K, Tuziguti K: Uber Vektordiagramme fur die gehirnelektrischen Erscheinungen des Menschen. Tohokushima J Exp Med 48, 73-86, 1944

Nauta WJH: The problem of the frontal lobe: a reinterpretation. J Psychiatr Res 8:167-187, 1971

Petsche H: Topography of the EEG: survey and prospects. Clin Neurol Neurosurg 79:15-28, 1976

Petsche H, Marko A: Das Photozellentoposkop, eine einfache methode zur bestimmung der feldverteilung und ausbreitung hirnelektrischer vorgange. Archives of Psychiatry 192:447-452, 1954

Remond A: Orientations et tendences des methodes topographiques dans l'etude de l'activite electrique du cerveau. Rev Neurol 93:399-410, 1955

Roth WT: Late event related potentials and psychopathology. Schizophrenia Bull 3:105-120, 1977

Shagass C, Roemer RA, Straumanis J, et al: Temporal variability of somatosensory, visual and auditory evoked potentials in schizophrenia. Arch Gen Psychiatry 36:1341-1351, 1979

Shagass C, Roemer R, Staumanis J, et al: Topography of sensory evoked potentials in depressive disorders. Biol Psychiatry 15:183-207, 1980

Shipton HW: A new electrotoposcope using a helical scan. Proceedings of the Electrophysiological Technology Association 2:2-11, 1956

Spitzer RL, Endicott J, Robins E: Research Diagnostic Criteria for Selected Group of Functional Disorders, 3rd edition. New York, Biometrics Research Division, New York State Psychiatric Institute, 1977

Stevens JR, Livermore A: Telemetered EEG in schizophrenia: spectral analysis during abnormal behavior episodes. J Neurol Neurosurg Psychiatry 45:385-395, 1982

Vaughn G, Ritter W: The sources of auditory evoked responses recorded from the human scalp. Electroencephalogr Clin Neurophysiol 28:360-378, 1970

Walter WG: Analytical means of studying the nature and origin in epileptic disturbances. Res Publ Assoc Nerv Ment Dis 26:237-251, 1947

Walter WG, Shipton HW: A new toposcopic display system. Electroencephalogr Clin Neurophysiol 3:281-292, 1951

Weinberger DR: Implications of normal brain development for the pathogenesis of schizophrenia. Arch Gen Psychiatry 44:660-669, 1987

Weinberger DR, Wyatt RJ: Structural brain abnormalities in chronic schizophrenia: computed tomography findings, in Perspectives in Schizophrenia Research. Edited by Baxter C, Melnechuk T. New York, Raven Press, 1980

Weinberger DR, Berman KF, Zec RF: Physiological dysfunction of dorsolateral prefrontal cortex in schizophrenia, I: regional cerebral blood flow (rCBF) evidence. Arch Gen Psychiatry 43:114-124, 1986

Wolkin A. Jaeger J, Brodie JD, et al: Persistence of cerebral metabolic abnormalities in chronic schizophrenia as determined by positron emission tomography. Am J Psychiatry 142:564-571, 1985

Chapter 4

Imaging Brain Function by Single-Photon Emission Computer Tomography

Michael D. Devous, Sr., Ph.D.

Single-photon emission computed tomography (SPECT) is the only currently available method for the three-dimensional measurement of regional cerebral blood flow in a clinical setting. Unfortunately, SPECT has for some time been viewed as the "poor stepchild" of positron emission tomography (PET). Recent developments in radiopharmaceuticals (the radioactively tagged compounds used to trace cerebral physiology) and imaging instruments have significantly altered this standing. SPECT now offers measurements of brain blood flow and receptor function which rival PET technologies in resolution and sensitivity. SPECT has the additional major advantage of being clinically affordable and capable of widespread distribution. It is the purpose of this chapter to outline the history of SPECT, to describe new radiopharmaceuticals and imaging instruments, and to discuss applications of SPECT in psychiatry.

These developments are so recent that very little direct application has been achieved. In fact, two of the new radiopharmaceuticals have only been available in the United States during the past year. Several highly sophisticated brain-imaging instruments using SPECT techniques have only recently been developed. We stand at the forefront of an era in which high-powered imaging technologies available only in major research institutions will be brought into widespread research and clinical utility in the hope of significantly improving research, diagnosis, and therapy in psychiatry.

147

History

The history of SPECT can be traced to two major developments. The first was the application of noninvasive techniques to measure brain blood flow. The second was the development of tomographic technologies for the measurement of brain structure. SPECT and PET both derive their basic principles from an intermixing of these two seminal developments.

Noninvasive measurements of brain function (biochemistry/physiology) have been sought since the earliest days of medicine. Since many psychiatric disorders are not associated with clearcut structural abnormalities, it was assumed that disturbances in brain physiology might be the cause of these disorders. Among the earliest tools used to assess brain function was the measurement of brain blood flow. Brain blood flow is important because of its role in providing nutrients and because it is tightly coupled to brain metabolism through the process of autoregulation. Kety and Schmidt (1948) employed nitrous oxide as a diffusible indicator of brain blood flow in humans. This was an insightful application of the Fick principle governing the relationship among the arterial delivery of a chemically inert substance, its cellular uptake, and its clearance into the venous system. By monitoring the difference between arterial input and venous outflow, cellular uptake could be determined. The latter is directly related to perfusion for compounds that are freely diffusible and not metabolized.

These early measurements required carotid injection and internal jugular sampling, and they could only measure whole-brain blood flow. Nitrous oxide was soon replaced by chemically inert radioisotopes as the diffusible indicator, because radiotracers could be detected in local brain regions by the use of collimated detectors. Thus, brain blood flow from regions smaller than the entire brain could be measured. Lassen and Monk (1955) used the Kety–Schmidt model with Kr-85, which required surgical exposure of the brain in order to detect the emitted beta radiations. It was rapidly replaced by the use of Xe-133 as the detectable radiotracer (Glass and Harper 1963), because Xe-133 emits gamma rays that can be detected through the intact skull. The use of Xe-133 led to techniques for measuring regional cerebral blood flow (rCBF) with multiple scintillation probes, mathematically separating flows to gray and white matter (Obrist et al. 1967, 1975; Risberg et al. 1975a). This advance led to a rapid development of two-dimensional measurement systems, with ever-increasing numbers of probes, and thus to subjection of an increasing number of brain regions to analysis, culminating in the 254-detector unit described by Sveinsdottir et al. (1977). Simultaneous improvements in detector sensitivity and curve-fitting algorithms permitted replacement of intra-arterial injections with either inhalation or intravenous injection of Xe-133 so that the determination of rCBF became a noninvasive procedure.

During the development of two-dimensional methods for assessing brain function, three-dimensional methods for measuring the internal structure of objects were also being developed. The concept of tomography (deriving three-dimensional information from two-dimensional data) takes its roots from the solution of a mathematical problem in astronomy, presented by Radon (1917) at the turn of the century. It was first applied in medicine by the Nobel laureates A. M. Cormack (1963) and G. N. Hounsfield (1973), who developed the first CT scanner, and almost simultaneously by Bracewell (1967), who used radio signals from space to reconstruct three-dimensional surfaces of astronomical objects. The basic principles of tomography have been applied across a broad range, from the study of the internal structure of atoms (Manuel 1982) to the study of oceans (Behringer et al. 1982). Kuhl and Edwards (1963) were the first to apply tomographic principles to reconstruct three-dimensional images of the distribution of radiotracers in humans, which ultimately led to the technologies we now call SPECT and PET. It was the marriage of three-dimensional imaging technology with radiotracer measurements of rCBF that permitted the first views of the physiologic behavior of the brain beneath the cortical surface.

Three tomographic technologies have been employed to measure rCBF: x-ray CT, PET, and SPECT. Most cost-effective of these may be SPECT, even though its limitations have been clearly delineated (Budinger 1980; Ter-Pogossian 1985). Many of these limitations have been addressed by instrumentation developments, described later in this chapter. Efforts to develop SPECT systems to measure rCBF with diffusible indicators such as Xe-133 include a rotating, 4-detector system (Tomomatic 64) designed by Stokely et al. (1980), and a ring-detector system (HEADTOME) designed by Kanno et al. (1981).

The first successful tomographic imaging of rCBF with diffusible noble gas indicators was by Yamamoto et al. (1977), employing Kr-77 and PET imaging. Drayer et al. (1978) and Meyer et al. (1981) have utilized stable xenon inhalation with x-ray CT to calculate rCBF and xenon partition coefficients. Unfortunately, these systems require the inhalation of xenon close to levels producing anesthesia, and some questions have arisen concerning the validity of the technique. Newer SPECT systems are capable of measuring the distribution of statically distributed radiopharmaceuticals (radiotracers that are trapped in the brain and whose distribution remains stable over a period of time), including I-123-labeled amines that reflect brain perfusion patterns (Winchell et al. 1980; Kung et al.

1983; Hill et al. 1982; Kuhl et al. 1982a). Most recently, our group and others have completed work that has led to the development of a SPECT system capable of high-resolution imaging of statically distributed radio-pharmaceuticals and quantitative measurements of dynamic radiopharmaceuticals such as Xe-133 (Lim et al. 1985).

Overview

SPECT is a method to determine the three-dimensional distribution of a radiotracer within the human body. The radiotracer (often dubbed "radiopharmaceutical") can be as simple as a radioactive element (e.g., Xe-133, T1-201) or as complicated as a labeled neurotransmitter antagonist (e.g., I-123-3-quinuclidinyl 4-iodobenzilate, or QNB). The radiopharmaceuticals for SPECT are distinguished from those used in PET in that the former emit a single gamma ray, while PET radiopharmaceuticals emit two gamma rays simultaneously in exactly opposite directions following annihilation of the emitted positron with a nearby electron. This distinction in gamma ray emissions leads to the distinction in instrumentation between SPECT and PET. Single-photon tomographs are designed to detect single photons (gamma rays) and to determine their point of origin based solely on their trajectory. PET makes valuable use of the dual photon emissions to determine point of origin based both on the trajectories of both gamma rays and on the timing with which the two photons arrive at the surface of the tomograph's detectors.

Early instrumentation to reconstruct single-photon data into three-dimensional images provided a resolution of 15–20 mm and required 20–60 minutes of imaging time to obtain data. Advances in detector technology have led to improvements in both resolution and sensitivity. State-of-the-art nuclear medicine imaging equipment (with resolution of about 12 mm), coupled with recent advances in radiopharmaceuticals, should be able to produce rCBF images in as little as 10 minutes. Very recent innovations in SPECT tomography have led to one system capable of 8 mm resolution and imaging times as short as 2–3 minutes for rCBF measurements.

Today, SPECT is capable of measurements of rCBF and of the muscarinic cholinergic receptor system. Measurements of dopaminergic and adrenergic receptor systems should be possible within the next few years. One of the major strengths of PET imaging is the measurement of glucose metabolism. No radiopharmaceutical for SPECT related to regional glucose metabolism yet exists. Fortunately, rCBF and glucose metabolism are tightly coupled in the brain under most circumstances; thus rCBF measurements reflect neuronal metabolism.

Advantages and Applications

The major advantage of SPECT is that the instrumentation involved and the radiopharmaceuticals employed are routinely available in most nuclear medicine departments. The radioisotopes are those commonly used for nuclear medicine procedures (Tc-99m, I-123, and Xe-133). They are available from commercial manufacturers, can be purchased on a "per dose" basis, and do not require an on-site cyclotron for their production. Similarly, many SPECT instruments can be obtained from commercial manufacturers at a reasonable price, and they do not require extensive technical support to operate. The implication of these circumstances is that SPECT imaging can be performed in a clinical environment on large numbers of patients at a reasonable cost. Two of the major hindrances to the advance of functional brain imaging through PET have been the lack of availability of systems in urban locations and the extreme cost of the studies. SPECT could relieve both of these difficulties.

To date, SPECT applications in psychiatry have been confined to the research arena. Since SPECT radiopharmaceuticals and instrumentation have only been available for a few years, the technique has not yet been applied in routine clinical care. However, research findings described later in this chapter imply that SPECT has the potential to be useful both in diagnosis and in monitoring therapy. It should continue to play a major role in psychiatric research that would expand with increased availability of high-resolution–high-sensitivity systems.

BASIC PRINCIPLES

Overview

Functional brain imaging by SPECT is a two-stage process. In the first stage a radiotracer is administered, while in the second stage the radiotracer distribution is determined by a tomographic instrument. In some cases these two stages occur simultaneously, such as in Xe-133 tomography of rCBF, while in others a considerable delay occurs between administration of radioisotope and imaging (e.g., imaging of radiolabeled receptor ligands). The basic principles underlying each of these stages are reviewed below.

SPECT is founded on the assumption that some chemical compounds distribute to the brain in a way that is reflective of brain physiology, and that these compounds can be bound to radioactive elements whose emissions can be externally detected. For example, consider the case of rCBF imaging. Without concerning ourselves with the detail of what radiopharmaceutical one might use, on general principles one can imagine SPECT imaging of rCBF performed with a compound that flows into the brain with the arterial blood and is transferred across the blood–brain barrier in a manner solely dependent on the concentration gradient. Processes such as active transport would thus not be involved. Areas receiving high arterial blood perfusion would receive large quantities of this compound, and areas receiving relatively little perfusion would receive smaller quantities of this compound. Thus, if we could stop the process instantaneously after delivery of the compound its distribution in brain tissue would reflect regional blood flow.

This process is exactly the one used to examine rCBF in animal studies with C-14 iodoantipyrine and tissue autoradiography. In fact, PET and SPECT both represent a noninvasive form of autoradiography.

With imaging techniques, however, external recording devices are used rather than radiographic film. The next step in our general scheme would be to determine the distribution of the compound at the instant of delivery to brain in proportion to blood flow. Since the compound is labeled with a radiotracer that emits gamma rays, our need is to determine the distribution of emitted gamma rays. To do this, we might surround the brain with detectors each of which would record the emitted gamma rays. This process is illustrated in Figure 1. In order to determine the distribu-

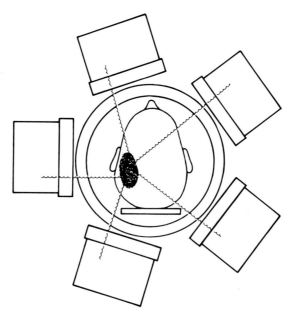

FIGURE 1. A schematic representation illustrating a multidetector system for single-photon emission computed tomography of the brain. Efficient and rapid tomography may be performed if substantial detector volume can be placed in close proximity to the brain to record the emitted gamma rays.

tion of emitted gamma rays we must be able to find in the brain the site of origin of a given gamma ray. Since they are uniformly emitted in all directions, a device in front of the detectors is required to distinguish gamma rays coming from different parts of the brain. This device is called a collimator and is simply a lead sheet thick enough to stop gamma rays from penetrating to the detector. The collimator contains long apertures

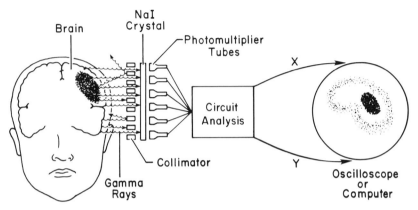

FIGURE 2a. Schematic diagram of the collimator/crystal/circuitry of a gamma camera observing gamma rays emitted from a radiopharmaceutical taken up in a localized portion of the brain. Gamma rays pass through parallel holes in the collimator to the detector for subsequent display on an oscilloscope or computer. Gamma rays approaching the collimator at angles not parallel with the collimator hole are reflected. The resultant image is a one-for-one mapping of the radioactivity underlying the collimator and crystal.

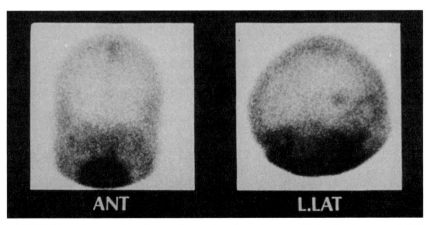

FIGURE 2b. Conventional two-dimensional nuclear medicine brain scans (ANT: anterior; L.LAT: left lateral). A series of such images taken at various angles around the brain can be combined to create tomographic cross-sections.

through which gamma rays pass unobstructed to the detector surface. Since nonaligned gamma rays are blocked by the collimator, it is assumed that a gamma ray detected on a given spot in the collimator comes from a part of the brain directly below the hole through which that gamma ray passed. This process is illustrated in Figure 2a. However, the collimated gamma ray can in fact come from any part of the brain on a line parallel with the collimator hole. Therefore, the collimated detected radiation only determines the line through the brain from which the gamma ray was emitted, not the exact point.

The detector actually covers a large area and the collimator is built with an array of holes, so that a series of lines representing radiation from the brain are imaged simultaneously. This process represents the conventional two-dimensional nuclear medicine image (Figure 2b). It is not different from images taken of liver, bone, or heart. This two-dimensional image, called a projection, represents a sum of all of the emissions along the lines represented by the collimator holes. Thus, it is a three-dimensional brain-activity distribution squashed down to a two-dimensional plane (the plane of the detector surface).

One way to expand two-dimensional information about the brain into a three-dimensional picture is to collect a series of two-dimensional images (projections) by moving the detector around the brain. In our mind's eye we could reconstruct a crude tomographic image of the distribution of activity by envisioning the three-dimensional location of an object from a series of two-dimensional pictures. Take for example, the process illustrated in Figure 3. Within the ellipse representing the brain is an area of high radiopharmaceutical uptake. This area is on the left side near the rear (Figure 3a). A two-dimensional image from the front of the head provides the distribution shown in Figure 3b. A "hot spot" representing the highly radioactive area is seen just to the left of midline. Another image from the left side of the head yields the distribution shown in Figure 3c. In this case a hot spot located near the back of the head is observed but we do not know whether it is on the left or right side. The image taken from the front of the head (Figure 3b) yields lateral coordinates, while the image taken from the side gives the anterior–posterior information (Figure 3c). However, combining the information from these two images tells us that there is a hot spot near the back of the head just left of the midline. Because these two-dimensional images also tell us something about the superior–inferior location of the hot spot we have some idea about where in the brain this radioactive hot spot lies.

We use the same principle in binocular vision every day to gain three-dimensional information, such as depth, about the world around us. Unfortunately, the structural distribution of blood flow, glucose metabolism, or receptor function is much more complex than our simple example.

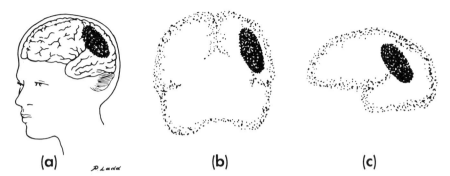

FIGURE 3. An area of increased radiopharmaceutical uptake is localized to the left posterior portion of the brain (a). An anterior view produces a nuclear medicine image with high uptake on the left superior side (b). A lateral image of the same radiopharmaceutical distribution indicates increased activity posterior and superior in the brain (c).

Therefore, two views are insufficient to capture the details of brain physiologic structure. To overcome this complication we add more and more views. Unfortunately, most of us are not capable of integrating in our heads tens to hundreds of two-dimensional views of the brain into a three-dimensional picture. Therefore, computer algorithms are employed to integrate all of these views into a single three-dimensional representation of the distribution of our radiopharmaceutical inside the brain. The mathematical tools employed in SPECT are identical to those employed in x-ray CT, and the detection systems are very similar to those used in PET.

There are a variety of methods available to reconstruct our projections into three-dimensional images, but the technology to display this three-dimensional information is quite limited at this time. Therefore, we traditionally redisplay three-dimensional data in two-dimensional images. However, instead of displaying the data as images of the brain surface (as in the projections we originally collected), it is displayed as cross-sections through the brain (see Figure 4a). Most commonly, transverse cross-sections are employed, although mathematically one could display the brain along any axis desired, including coronal, sagittal, and various oblique views. A considerable effort is under way to develop technical means to display all of the three-dimensional data collected. These include computer graphic techniques that give images a three-dimensional appearance, as illustrated in Figure 4b. Holographic images and virtual images obtained from vibrating mirrors are currently under consideration as sources of "true" three-dimensional images. The cost of these display modalities is currently too high, however, to make them practical for routine use.

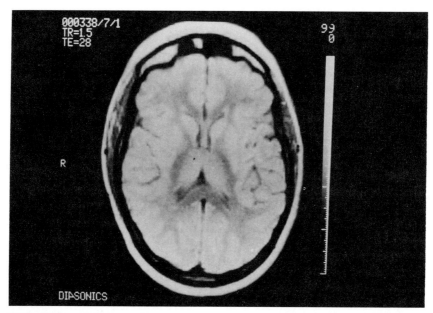

FIGURE 4a. A high-resolution magnetic resonance image of the brain in transverse cross-section. This is the most conventional image display format used in tomographic imaging. Volume imaging devices such as most SPECT units and some PET units are capable of displaying image cross-sections at other angles (e.g. coronal, sagittal).

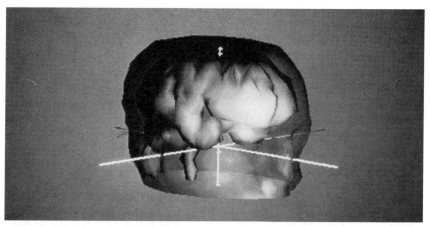

FIGURE 4b. A computer graphic technique using surface shading to display three-dimensional tomographic data in a "three-dimensional" perspective. These data were derived from transverse cross-sectional CT images. Courtesy of Daniel Schlusselbeg, M.D., Department of Radiology, University of Texas Health Science Center at Dallas.

There is a strong (though not absolute) structure/function relationship in the brain, and therefore it is important that functional brain images display as much anatomic detail as possible. In SPECT and PET ongoing efforts to improve spatial resolution have dominated instrumentation development. PET has led the way in this arena and continues to offer the greatest spatial resolution of the emission tomographic techniques. Recent developments in SPECT instrumentation have led, however, to images with resolution nearly comparable with current PET images. In this context, the best spatial resolution yet achieved with PET is 5 mm, and with SPECT it is 8 mm. The effect of resolution on image quality was nicely demonstrated by a computer simulation performed by Phelps et al. (1982), and shown in Figure 5. The improvement in anatomic definition provided by successively finer resolution is clearly illustrated.

Tomograph Construction

We have already indicated that SPECT detector systems involve a radiation-detecting device and a collimator. Traditionally, nuclear medicine

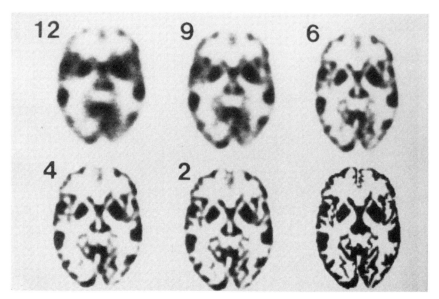

FIGURE 5. A computer simulation illustrating the effects of detection system resolution on images. An "original" brain cross-sectional image (lower right) would be degraded to images of the indicated resolution, where the numerical values are in mm. Reproduced with permission from Phelps et al; J Comput Assist Tomogr 6:551-565, 1982.

detectors are made of sodium iodide crystals which respond to incoming gamma rays by emitting light. The location of the emitted light can be detected by an electronic circuit composed of photomultiplier tubes. The intensity of the light corresponds to the energy of the incoming gamma ray, which allows discrimination of primary photons from lower-energy scattered radiation. By combining position and energy information, two-dimensional images of the distribution of radiopharmaceuticals have been obtained in nuclear medicine for many decades. The device composed of a single crystal and a lead collimator is conventionally called the Anger camera, named after its inventor Hal Anger (1958; see Figure 6). The simplest SPECT instrument can be viewed as an Anger camera (or gamma camera) that rotates about the patient. In fact, some of the earliest SPECT images were obtained from a conventional nuclear medicine Anger camera (incapable of rotation) by rotating the patient on a chair in front of the camera (Figure 7). Rotating gamma cameras have become very popular in nuclear medicine departments and have a widespread distribution even today. Currently, such systems are capable of 12–14-mm resolution and are rather insensitive (Figure 8). Kuhl et al. (1976) expanded this tech-

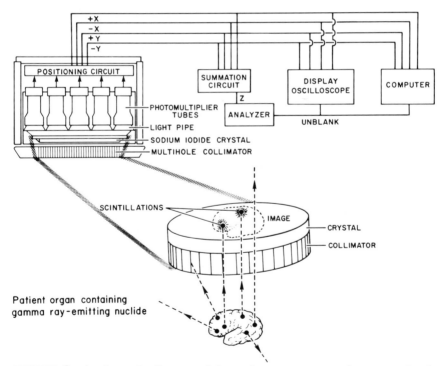

FIGURE 6. A schematic diagram of the major components of a conventional Anger camera (gamma camera).

FIGURE 7. An early method for SPECT imaging was to rotate the subject in front of a fixed position gamma camera. Reproduced with permission from Keyes, in Computed Emission Tomography. Edited by Ell PJ, Holman BL. New York, Oxford University Press, 1982.

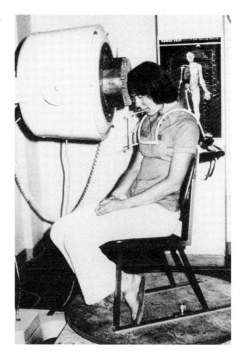

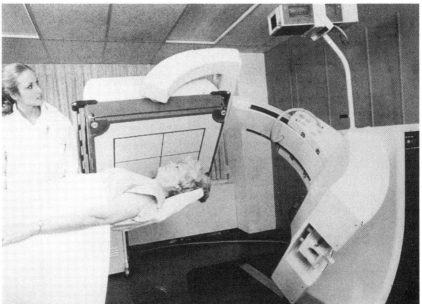

FIGURE 8. Modern rotating gamma camera. Photograph courtesy of Technicare Inc.

nology in order to construct the first dedicated SPECT unit, called the Mark IV, which was composed of four Anger cameras mounted on a rotating gantry (Figure 9). Specialized collimators enabled this unit to be placed close to the head, thereby improving image quality. This unit was never manufactured commercially.

In addition to rotating gamma cameras now in wide use and the Mark IV, two other SPECT tomographs have been developed. One of these (Tomomatic 64, Medimatic A/S, Copenhagen) is capable of both dynamic (diffusible tracers) and static (fixed tracers) tomography (Stokely et al. 1980; Figure 10a). It is the only SPECT unit capable of tomographic rCBF measurements derived from the cerebral transit of Xe-133. For this reason it is sometimes abbreviated DSPECT, for dynamic single-photon emission computerized tomograph.

This imaging unit contains four banks of individual sodium iodide detectors arranged in a hollow square configuration that rotates about the patient at 6 rpm (Figure 10b), producing a complete set of projections every 10 seconds. The collimation on this unit was designed for the high sensitivity required to make rapid measurements of the transit of Xe-133 through the brain. These collimators detect only three to five slices across the brain with an interslice separation of 4 to 2 cm. In order to achieve the high sensitivity required for Xe-133 measurements, these collimators have large holes and thus do not define the line from which the gamma rays come with great accuracy. The result of this high-sensitivity collima-

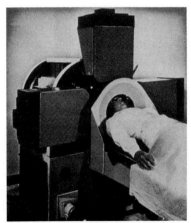
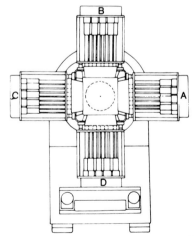

FIGURE 9.   The Mark IV SPECT system developed by Kuhl et al. Reproduced with permission from Kuhl et al; Radiol 121:405-413, 1976.

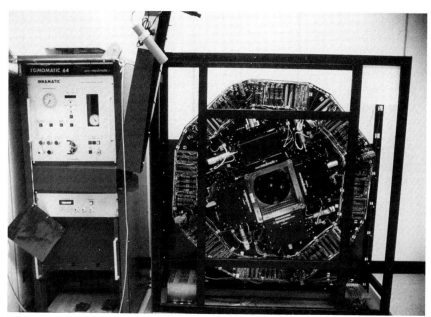

FIGURE 10a. The Tomomatic 64 dynamic SPECT system (with covers removed), developed by Stokely et al. The xenon delivery system is on the left and the rotating tomograph is on the right.

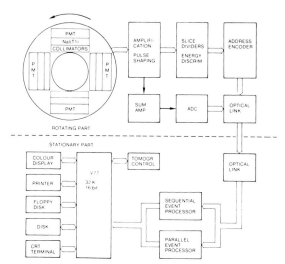

FIGURE 10b. Schematic diagram of the Tomomatic 64 demonstrating data acquisition on the moving part (top) linked optically to data analysis and reconstruction portions (bottom). Reproduced with permission from Stokely et al; J Comput Assist Tomogr 4:230-240, 1980.

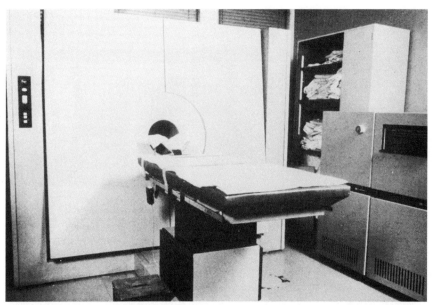

FIGURE 11a. The Harvard multidetector scanning brain system (previously known as the Cleon 710), a high-resolution, low-sensitivity, single slice SPECT system. Reproduced with permission from Ell PJ, in Computed Emission Tomography. Edited by Ell PJ, Holman BL. New York, Oxford University Press, 1982.

tor design is that this system has poor resolution (17 mm). However, it is the only SPECT unit capable of dynamic tomography, and the entire procedure can be completed in 4 minutes. The construction details of this tomograph have been described by Devous et al. (1985b). A second collimator design has been created for this tomograph which permits high-resolution, static radiopharmaceutical imaging. These collimators greatly decrease the sensitivity of the system but yield images of 12-mm resolution, confined to three transverse cross-sectional slices.

Although only two such instruments have been installed in the United States (our laboratory and the University of Iowa Medical Center), 20–30 such units are operational throughout Europe and Japan. In contrast, literally hundreds of rotating Anger camera SPECT units have been installed throughout the United States.

The only other commercially available, dedicated SPECT unit was originally developed and marketed collaboratively between Harvard University and Union Carbide (Cleon or Harvard Multidetector Scanning Brain System, Figure 11a; Stoddart and Stoddart 1979). It employs a unique arrangement of moving detector heads which define only a single

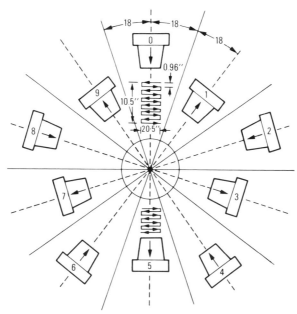

FIGURE 11b.   Schematic diagram illustrating the detector motions employed in this SPECT unit. Reproduced with permission from Moore, in Computed Emission Tomography. Edited by Ell PJ, Holman BL. New York, Oxford University Press, 1982.

tomographic transverse cross section. This unit has the highest resolution of currently available SPECT systems, but is relatively insensitive. A schematic diagram is shown in Figure 11b. Both head and body tomographic units were developed.

Our group has recently been involved in the development of a new SPECT system, called the PRISM, a schematic diagram of which is shown in Figure 12a (Lim et al. 1985). This has only recently become commercially available. PRISM consists of three rectangularly shaped Anger cameras mounted on a rotating plate. Each camera is capable of radial translation and thus can follow any orbit shape (circular or elliptical). These detectors have a wide rectangular field of view (40 × 20 cm) and thus accommodate both head and body imaging. Another advance employed is the use of fan-beam collimation, in contrast to most SPECT units that employ parallel-beam collimation (that is, all of the holes in the collimator have been drilled parallel to each other). Fan-beam collimation, similar to the technology employed in x-ray CT, affords enhanced resolution and sensitivity. This system has been designed for very rapid rotation for dynamic imaging, and high-resolution slower rotation for static imaging. Unlike the

PARALLEL BEAM IMAGING

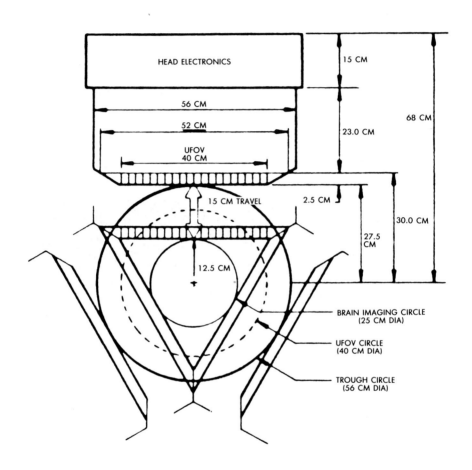

3X
Sensitivity

FIGURE 12a. Schematic diagram illustrating the detector formations for the PRISM SPECT unit. This unit is capable of either high-resolution static scanning or high-sensitivity dynamic scanning, and images the whole brain providing cross-sectional data at any angle.

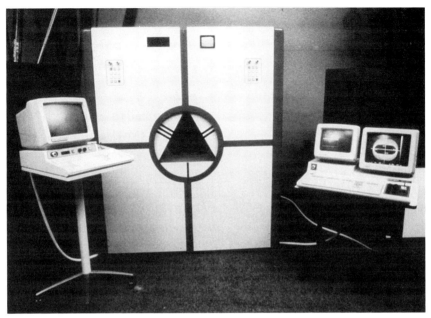

FIGURE 12b. The PRISM scanner with its computer display system and control module. Illustrations furnished courtesy of Technicare Inc.

Tomomatic and Cleon SPECT units, this system images contiguous sections of the brain that can be displayed in any angular orientation from any portion of the brain. The intrinsic resolution of this system (resolution of the individual Anger camera heads) is 3.4 mm, and its applied resolution (that is, resolution in patients) is 8–9 mm. Poorer resolution (13–17 mm) is achieved in the dynamic mode because of the necessity to take very rapid SPECT images of the inert gas tracers. A prototype PRISM system has been operating since early 1985 (Figure 12b). It began clinical use in our laboratory in late 1987. This system represents a major enhancement of SPECT tomography, and it provides the first unit that is truly competitive with PET.

A comparison of rotating gamma camera SPECT units, the Tomomatic 64, the Cleon, and the PRISM is presented in Table 1. The resolution and sensitivity of these systems are compared for both static and dynamic radiopharmaceuticals. Imaging times were compared among the tomographs only for statically distributed radiopharmaceuticals, since that is the only mode of operation they all have in common. The estimated times are based on the injection of 5 mCi of I-123-labeled iodoamphetamine, a currently available static brain-imaging agent. Static radiopharmaceuticals permit longer imaging times and thus achieve

TABLE 1.   Comparison of Brain-Imaging Parameters with SPECT Instruments

Instrument	Time (min)*	Number of Slices	Slice Orientation	Resolution
Rotating gamma camera	40	variable†	any†	12 mm
Mark IV	6	1	transverse	17 mm
Harvard Multidetector Scanner	20	1	transverse	10 mm
Tomomatic 64	16	3	transverse	12 mm
PRISM	8	variable†	any†	8 mm

* Estimated imaging times are based on an assumed dose of 5 mCi I-123 iodoamphetamine and production of cross-sectional images of equivalent count density.

† The number and orientation of cross-sectional images obtained are under user control since the whole brain is imaged.

higher resolution since the radiopharmaceutical is not redistributing. Dynamic radiopharmaceuticals must be imaged quickly and repeatedly. Repeat measurements of the redistribution of the dynamic radiopharmaceutical are used to calculate rCBF employing a modification of the Kety–Schmidt model (Kanno and Lassen 1979). This process is described in greater detail below.

Radiopharmaceuticals

Radiopharmaceuticals for SPECT imaging fall into four categories. These are: 1) diffusible indicators, 2) I-123-labeled lipophilic agents, 3) Tc-99m-labeled lipophilic agents, and 4) I-123-labeled neuroreceptor ligands.

Diffusible tracers do not chemically interact with brain parenchyma and freely traverse the blood–brain barrier. For SPECT imaging only Xe-133 is routinely available. This isotope of the noble gas xenon has been used routinely for more than two decades for two-dimensional measurements of rCBF using probe systems and the Kety–Schmidt model. Only the Tomomatic 64 is capable of dynamic SPECT measurements with Xe-133 at this time, although the PRISM system will be capable of such measurements in the near future. Xe-133 is readily available and inexpensive. Its major disadvantage is that the energy of its emitted gamma ray is low (80 keV) and thus is difficult to distinguish from scattered gamma rays that produce "noise" in tomographic reconstructions. The physical half-life of 5.3 days permits short-term storage for use as needed. It is typically administered by inhalation in doses of 10 mCi/liter during a one-minute rebreathing period. The principal radiation dose is to the lungs (0.1 to 0.2 rads) with a total-body dose of approximately 0.01 rad (McAfee et al. 1975). The highest dose is received by the upper airway mucosa (1–5 rads/procedure). This dosimetry limits the application of this technique to 5–10 studies per patient over a lifetime.

The use of a diffusible indicator such as Xe-133 is clearly distinguished from the "statically distributed" radiopharmaceuticals because one must apply a mathematical model to its uptake and clearance in order to measure rCBF. This is both an advantage and disadvantage. The modeling procedure yields quantitative measurements of rCBF that can be compared both among patient groups and within the same individual on several occasions. The statically distributed radiopharmaceuticals such as I-123 iodoamphetamine (IMP) represent the relative distribution of rCBF, but cannot easily be quantitated.

The procedure of fitting data from tomographic images to a mathematical model of inert gas tracer distribution (such as the Kety–Schmidt model) requires a series of tomographic images taken over a short period of time (typically four minutes) and limits the amount of activity obtained in each image. Limited activity leads to images of poorer resolution than those obtained with statically distributed radiopharmaceuticals.

RCBF calculations are based on the Kety–Schmidt model for single-compartment tissue perfusion. When an inert-gas radioactive tracer is employed in this model, perfusion is determined by observing time variations in the counting rates of specific tissues (for example gray matter and white matter) following tracer administration. In the tomographic approach, the tissue under observation is the volume element (voxel) determined by the reconstruction algorithm. For example, if the tomograph resolution is 1.7 cm and the transverse cross section is 2 cm thick, then the minimum voxel size is $1.7 \times 1.7 \times 2$ cm $= 5.8$ cc. This typically will include both gray and white matter.

Kanno and Lassen (1979) modified the Kety–Schmidt model to take into account the use of Xe-133 with its low photopeak energy and the statistical limitations of dynamic tomography. They developed what is called the double-integral method, which permits reasonably accurate quantitation of gray-matter rCBF, but very poor quantitation of white-matter flow. This model is heavily dependent upon the total observed radioactivity, and thus it provides good definition of areas of ischemia. Unfortunately, for a very similar reason the model is insensitive to small differences in activity at high perfusions and tends to overestimate high flows. The difficulties and benefits associated with this particular model have been described in detail by Celsis et al. (1981) and Smith et al. (1984). The application of this technique to the study of normal volunteers, its reliability and reproducibility, and its relationship to other methods of rCBF imaging have been described by Devous et al. (1986b).

In the early 1980s two I-123 radiopharmaceuticals were developed for SPECT determination of rCBF. I-123 is a useful imaging radiopharmaceutical because it has a half-life of 13 hours, and a gamma ray energy of 159 keV (nearly double that of Xe-133), permitting improved photopeak detection and resolution. Both compounds label I-123 to an amine structure. The first is iodoamphetamine (IMP), developed by Winchell et al. (1980), and the second is a diamine (HIPDM), developed by Kung et al. (1983). Only IMP is commercially available at this time. Kuhl et al. (1982a) have demonstrated that the initial uptake of IMP is directly proportional to rCBF. Devous et al. (in press) demonstrated that both IMP and HIPDM are related to rCBF up to 60 minutes after injection but that IMP begins redistribution between 60–90 minutes after injection. In contrast, HIPDM remains related to rCBF for at least 90 minutes after injection.

The time during which these agents are stable is important for successful application in routine rCBF SPECT. The instrument most widely available for SPECT imaging, the rotating gamma camera, has low sensitivity leading to imaging times ranging from 40 to 60 minutes. Thus, the distribution of the radiopharmaceutical must be stable during that time period. This is just barely true for IMP, but appears to be acceptable for HIPDM.

The distribution of these agents can only be quantitated if arterial blood samples are obtained during the early injection phase (Kuhl et al. 1982a; Lucignani et al. 1985). To quantitate rCBF from these agents one must use a model similar to those used for invasive rCBF measurements. These would include C-14 iodoantipyrine and autoradiography or radioactively labeled tracer microspheres for rCBF determinations from individual tissue samples. A model for this process has been suggested (Sumiya et al. 1985), but remains to be verified.

The actual process by which these two radiopharmaceuticals distribute in brain is not well understood. Upon injection they are lipophilic and cross the blood–brain barrier in direct proportion to regional perfusion. After entering the brain parenchyma it is believed that they undergo a structural or conformational change exposing anionic surfaces, significantly reducing their lipophilicity, and temporarily trapping them within the brain cells. This trapping mechanism is not permanent, and they are removed or redistributed from the brain with time. It appears that they are not significantly metabolized by the neurons (Kuhl et al. 1982a; Lucignani et al. 1985; Holman et al. 1983, 1984).

The third class of radiopharmaceuticals are those labeled with Tc-99m. Tc-99m has been the mainstay of nuclear medicine procedures for many years since it is commercially available, inexpensive, easy to handle, and has very favorable dosimetry. Thus, it can be administered to patients in much larger quantities than I-123 if it can be bound to appropriate ligands. Unfortunately, technetium chemistry is very complex and the development of iodine-labeled agents has usually preceded those of technetium because of the much simpler chemical syntheses involved. This has certainly been true for rCBF radiopharmaceuticals, since the first reports of Tc-99m-labeled rCBF agents appeared three years after those for I-123.

Three different groups have recently succeeded in binding Tc-99m to lipophilic ligands which cross the blood–brain barrier and distribute in proportion to rCBF. The initial compounds were poorly retained in the brain and were rapidly washed out, making them useless for imaging with rotating gamma cameras (Kung et al. 1984; Volkert et al. 1984; Lever et al. 1985). Later derivatives of these initial compounds have longer retention times, permitting imaging by conventional technology. One of these (Tc-99m HMPAO) was developed by Volkert et al. (1984) and has been used in humans in Europe (Holm et al. 1985). This compound was distributed for Phase I clinical trials in the United States early in 1986. A second compound (Tc-99m NEP-DADT) was developed by Burns and colleagues (Lever et al. 1985); animal studies appear promising, and Phase I clinical trials have been planned. These compounds distribute in a manner very similar to the I-123-labeled amines. Their major advantage is that the radioisotope to which they are tagged is widely available and less expensive. In addition Tc-99m dosimetry permits the administration of much higher doses (15–20 mCi/patient/procedure) and thus should dramatically shorten imaging times.

Normal rCBF images from Xe-133, I-123-IMP, and Tc-99m-HMPAO are shown in Figure 13. Clearly, the Xe-133 image suffers from poor resolution and limited gray/white-matter distinction (Figure 13a). However, the quantitative nature of these images (image values represent ml/min/100 g) is a significant advantage. The IMP image (Figure 13b) was obtained with the Cleon, and the HMPAO image (Figure 13c) with the high-resolution collimators for the Tomomatic 64. Both images demonstrate improved resolution and gray/white-matter distinction, but rCBF cannot easily be derived from the voxel values.

The final class of SPECT imaging agents are neurotransmitter ligands. Eckelman et al. (1984) have produced I-123-labeled QNB, a muscarinic cholinergic agonist. Although some difficulties with the distribution of various isomers created during the synthesis have been delineated (Gibson et al. 1984; Eckelman et al. 1985), it appears that this agent will be

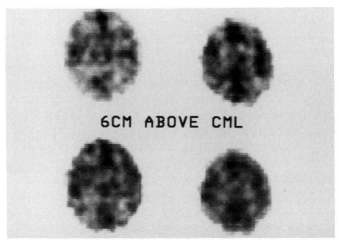

FIGURE 13a. Four examples of normal Xe-133 rCBF images. Images are oriented so that left is to reader's left, and anterior is up. Note the nearly continuous ring of high flows in the cortex, and the inappropriately high levels in the white matter regions medially. This technique yields reasonable data for gray matter flows but substantially overestimates white matter rCBF.

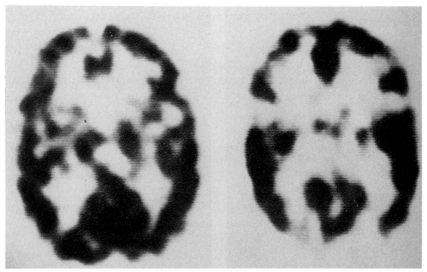

FIGURE 13b. Examples of rCBF obtained with the Cleon 710 SPECT unit and I-123 iodoamphetamine. The image on the left was obtained with the subjects's eyes open, while the image on the right was obtained with the eyes closed. Reproduced with permission from Hill et al., in Computed Emission Tomography. Edited by Ell PJ, Holman BL. New York, Oxford University Press, 1982.

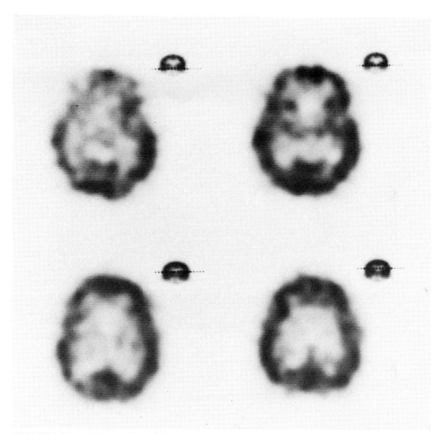

FIGURE 13c. Examples of brain SPECT rCBF images from a normal individual using a rotating gamma camera and Tc-99m HM-PAO. The levels from which each slice is obtained are indicated by the smallish figures in the upper right quadrants. Photograph furnished courtesy of Richard A. Holmes, M.D., University of Missouri.

useable for receptor imaging. Its earliest application in humans is illustrated in Figure 14 (Holman et al. 1985). Dopaminergic receptor imaging has been successfully accomplished with PET using C-11- or F-18-labeled spiperone and C-11-labeled raclopride. These positron emitters have been replaced by I-125 in recent efforts, and very recently I-123 FLA961 has been used to image D2 receptors in man (Crawley et al. 1986). Research is under way to develop adrenergic receptor ligands labeled with I-123 as well. Each of these receptor agents will only be available in research settings for the foreseeable future. It is not clear at this time whether there is sufficient clinical demand to encourage commercial manufacturers to produce such agents for routine distribution. In addition, they are all

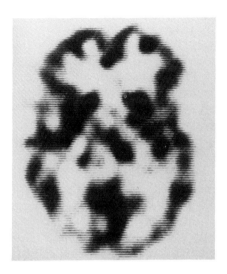

FIGURE 14. A high-resolution SPECT study (Cleon 710) of the distribution of muscarinic cholinergic receptors in a normal volunteer using I-123 labeled 3-quinuclidinyl 4-iodobenzilate (QNB). Reproduced with permission from Eckelman et al; Science 223:291-293, 1984.

currently labeled with I-123 which has limited availability. Advances to technetium-labeled receptor ligands would greatly improve the application of receptor imaging through SPECT.

Image Interpretation

Image data can be analyzed in two ways: 1) quantitative values from specific brain regions can be determined and 2) qualitative interpretations (visual inspection) of images by experienced observers can be obtained. Both visual interpretation and quantitative analyses require a known relationship between the functional image and anatomic structure in order to compare data in the same patient on several occasions, or to compare data among patient groups. In order to relate functional imaging to anatomic structure, patients must be positioned carefully, and a method must be employed to locate the functional images within the structural boundaries of the brain. The accuracy with which functional images and anatomic structure can be related determines the reliability with which the data can be interpreted. No uniformly accepted procedure has yet been developed. Most commonly, skull x-rays or MRI scans, are obtained for overlap with functional images in each individual.

In SPECT, quantitative analyses are limited at this time to dynamic Xe-133 rCBF imaging. Normal values shown in Table 2 have been obtained in individuals ranging in age from 20 to 70 years and of both sexes (Devous et al. 1986b). The relationship between these rCBF values and the indicated anatomic structures must be viewed in the context of the limited

TABLE 2. Normal Values of Regional Cerebral Blood Flow (rCBF) Measured by Various Techniques

Technique	Flow (ml/min/100 g)*				Reference
	Frontal	Parietal	Temporal	Occipital	
Xe-133 tomography	69±12	78±13	68±12	74±13	Devous et al. 1986a
Xe-133 16 probes	84±15	73±14	80±14	78±11	Meyer et al. 1978
Xe CT 35%	76±12	71±11	76±13	78±12	Amano et al. 1982
13-NH₃ positron	74±10	76±10	—	—	Yamamoto et al. 1977
H₂O-15 positron	55±10	—	61±10	63±17	Baron et al. 1981

* mean ± standard deviation

resolution of this device (17 mm) and with an understanding that the data are from one transverse cross-sectional slice located 6 cm above and parallel to the cantho-meatal line (CML). Even so, these data allow the determination of abnormalities in patient groups by between-group comparisons as long as patient positioning and imaging procedures are determined reliably.

Quantitative rCBF data can be derived by one of two methods (Stokely et al. 1982). The first method is an automated scheme in which regions of interest (ROI) corresponding to general anatomic zones are placed interactively over rCBF images. The ROI is taken from an anatomic atlas (An Atlas of the Human Brain for Computerized Tomography, Matsui and Hirano 1978) to correspond to sections parallel to the cantho-meatal line (CML), and at either 2 or 6 cm above it, as appropriate. Because of limited resolution and inconsistencies in brain position relative to external landmarks, these anatomic zones only represent approximate correlations with real structures. For the slice 2 cm above the CML, ROI include inferior temporal and cerebellar tissues bilaterally. At 6 cm above the CML, ROI include frontal, parietal, superior temporal, occipital, central,

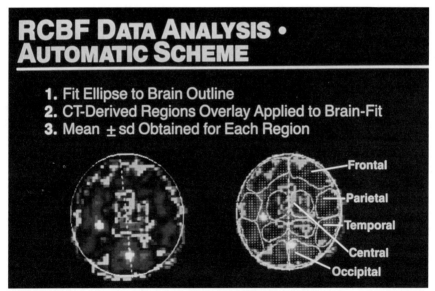

FIGURE 15. An automatic computer assisted data analysis routine employed to analyze Xe-133 DSPECT rCBF images. This scheme derives quantitative values from 10 subregions and 2 hemispheres for the slice 6 cm above the CML, and 4 subregions for the slice 2 cm above the CML. The only operator intervention required is to fit the outline of the brain to an ellipsoidal shape.

and hemispheric zones bilaterally. The rCBF image is fit with an ellipse by interactive identification of the major and minor axes (Figure 15). The ellipse data are then used to adjust the size and position of the atlas-based ROI which are stored in an overlay plane. Mean rCBF values and standard deviations are reported for each ROI. This method involves minimal observer bias and thus provides an objective analysis scheme.

In some cases ROI are required that do not conform to predescribed anatomic zones. For this reason a second analysis scheme was developed that involves manual drawing of selected ROI (Figure 16). This scheme may be employed in one of three modes. In the first, data may be derived for hand-drawn regions directly from rCBF images. In the second, the user may request that a selected ROI be reproduced in mirror-image symmetry in the hemisphere contralateral to the original placement. This application is useful for left–right asymmetry measurements. In the third mode, an ROI may be reproduced in a second image. This procedure may be used to compare values in a patient before and after some intervention, or to compare values in a patient to data from a composite image representing a group of patients or a normal population. The latter two schemes require

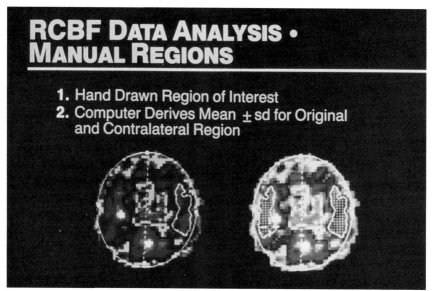

FIGURE 16. Alternative to the automatic scheme illustrated in Figure 15, users may draw regions of interest manually to correspond to specific anatomic zones, areas of reduced perfusion, or other criteria. Such regions may be matched symmetrically in the contralateral hemisphere or may be reproduced in other rCBF images, e.g. a composite image of normal rCBF.

fitting an ellipse to the involved images as in the automated analysis scheme.

Since rCBF is coupled to neuronal metabolism, one must consider mental activity at the time of the measurement. Numerous investigators have debated this problem largely in the context of two-dimensional measurements of rCBF with probe systems and Xe-133. No standard exists for a so-called "control" or "resting" state. In our laboratory subjects are studied supine with eyes and ears open. The room is dimly lit and background noise originates primarily from fans cooling the tomograph. Subjects are allowed approximately two minutes for adaptation, and little communication occurs between the operator and subject after the study begins.

We have chosen to study patients with eyes and ears open in order to provide a baseline of auditory and visual "noise." We noted in early studies that subjects studied in this environment demonstrated very symmetric and reproducible rCBF patterns. rCBF symmetry and reproducibility associated with our study conditions were later confirmed in a larger group of normal volunteers (Devous et al. 1986b). It may be that subjects studied under conditions of auditory and visual sensory deprivation focus their attention in a way that leads to specific regional neuronal activation. Certainly, the cognitive state most commonly experienced in everyday life is that with continuous baseline levels of auditory and visual input. In contrast, subjects studied in total darkness with ears plugged demonstrated greater intersubject variability. Phelps et al. (1981) have noted similar consequences of sensory deprivation in PET measurements of glucose metabolism.

At present, no functional brain-imaging test, either in SPECT or PET, based upon quantitative data from an individual brain region can be used to distinguish an individual patient from normal unless a severe structural abnormality is also present (as in the case of stroke or tumor). However, functional imaging techniques have been used to follow changes in brain function with time and in response to therapy, and to enable investigation of the differences in cerebral function among patient groups and normal volunteers. Improved resolution and improved quantitation schemes might permit SPECT to be used as a diagnostic tool to distinguish individual patients from normal and perhaps for their classification into discrete diagnostic categories. Data presented later in this chapter indicate that such discrimination may be possible in schizophrenic patients.

Visual interpretation of images has long been the predominant means of analysis in radiology and in nuclear medicine. This continues to be a useful procedure in SPECT. Normal rCBF images are very symmetric. Image asymmetry can often be detected by the eye much more readily than by available quantitative schemes. Indeed, quantitative schemes usually assume a known area of interest based on anatomical structures. Functional abnormalities may show up in regions which overlap more than one preselected anatomic region of interest, or may be smaller than the regions chosen for objective analyses. The subjectivity of visual image interpretation can be minimized by using multiple observers under blinded conditions who have considerable training in image analyses. Such analyses successfully distinguish patients with frontal lobe abnormalities from normal controls and other patient groups, and they also distinguish patients who undergo rCBF changes following cognitive activation or pharmacologic stimulation from those not responding.

Practical Considerations

It is the purpose of this section to compare costs, relative values of commercially available units, and availability of systems with respect to the utility of SPECT in psychiatric studies. SPECT is the only hope in the foreseeable future for tomographic imaging of brain function in a widespread, clinically applicable environment. PET is too expensive and too limited to reach widespread use in the next 10 years. (This assertion is hotly debated; see for example Ter-Pogossian 1985; Powers and Raichle 1985; Wagner 1985.) In that light, it is encouraging to note that commercial manufacturers have developed several SPECT systems capable of reasonable-to-high resolution and moderate-to-high sensitivity.

The costs of these systems are moderate. Rotating gamma camera-based SPECT systems range in cost from $130,000–230,000. Dedicated SPECT systems, such as PRISM, will cost on the order of $500,000. These costs are still much lower than those associated with PET, MRI, or CT. For rCBF imaging the data available through SPECT will be comparable or even better than that available through PET. Thus, SPECT systems for rCBF measurements should be available, practical, and cost effective in the immediate future.

There is no theoretical reason to limit SPECT systems to university research facilities. In fact, one of the major values of SPECT is that it is as easily performed in a community hospital as in a university setting. One might thus anticipate that research in psychiatry will proceed at a much faster pace with the availability of SPECT than it has through PET because many more investigators and clinicians will have access to this technology. As has always been true in technologically driven modalities, increasing application will inspire manufacturers of both instruments and radiopharmaceuticals to increasing improvements that will make further applications possible. Thus, it becomes the obligation of the basic and clinical research communities to determine the ultimate value of SPECT in psychiatry.

APPLICATIONS IN PSYCHIATRY

Research Applications

The applications of SPECT imaging to psychiatry originate in the history of two-dimensional rCBF determinations with Xe-133 and probe systems. Although it is currently possible to image rCBF with radiopharmaceuticals other than Xe-133, these agents have been available such a limited period of time that no research has been published employing them beyond simple demonstrations of their utility. SPECT imaging with labeled receptor agents is even newer. Only four publications exist demonstrating that muscarinic cholinergic receptor imaging can be accomplished with SPECT (Eckelman et al. 1984, 1985; Gibson et al. 1984; Holman et al. 1985). Therefore, the following SPECT information concerns primarily Xe-133 rCBF imaging. PET and two-dimensional probe studies of rCBF, glucose metabolism, or oxygen metabolism are also extensively reviewed since they provide information pertinent to current or potential SPECT applications.

The following sections deal with studies in normals, the effects of cognitive or pharmacologic activation, the relationships between structure and function in SPECT imaging, and SPECT imaging in various pathologies of interest to psychiatry including affective disorders, schizophrenia, and dementia. Readers should keep in mind that the first research use of SPECT in psychiatry occurred less than five years ago, that PET has been applied to psychiatric disorders for approximately a decade, and that two-dimensional rCBF measurements have been used to study psychiatric disorders for nearly 40 years. Thus, SPECT should be viewed as a technology with great research and clinical potential that is as yet in its infancy.

Studies in Normal Subjects

The first measurements of cerebral blood flow in normal subjects were performed by the inert gas washout technique of Kety and Schmidt (1948). These measurements were reported as mean whole-brain blood flows that ranged between 50–60 ml/minute/100 g (Heyman et al. 1951; Scheinberg and Stead 1949). Such values represent a mixture of gray- and white-matter flows from large brain volumes. In the late 1960s the multicompartment model was developed and values for both gray- and white-matter blood flows appeared in the literature (Obrist et al. 1967). Wilkinson et al. (1969) reported an average gray-matter flow of 87 ml/min/100 g and an average white-matter flow of 22 ml/min/100 g. As multiprobe technology developed, rCBF values from various brain regions began to appear in the literature.

rCBF measurements derived from tomographic imaging techniques appeared in the late 1970s. By the early 1980s, rCBF in normal subjects had been reported by investigators using the inert-gas washout technique with dynamic tomography and Xe-133 (Bonte and Stokely 1981; Devous et al. 1985b), positron tomography with a variety of radiotracers (Yamamoto et al. 1977; Baron et al. 1981; Frackowiak et al. 1980; Lenzi et al. 1981; Madsen et al. 1981), and x-ray CT with stable xenon gas (Amano et al. 1982). rCBF values obtained using these techniques are compared in Table 2. Gray-matter flows generally range between 70–90 ml/min/100 g for each technique without substantial differences among regions (Table 2). The only major departure occurs when H_2O-15 is employed with PET to measure rCBF. Since the water partition coefficient is related to flow in a nonlinear fashion, this particular tracer yields low rCBF gray-matter values.

Normal rCBF images for the Xe-133 technique, and for I-123-IMP, and Tc-99m-HMPAO using high-resolution SPECT are compared in Figure 13. Patients are placed in the tomograph so that three cross-sectional images are obtained at 2, 6, and 10 cm above and parallel to the cantho-meatal line for the rCBF images obtained from dynamic SPECT with Xe-133. The orientation of these images is such that anterior is up and subject's left is to the reader's left. These images can be displayed either in a linear gray scale or in a quantitative color scale in which the light intensity or color corresponds to blood flow in ml/min/100 g of tissue. The images in Figure 13 are displayed in a gray scale in order to compare them to the high-resolution SPECT images obtained with I-123 IMP. Low-resolution images are often more favorably displayed in color because greater contrast is obtained. Color displays can also be misleading and must therefore be used with caution.

Transverse cross sections (slices) obtained 2 cm above the CML provide rCBF values from inferior temporal and cerebellar flows and can demonstrate inferior frontal rCBF regions. Unfortunately, the inferior frontal regions are often contaminated by Xe-133 scatter from the nasal passages. Slices are 2 cm thick and thus may include inferior portions of basal ganglia and superior portions of mid-brain (Figure 17a). Frontal, parietal, superior temporal, occipital, and central gray-matter regions are represented in the slice 6 cm above the CML. A nearly continuous ring of cortical gray-matter flow is typically observed just inside the low-flow perimeter of scalp and skull (Figure 17b). In some individuals this ring may be broken, most commonly in the posterotemporal regions and/or in the frontal regions, yielding a "Maltese cross" appearance. In addition, high flows corresponding to central gray matter are observed in most normal individuals.

The slice 10 cm above the CML includes the superior cortical surface

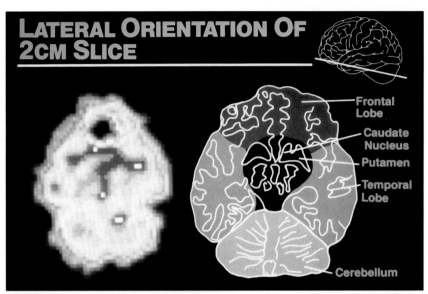

FIGURE 17a.   rCBF image and schematic anatomic drawing 2 cm above and parallel to the CML. The orientation of this slice is left to left, and anterior up. The color scale shows lowest flows in blue through highest flows in red and white. Note the artifact (black hole) in the anterior portion of the image caused by scatter of Xe-133 from the nasal sinuses.

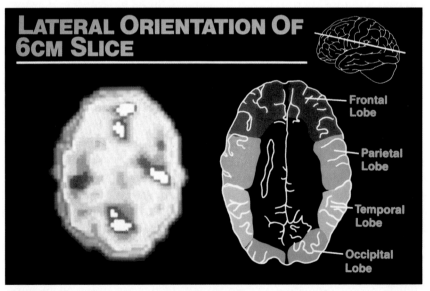

FIGURE 17b.   rCBF image and schematic anatomic drawing of the transverse cross-section 6 cm above the CML. Note the nearly continuous cortical ring of high gray matter flows with lower flows centrally.

of the frontal and parietal lobes. Because of its thickness and intermixing of skull and scalp flows, it is seldom of diagnostic significance. Since the slice separations in this tomographic device are fixed, that part of the brain interposed between slices can only be observed by moving the subject and repeating the study. Recent modifications have been made in some versions of this scanner which permit the study of five separate slices.

In our laboratory, highest flows are normally observed in the parietal lobes. The visual cortex when taken as a separate region of interest within the occipital lobe has the highest flow of any normal structure (81 ± 16 ml/min/100 g) because our subjects are studied with their eyes open. The environment in which measurements are made will alter "normal" rCBF values.

Under these conditions, hemispheric asymmetry in rCBF is minimal. In general, flow to the right hemisphere is greater than to the left (see Table 3). Right flow was significantly greater than left flow in superior temporal, occipital, central, and hemispheric regions when measured in 97 normal volunteers in our laboratory conditions. Quantitatively, this asymmetry was very small, ranging only from 0.7 to 3.4 ml/min/100 g among regions. However, the reverse was true in the frontal and inferior temporal lobes. No statistically significant asymmetry was demonstrated in the parietal lobes or in the cerebellum.

TABLE 3. Hemispheric Asymmetry in Regional Cerebral Blood Flow

Area	Flow (ml/min/100 g)*			p†
	Left	**Right**	**R–L**	
Frontal	72 ± 11	71 ± 10	-1.4 ± 3.7	.022‡
Parietal	79 ± 11	79 ± 12	0.7 ± 4.6	.200
Superior temporal	70 ± 11	71 ± 10	1.2 ± 3.7	.046**
Inferior temporal	75 ± 10	73 ± 10	-1.8 ± 5.2	.038‡
Occipital	73 ± 10	76 ± 12	3.1 ± 5.4	.002**
Central	73 ± 12	77 ± 14	3.4 ± 4.9	.001**
Hemisphere	72 ± 10	73 ± 11	1.3 ± 1.9	.001**
Cerebellum	75 ± 11	75 ± 9	-0.4 ± 3.5	.267

*mean ± standard deviation
†p value for paired t test of L/R asymmetry by region in 31 normal volunteers
‡statistically significant difference, left>right
**statistically significant difference, right>left

White-matter flows measured by most techniques range between 20–30 ml/min/100 g. However, values measured with Xe-133 tomography are significantly higher (59 ml/min/100 g). In part, this results from the algorithm's choice of 1.0 for both gray- and white-matter partition coefficients (a choice not under operator control). In normal subjects the gray-matter partition coefficient is 0.8 and for white matter it is 1.5. A computer simulation study (Smith et al. 1984) demonstrated that errors in the partition coefficient can lead to errors in white-matter flow ranging from 7–67%. In particular, a 40% overestimation of white-matter flow results from assuming a gray-matter coefficient of 1.0 relative to a correct choice of 0.8. This overestimate is further aggravated by scatter of Xe-133 gamma rays from other regions. Such scatter contributes more significantly to observed counts in low-flow areas such as white matter than in high-flow areas such as gray matter.

The reproducibility of rCBF values measured by dynamic SPECT of Xe-133 washout was studied by performing repeat measurements in normal volunteers. Second studies were performed from one hour to 10 days after the first study. When background corrections were made for residual Xe-133 activity in the head and lungs, no statistically significant differences in flow values were found between the first and second study. Thus, this technique provides reproducible results in normal subjects when studied under the conditions described above.

The effects of age and sex on SPECT-determined rCBF values are illustrated in Figure 18. We studied 97 normal volunteers (56 males and 41 females) ranging in age from 20–59 years. There was a small but statistically significant decline in rCBF with age for both sexes, and females had higher flows than males at all ages.

Our results do not differ significantly from published rCBF values obtained by two-dimensional measurements of Xe-133 cerebral transit with probe systems except in one regard. It has often been reported by investigators using probe systems that frontal lobes have the highest flows (so-called hyperfrontality; Lassen et al. 1978). Hyperfrontality is not generally observed in tomographic studies of rCBF, whether performed by SPECT, PET, or x-ray CT (Table 2). In probe studies, more cortical gray-matter mass is integrated in the collimator view of the frontal lobes than is observed in laterally oriented lobes, and this frontal region is also contaminated by Xe-133 scatter in the sinus cavities. A tomographic imaging approach does not suffer from the deep gray-matter integration problem and minimizes scatter contamination. Therefore, the discrepancy between probe studies demonstrating hyperfrontality and tomographic studies may be the result of a technical artifact associated with probe studies.

Very preliminary SPECT images depicting the distribution of muscarinic cholinergic receptors in the brain using I-123 QNB have been pub-

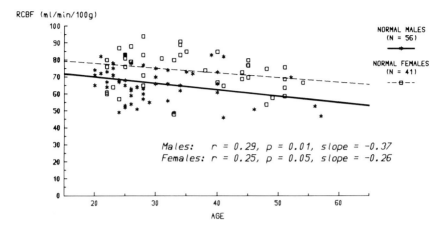

FIGURE 18. Regional cerebral blood flow in normal volunteers plotted as a function of age (range 20 to 59 years) and sex. Note that there is a slight decline in rCBF with age for both sexes, and that rCBF is higher in females than males at all ages. Reproduced with permission from Devous et al; J Cereb Blood Flow Metab 6:95-104, 1986.

lished by Eckelman et al. (1984) and Holman et al. (1985). They observed uniform cerebral uptake of I-123 QNB in one normal subject. Uptake was slow and continued to increase throughout the 15 hours during which the subject was imaged (approximately 3 times as much brain activity at 15 hours as at 2 hours). Very little activity was observed in cerebellum, where few muscarinic cholinergic receptors are located. In fact, the ratio of cerebellum/caudate activity was .07, 15 hours after injection, which compares favorably with the cerebellum/caudate ratio of concentration of muscarinic acetylcholine receptor sites (cerebellum/caudate = .02; Wastek and Yamamura 1978). An example is shown in Figure 14. While these preliminary studies support the concept of SPECT receptor imaging, much work is required before their value can be established.

Effects of Sensory Stimulation. Autoradiographic techniques have been used to study brain regions associated with somatosensory, visual, and auditory stimulation in great detail. Noninvasive techniques to measure the distribution of radiotracers in humans have similarly been employed. Initially, two-dimensional probe systems were used to measure rCBF in response to sensory stimulation. Such studies have now been extended by using PET to obtain three-dimensional representations of rCBF or regional glucose metabolism.

Several studies of visual stimulation have been conducted. Greenberg et al. (1981) examined the effects of visual hemi-field stimulation. Subjects were instructed to fix on a small light located in the center of a plexiglass hemisphere that was dimmed at random. The location of the hemisphere could then be used to limit the subject's vision to the hemifield desired. The stimulus consisted of a well-illuminated, slowly moving, high-contrast black and white pattern of small lines at various orientations, and abstract color images presented to one visual hemi-field. The visual stimulus caused an increase in glucose utilization that was 8% greater in the contralateral than in the ipsilateral visual cortex. Normal asymmetry without stimulation was only 0.5%. In another study Phelps et al. (1981) examined both the effects of stimulation and deprivation. Stimulation was carried out at several levels of intensity, the first consisting of a bright white light, the second a 2-Hz alternating black and white checkerboard pattern, the third a complex stimulation consisting of outdoor scenes. White-light stimulation produced a 12% increase in glucose utilization in the primary visual cortex and a 6% increase in the association cortex. The alternating checkerboard pattern produced a 29% increase in primary cortex and 27% increase in associative. The complex outdoor scene produced a 45% increase in primary and 59% increase in association cortices. Kushner et al. (1982) examined the effects of restricting the spatial extent of the visual stimulus to the central 20° (macular region) of the left hemi-field and the peripheral 60° of the right hemifield. This resulted in approximately 20% higher metabolism in the right posterior striate cortex (macular vision) and approximately 10% higher metabolism in the left anterior striate cortex (peripheral vision).

In a somewhat simpler study using SPECT, Devous et al. (1985b) measured rCBF with the Xe-133 inhalation in 13 subjects studied either in total darkness with eyes closed and masked, or in a brightly lit scene with tomograph operators moving about randomly. With visual stimulation, rCBF increased in the visual cortex as expected (see Figure 19). Whole-brain blood flow increased slightly from 71 to 75 ml/min/100 g (not significant), and central gray-matter flow increased, reaching statistical significance only on the left side. This is an interesting result since Reivich et al. (1981) reported decreased metabolic activity in the thalamus in patients with visual field defects due to vascular disease. The response of central gray matter may be related to the fact that the pulvinar has numerous connections with striate and extrastriate visual cortical areas.

These studies have shown 50% of the input from each eye goes to each visual cortex, that the magnitude of blood flow or glucose utilization of the visual cortex is a function of both stimulus complexity and rate, and that, as expected from animal studies, the metabolic topography of the human visual cortex is related to the site and size of retinal stimulation. Similarly, studies in patients (Phelps et al. 1981; Reivich et al. 1981) have

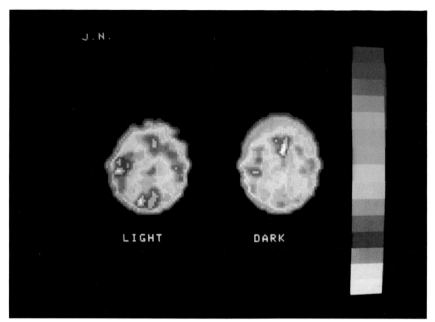

FIGURE 19. rCBF images in an individual studied in a brightly lighted environment with eyes open and ears unplugged (left) or in a darkened environment with eyes covered (right). The most significant difference between these images is the high perfusion to the visual cortex (bottom of image) in the light condition relative to the dark condition.

demonstrated that lesions of the visual system produce functional abnormalities that correlate with the patient's clinical symptoms even though there may be no evidence of anatomical lesions on x-ray CT.

Emission tomographic studies of auditory stimulation have also largely confirmed our knowledge about the cortical auditory system derived from studies of patients with focal brain damage. Such studies indicate that the primary auditory cortex in humans is located on the transverse temporal plane within the Sylvian fissure, which when stimulated produces auditory sensation referred most commonly to the contralateral ear. The secondary auditory cortex extends laterally and posteriorly along the supratemporal plane comprising part of Wernicke's area in the left hemisphere.

PET measurements of glucose metabolism were used to evaluate subjects listening to a tape-recorded factual story presented through earphones to only one ear. Attentiveness to the task was assessed by recall testing at the end of the study and subjects were told they would be paid in proportion to how well they tested. Such auditory stimulation resulted in a 7% higher metabolic rate in the temporal cortex contralateral to the stimulated ear, which is consistent with literature suggesting the predominance of crossed pathways in the human auditory system. A replication of this study with a higher-resolution PET tomograph demonstrated activation of several cortical regions with complex verbal stimuli. The primary auditory cortex in the transverse temporal gyrus contralateral to the ear stimulated was significantly activated while all other regions that underwent significant activation were located in the left hemisphere regardless of the ear stimulated, including the left posterior superior temporal cortex (Wernicke's area), the left inferior frontal cortex (Broca's area), the left inferior parietal region, and the left superior motor cortex. The only region in the right hemisphere activated independent of the ear stimulated was located in the posterior inferior parietal cortex.

Mazziotta et al. (1982, 1984) have reported two studies of auditory stimulation with PET glucose measurements that indicate a correlation between the distribution of glucose utilization and the content of the stimulus, and in some cases the strategy used by the subject to solve the task. When the auditory stimulus was the verbal delivery of a factual story (4 subjects), significant activation was seen in the left frontal cortex, and bilaterally in the posterior and transverse temporal cortices (6–25% increases in glucose utilization), independent of which ear was stimulated. The tonal memory test and timbre test were also administered to a series of subjects in this study. Subjects using a nonanalytic strategy for remembering the sequence of tones had higher metabolic rates in the right frontal and parietotemporal regions. Subjects who used an analytic approach developed higher metabolic rates in the left posterior superior temporal cortex. Thus, the metabolic changes observed in this study were a function of the analysis strategy employed rather than the side of stimulation. In general, verbal stimuli caused asymmetric increases in glucose utilization in the left hemisphere in right-handed individuals, while nonverbal stimuli (e.g., musical chords) activated primarily right hemispheric areas particularly in the inferior frontal, parietal, and superior temporal regions. It is important to keep in mind that the stimuli used in these studies were very complex and involved multiple cognitive functions. Therefore, interpretation of these results must be made with caution.

Somatosensory stimulation has also been investigated. Ingvar et al. (1976) reported that painful stimulation of the right forearm caused increases in frontal blood flow. Buchsbaum et al. (1983) have employed this strategy and PET in controls, schizophrenics, and patients with affective disorders to study the distribution of glucose metabolism. Under these circumstances, both normals and patients showed a significant increase in glucose use in anterior regions, although the anterior–posterior gradient was smaller in patients.

Visual, auditory, and somatosensory evoked potentials have long been used with electroencephalographic measurements to investigate brain physiology and pathophysiology. Recent instrumentation developments now permit topographic mapping of EEG, and therefore it may be possible to cross-correlate electrical neuronal activity with metabolic neuronal activity by simultaneous acquisition of topographic EEG data and emission tomographic measurements of glucose metabolism or rCBF. A preliminary report of just such a comparison has been prepared by Buchsbaum et al. (1982a).

Responses to Cognitive Activation.   As is the case with sensory stimulation, cognitive activation of the brain may produce either discrete or generalized responses in neuronal metabolism depending upon the nature of the task. These changes are reflected either in measurements of glucose metabolism or rCBF since both are tightly coupled under normal physiologic conditions and even under most pathophysiologic circumstances. For example, numerous investigators have discovered that the left posterior inferior frontal region (Broca's area) undergoes increased rCBF during speech in right-handed volunteers while the posterior regions of the right hemisphere show similar increases during visual/spatial problem solving (Halsey et al. 1977; Risberg and Ingvar 1973; Ishihara et al. 1977; Risberg et al. 1975b, 1977; Meyer et al. 1977). In addition, Meyer (1978) has shown that anterior frontal regions, particularly those of the left hemisphere, undergo rCBF increases during concentration, attention, and apprehension. This is particularly marked when solving a new task, while habituation to such tasks blunts the response (Risberg et al. 1977).

This points out the extreme importance of study design, subject involvement, and extraneous stimuli. For example, Risberg et al. (1975b) found that a verbal analogy test gave larger flow increases over Wernicke's region while nonverbal perceptual tests (Street test) resulted in increases to right frontal and parietal regions when studies were conducted in 12 volunteers who were highly motivated because their monetary compensation was proportional to their test scores. In another group of 12 subjects who were offered no monetary reward, much smaller and statistically insignificant asymmetries resulted for the same activation procedures. Similarly, Maximilian (1982) measured the responses to a simple task of listening to a word list and discriminating words with a certain meaning. No flow changes occurred during the task presumably because of its simplicity and small demand on neuronal metabolism.

Meyer at al. (1980) examined rCBF changes in normal volunteers between a resting state with eyes closed and quiet darkness, and an activation state in which subjects performed multiple psychophysiologic tasks including motor and sensory speech, calculation, and audiovisual stimulation. During activation left-hemispheric flow values increased by 11% and that of the brain stem–cerebellar regions increased by 20%. Bilateral frontal, pre-central, Sylvian-opercular, posterior temporal, and inferior temporal activations were also observed. This activation process elicited similar responses in both young and older volunteers even though numerous investigators have demonstrated declines in rCBF with advancing age. Other two-dimensional measurements of rCBF have also confirmed a general activation of metabolism and blood flow during cognitive activity relative to resting baseline conditions (Ingvar and Risberg 1967; Prohovnik et al. 1980; Risberg and Ingvar 1973).

PET measurements of regional glucose metabolism have also been used to assess responses to cognitive activation. For example, Gur and Reivich (1980) compared glucose metabolism rates in individuals undergoing either a verbal task adapted from the Miller's analogies test or a spatial task adapted from Street's Gestalt completion test. The verbal task led to increases in rCBF as expected in the left hemisphere while the spatial task produced right-hemispheric increases in 17 of the 36 subjects, and reversed asymmetry in 17 subjects, suggesting that the spatial task could be solved by either hemisphere while the verbal task was more consistently localized. Subsequently, this same group (Gur et al. 1982) replaced the Street test with a spatial, line-orientation task developed by Benton. Under these circumstances, the anticipated verbal-to-left hemisphere and spatial-to-right hemisphere lateralizations were obtained. In addition, it was found that these responses were influenced by handedness and gender.

Later, Reivich et al. (1985) examined regional glucose metabolic responses under very similar conditions focusing on regions including superior temporal (ST), inferior parietal (IP), and frontal eye fields (FEF). They found that subjects undergoing the verbal task did not differ in overall metabolic rate from those undergoing the spatial task, and in both groups there was a significantly higher right-hemispheric metabolic rate, perhaps related to the concept of right-hemispheric predomination in attentional processes (Heilman and Van Den Abell 1979; Mesulam 1981). The two groups did differ in lateralization of metabolic activation in the primary target areas (ST and IP) with greater right-hemispheric activation for the spatial task and greater left-hemispheric activation for the verbal task. Interestingly, the two groups also differed in FEF laterality, with the effect in the same direction (right-hemispheric dominance). Statistically significant differences were not observed in control regions including inferior temporal, auditory and visual association cortices, frontal poles, and inferior frontal cortex.

The FEF results are interesting in that they provide a demonstration that lateralized metabolic activity produced by different types of cognitive tasks (e.g., verbal and spatial) lead to lateralized metabolic activity in a motor region. This is consistent with Trevarthen's hypothesis (1972) that cognitive activation will mimic the effects of lateralized sensory stimulation in the functionally asymmetric brain and produce a contralateral orienting response.

This group has also analyzed data from young, right-handed, male volunteers studied under either stimulated conditions (visual stimulation with a light-dimming sequence or auditory stimulation with monitoring for a particular word) or in an unstimulated condition with both visual and auditory input oblated (Greenberg et al. 1981). In these studies attention was focused on changes in the inferior parietal lobe. The superior temporal lobe was used as an adjacent control region not implicated in a lateralization of attentional processes. The cerebellum was used as a remote control region involved in sensory and motor aspects of these tasks but not in their attentional functions. Subjects were rewarded monetarily for their performance in order to assure attentional involvement. Metabolic rates in stimulated subjects were higher in right IP regardless of the type of stimulation whereas nonstimulated subjects showed no IP asymmetries. In addition, no asymmetries were noted in stimulated subjects in temporal or cerebellar control regions. This study further implicates the right inferior parietal lobe in attending to external sensory stimulation.

SPECT measurements of rCBF have been used in our laboratory to examine in normal volunteers responses to a variety of cognitive states. Cognitive tasks examined in comparison to our control state include responses to Miller's analogies, Benton line-orientation task, the Wisconsin Card Sort, simple arithmetic problem solving, and word finding in prosodic/aprosodic readings. Tasks in the first three categories were presented visually in a slide format. Subjects responded by simultaneously pressing keys on a response input board with the same finger of both hands. Arithmetic problems were presented orally by one of the investigators standing at the foot of the patient bed. Word recognition during prosodic/aprosodic readings was accomplished by bilateral auditory input through earphones. Preliminary analyses of these data indicate right parietal activation during the line-orientation task, bilateral (but left-dominant) activation during the analogy task, and mild left activation during the arithmetic task. Results of the Wisconsin Card Sort studies are described in detail below (see Schizophrenia). Little response was observed in the prosody/aprosody study, perhaps due to the low level of difficulty associated with the task.

Pharmacologic Activation.   Another strategy for examining cortical function is to stimulate the brain pharmacologically. Cognitive activation can be viewed as an internal stimulation or probing procedure, and pharmacologic activation as an external or extrinsic activating procedure.

Our group and others have used acetazolamide (Diamox) as a pharmacologic stimulator of rCBF (Vorstrup et al. 1984; Hauge et al. 1983; Laux
and Raichle 1978; Devous et al. 1986a), while others have used hyper-
ventilation and 5% CO_2 inhalation as a means to alter rCBF (Grubb et al.
1974; Meyer 1978; Melamed et al. 1975). All three procedures lead to
changes in local cerebral CO_2 content which stimulates rCBF responses
proportional to CO_2 content through autoregulatory mechanisms. Diamox
stimulation, achieved by giving 1.0 g intravenously 10–20 minutes before
imaging, produces a $33 \pm 3\%$ symmetric and uniform rCBF increase. As
described below, such a procedure can be used in patients to determine if
low-flow areas observed at rest retain vasodilatory capacity, or to determine if areas with normal resting flow have normal perfusion reserve
(Devous et al. 1986a).

We have also examined regional neuronal responses to manipulations
of the cholinergic receptor system by administering arecoline, a central
cholinergic agonist. These experiments are described in greater detail in
the section on affective disorders (below). One can envision multiple
protocols designed to assess regional brain responses to pharmacologic
manipulation of either receptor pathways or metabolic mechanisms.

Affective Disorders

Noninvasive measurements of brain physiology including SPECT, PET,
topographic EEG mapping, NMR, and CT have in general been more
widely applied in the study of schizophrenia than in affective disorders.
However, there are currently several hypotheses concerning the origin of
affective pathology which imply different regional brain dysfunction. In
particular, patients with endogenous (Spitzer et al. 1978) or melancholic
(APA 1980) features have impairment of higher cortical functions as
evinced by electrophysiologic (Flor-Henry and Koles 1980; Flor-Henry
1979), neurophysiologic (Hommes and Panhuysen 1971; Gruzelier and
Venables 1974; Myslobodsky and Horesch 1978), and neuropsychologic
(Wexler 1980; Bruder et al. 1981) studies without clear delineation of
the specific neurochemical, cognitive, or neurophysiologic impairments
involved. There is also strong evidence that mood disorders have underlying biochemical mechanisms. Studies of neuroendocrine responses (Carroll et al. 1981), changes in monoamine metabolism (Koslow et al.
1983), alterations in diurnal rhythms for various body functions (Wehr
and Wirz-Justice 1982), and the often dramatic response of patients to
psychoactive medications (Charney et al. 1981) support the concept of a
biochemical basis to the expression of mood. Unfortunately, most investigations designed to determine which brain structures might be involved
in regulating affect have been unsuccessful. This could be a consequence

of the biological heterogeneity of these disorders or to the limited spatial resolution of the techniques used for investigation. Fortunately, recent studies with PET and SPECT are beginning to shed some light on this important area.

Two hypotheses of depression with anatomic correlates are 1) involvement of the nondominant cortex and 2) the catecholamine function of the limbic reward systems. Right-hemispheric dysfunction has been studied by taking advantage of naturally occurring lesions, administering carefully selected neuropsychologic tasks, and examining left–right differences in EEG and evoked potentials (Flor-Henry 1979; Ross and Rush 1981). Risberg (1980) examined 70 patients with affective disorders using Xe-133 and two-dimensional probes; he found normal flow distributions in depressed patients and little correlation between rCBF and the mental state of the patient as rated by a psychiatrist. In a serial study of 13 patients undergoing electroconvulsive therapy (ECT), however, the 7 patients with the "best" therapeutic results showed stable and normal pre-ECT rCBF levels, while those with less improvement showed lower pretreatment rCBF levels. Matthew et al. (1980), using similar methods, studied 13 patients with major depressive disorder (MDD). He found significantly lower flow in the left hemisphere compared to age-matched controls, and a tendency toward decreased right-hemisphere flow. Importantly, rCBF values in both hemispheres correlated with the level of depression as assessed by the Hamilton Rating Scale for Depression (HRS-D). This study did not involve severe melancholic depressions since the mean HRS-D was only 25.

In contrast, Uytdenhoef et al. (1983) found increased left-frontal and decreased right-posterior flow in patients with MDD. This group later reported (Charles et al. 1983) that those patients with normal rCBF patterns were dexamethazone nonsuppressors, while those with high left-frontal flows and low right-posterior flows were suppressors. In addition, they found that they could diagnose 8 of the 16 major depressive patients by the dexamethazone suppression test (DST) alone, and 15 of the 16 by a combination of the DST and rCBF data.

Gur et al. (1984) measured rCBF at rest and during the performance of a verbal and a spatial task in 14 medicated depressives and 25 matched controls. In resting studies, patients and controls did not differ in overall flows or in anterior–posterior gradients. However, differences between patients and controls did occur during cognitive activity and these differences depended upon sex. Depressed female patients had higher-than-normal flows under all conditions, while depressed male patients had lower-than-normal flows at rest which increased to normal during cognitive activation. This latter group had increased anterior flows during the verbal task but not during the spatial task. The distinction between observations in this study and that of Matthew et al. (1980) may be related to the fact that these patients were all receiving antidepressant medication.

Very few PET studies of depression have been reported. Kuhl et al. (1983) found normal whole-brain glucose metabolism in depressed patients, but found a specific reduction in the glucose metabolic rate of the inferior left frontal cortex. Buchsbaum et al. (1984) discovered that both schizophrenic and depressed patients had a smaller anterior–posterior gradient of glucose metabolism particularly at superior levels when compared to normal controls. This reduced gradient was more a result of increased posterior glucose utilization than decreased frontal utilization. All subjects were studied during the administration of electrical shock to the right forearm. Most recently, Baxter at al. (1985) examined subjects with unipolar depression ($N = 11$), bipolar depression ($N = 5$), mania ($N = 5$), bipolar mixed states ($N = 3$), and normal controls ($N = 9$). They found that bipolar depressed and mixed patients had supratentorial whole-brain glucose metabolic rates that were significantly lower than in other groups and that such rates for patients with bipolar depression increased as the patients proceeded from depression or mixed states to euthymic or manic states (similar results have been obtained with SPECT in our laboratory, see below). In addition, patients with unipolar depression had a significantly lower ratio of metabolic rate of the caudate nucleus to metabolic rate of the hemisphere in comparison to normal controls and bipolar patients.

SPECT studies of affective disorders have originated solely in our laboratory. In an early study (Rush et al. 1982) four patient groups were examined: unipolar endogenous (UPE, $N = 10$), bipolar depressed (BPD, $N = 6$), unipolar nonendogenous (UPNE, $N = 4$), and bipolar mixed or manic (BPMM, $N = 6$). Twenty-one of these subjects were evaluated at two points in time: when acutely ill and 3–12 weeks later when clinically remitted (mean time between measurements: 40 ± 21 days). The Hamilton Rating Scale for Depression (HRS-D) was used to evaluate severity of illness at each point. During the initial measurements patients were free of all psychotropic medications for at least 7 days. Patients were under treatment during the second evaluation and, for those receiving electroconvulsive therapy, the second evaluation was conducted at least 2 days and typically 5 days after the last ECT treatment.

Mean rCBF was lower for the unipolar endogenous group ($t = 2.01$, $p < 0.05$) and higher for the bipolar mixed or manic group ($t = 2.97$, $p < 0.01$) relative to controls. The bipolar depressed group did not differ from controls ($t = 0.09$, $p < 0.50$). Flow in unipolar nonendogenous patients was higher than controls, but the small sample size precluded meaningful statistical evaluation. A significant increase in whole-brain flow was found with treatment and a complete clinical response (HRS-D less than 6) in the unipolar endogenous group (paired t test, t = 2.62, p < 0.04). The type of treatment (ECT versus medication) was unrelated to this finding. RCBF changes in treated depressed bipolars were more heterogeneous, with 3 subjects showing increases and 3 decreases. Interestingly, 2 of the 3 with decreases subsequently relapsed during the following two months. These data suggest that 1) whole-brain cerebral blood flow is low in severely depressed UPE patients compared to controls and compared to themselves when in clinical remission, and 2) whole-brain flow is elevated in BPMM patients compared to controls.

There was also a significant difference in right–left asymmetry ($\chi^2 = 7.26$, p < 0.01) between normals and patients (exclusive of the unipolar nonendogenous patients). Most controls (14/16) had slightly greater flow to the right hemisphere when at rest with eyes open while 13/22 UPE, BPMM, and BPD patients had slightly greater flow to the left hemisphere when acutely ill.

More recently, these studies were extended to include regional analyses in 29 normal volunteers, 22 unipolar endogenous patients, 9 unipolar nonendogenous patients, and 13 bipolar depressives (Devous et al. 1984). rCBF was quantitated in 14 brain regions by an automated fitting routine and anterior–posterior gradients were assessed by subtracting parietal lobe or temporal lobe flows from frontal lobe flows. Both gradients and regional flows were compared among groups and left–right asymmetries were evaluated for occipital, temporal, parietal, frontal, and hemispheric regions. The demographic data, Hamilton Rating scores, and dexamethazone suppression results are shown in Table 4. Comparisons of rCBF in patients relative to controls are shown in Table 5,

TABLE 4. Demographic Data and Test Results in Normal Volunteers and in Depressed Patients with Regional Cerebral Blood Flow Measurements

	Controls	UPE	UPNE	BPD
Age	33 ± 11	41 ± 14	39 ± 10	40 ± 15
Sex (F/M)	20/11	13/8	6/3	6/6
HRS-D	3 ± 1	24 ± 12	18 ± 4	27 ± 8
DST (% NS)	4%	68%	11%	70%
N	29	22	9	13

HRS-D: Hamilton Rating Scale for Depression
DST (% NS):   % Nonsuppressors on the dexamethasone suppression test
UPE: Unipolar endogenous depressed patients
UPNE: Unipolar nonendogenous depressed patients
BPD: Biopolar depressed patients

TABLE 5.   Regional Cerebral Blood Flow in Depressed Patients and Normal Controls

		Controls (N = 29)	UPE (N = 22)	UPNE (N = 9)	BPD (N = 13)
Frontal	L	72 ± 11	67 ± 11	77 ± 14	78 ± 10
	R	71 ± 10	67 ± 12	74 ± 13	77 ± 13
Parietal	L	79 ± 11	74 ± 14	83 ± 16	88 ± 14*
	R	79 ± 12	71 ± 12*	81 ± 19	80 ± 11
Temporal	L	70 ± 11	64 ± 11	70 ± 10	78 ± 12*
	R	71 ± 10	64 ± 10*	71 ± 11	74 ± 10
Occipital	L	73 ± 10	69 ± 14	74 ± 13	80 ± 10
	R	76 ± 12	70 ± 14	79 ± 14	84 ± 12
Hemisphere	L	72 ± 10	67 ± 12	75 ± 13	79 ± 10*
	R	73 ± 11	68 ± 12	77 ± 14	78 ± 10
(R–L) Parietal		0.7 ± 4.7	− 3.2 ± 5.5*	− 1.9 ± 3.4	− 8.8 ± 13.6*
(R–L) Temporal		1.2 ± 3.7	0.3 ± 3.7	0.9 ± 3.1	− 3.5 ± 6.7*

UPE: Unipolar endogenous
UPNE: Unipolar nonendogenous
BPD: Bipolar depressed
* $p < 0.05$ relative to controls

TABLE 6.   Regional Cerebral Blood Flow in Unipolar Endogenous (UPE) and Bipolar Depressed (BPD) Patients

Area		UPE (N = 22)	BPD (N = 13)
Frontal	L	67 ± 11	78 ± 10**
	R	67 ± 12	77 ± 13*
Parietal	L	74 ± 14	88 ± 14*
	R	71 ± 12	80 ± 11
Temporal	L	64 ± 11	78 ± 12**
	R	64 ± 10	74 ± 10*
Occipital	L	69 ± 14	80 ± 13
	R	70 ± 14	84 ± 12**
Hemisphere	L	67 ± 12	79 ± 10**
	R	68 ± 12	78 ± 10*

* $p < 0.05$
** $p < 0.01$

while intercomparisons of endogenous unipolars and bipolar depressives are shown in Table 6. Unipolar patients demonstrated significantly lower flow in the right temporal and parietal lobes relative to normals. Nonendogenous patients were not significantly different from normal controls or from any other patient group, possibly due to their small number ($N = 9$). Bipolar depressives had significantly higher flows than normals in the left parietal and temporal lobes, and in the left hemisphere. In addition, bipolars demonstrated increased flows relative to unipolar endogenous patients in all regions, except in the right parietal lobe where there was a trend toward increased flows ($p = 0.08$). Anterior–posterior gradients were not different from normal controls in this group.

Right–left asymmetry in normals was small (left minus right: -1.2 ml/min/100 g in temporal lobes, -0.7 ml/min/100 g in parietal lobes). Significant reversal (left greater than right) was found in the parietal lobe for UPE (3.0 ml/min/100 g, $p = 0.01$); and bilaterally in temporal (4.4, $p = 0.001$) and parietal (8.6, $p = 0.002$) lobes for BPD. Nonendogenous patients were not different from normals or other patient groups. Analyses of regional flow values for treatment effects or correlations with symptom severity are in progress but have not been completed at this time.

Schizophrenia

Perfusion and metabolism have been studied in schizophrenia more extensively than in any other psychiatric disorder. Soon after the development of the nitrous oxide technique, Kety and Schmidt (1948) found that whole-brain blood flow did not differ significantly between normal controls and schizophrenic patients. However, somewhat prophetically, Kety suggested that regional differences might be found when appropriate techniques were developed to make such measurements., Twenty-six years later, Ingvar and Franzen (1974) reported a reduction of frontal rCBF in schizophrenic patients relative to normal controls using intra-arterial Xe-133.

Summarizing a series of papers, Ingvar (1980) stated that resting rCBF varied with the presence of positive or negative symptoms. Highest flows were found in patients with productive schizophrenias (in the acute state of psychosis, with hallucinations, sensations of apprehension, and catatonic excitement). Lower rCBF was associated with patients with negative symptoms (inactivity, hebephrenia, autism). Increases in cognitive disturbances such as hallucinations correlated positively with postcentral flows and negatively with frontal flows. Ingvar hypothesized that these perfusion abnormalities were secondary to one or several defects in certain subcortical/cortical projection systems, possibly including the catecholeminergic projections to the cortex. Similarly, Buchsbaum et al. (1982b) in reporting decreased frontal glucose metabolism in schizophrenic patients suggested that this defect might reflect a cortical/subcortical dopaminergic dysfunction.

Matthew et al. (1981) showed diffuse rCBF reductions which were statistically significant only in the right frontal area, while Ariel et al. (1983) found a diminished anterior–posterior rCBF gradient. In a later report, Matthew et al. (1982) described an inverse correlation between postcentral rCBF and hallucinatory behavior. This result directly contrasts with that of Ingvar (1980), possibly because of the significant difference in age and duration of disease between Ingvar's patient population and Matthew's. In addition, the very young ages of the patients studied by Matthew et al. (1981, 1982) might explain the lack of clear-cut frontal hypoperfusion found by most other investigators.

A global study of rCBF and oxygen utilization conducted by Hoyer and Oesterreich (1975, 1977) included schizophrenic patients subtyped according to clinical symptoms. They found highest flows in patients with productive schizophrenias and acute psychoses, and reduced rCBF and oxygen utilization in patients with nonproductive schizophrenia. These findings strongly implicate the relationship between cerebral function and symptomatology.

In contrast, Gur et al. (1983) and later Berman et al. (1984) did not find differences between schizophrenics and normal subjects in resting rCBF values. However, Gur et al. (1983) did report significantly altered hemispheric activation patterns in schizophrenic patients during the performance of cognitive tasks. Schizophrenic patients differed from controls by demonstrating symmetric increases in rCBF for a verbal task and relative left-hemispheric increases for a spatial task. Controls had larger left-hemispheric flows for the verbal task, and right-hemispheric increases with a spatial task.

Berman et al. (1984, 1986) found that schizophrenic patients had smaller increases in frontal rCBF than normal controls while performing a version of the Wisconsin Card Sort task (WCST). This group examined chronic schizophrenic patients by measuring rCBF at rest, while performing the WCST, and while performing a number-matching task that controlled for aspects of the WCST not specifically related to frontal lobe function (Weinberger et al. 1986). They found a lack of activation of the frontal lobes during the WCST in unmedicated patients when compared to normal controls. This lack of activation was only clearly distinguished from normal controls when compared to rCBF measurements during the number-sequencing task. They felt that this control task was important because rCBF values obtained at rest were highly variable. They also compared these results to a similar study in neuroleptic-treated schizophrenic patients in order to determine if the presence of active symptoms was a predominant factor in poor frontal lobe activation in the medication-free group. They found that medication-free and neuroleptic-treated patients did not differ significantly in their response to the Wisconsin Card Sort, suggesting that these impairments were stable traits of the illness independent of medication status. These data confirm that frontal hypoperfusion in schizophrenics is also associated with active processing dysfunction.

Berman et al. (1984, 1986) also studied medication-free patients while performing two versions of a continuous-performance task (CPT). The purpose of this second study was to examine whether a task which requires attention, arousal, motivation, vigilance, performance, and mental effort, but which is not specific to frontal lobe activation, would lead to similar results. They found that schizophrenic patients did not differ from normal controls in rCBF variables while performing CPTs. These results suggested that disturbances in nonspecific attention performance cannot account for the WCST findings. They also noted that compared to normal subjects, medication-free patients with chronic schizophrenia performed as poorly on the CPTs as on the WCST, yet they did not show frontal impairment during the former. Thus, engaging in a difficult task on which one does poorly does not of itself produce frontal dysfunction.

There have been only a few PET studies conducted in schizophrenic patients. Buchsbaum et al. (1982b) reported significantly decreased glucose utilization in the frontal cortex and left subcortical gray matter in eight schizophrenic patients compared to six normal controls. Similarly, Widen et al. (1981) found decreased frontal-to-temporal cortical ratios of glucose utilization in nine schizophrenic patients. More recently, Buchsbaum et al. (1984) reported that patients with schizophrenia and patients with affective disorders had a decreased antero–posterior glucose gradient. These later patients were studied during somatosensory stimulation with a painful shock to the forearm, in contrast to his earlier study in which patients were studied at rest. They found that this decreased gradient was more the result of increased posterior glucose utilization than decreased frontal utilization. Farkas et al. (1984) also found decreased frontal glucose utilization relative to posterior regions in schizophrenics.

In an earlier report Farkas et al. (1980) reported a longitudinal study of a single schizophrenic patient. The patient had intense auditory and somatesthetic hallucinations prior to neuroleptic therapy. At this time, there was a 40% depression in frontal cortex glucose utilization, and a higher-than-normal glucose utilization in the right temporal and somatosensory cortices. Neuroleptic treatment for four months produced moderate recovery with an improvement in glucose utilization, although the latter remained 25% below normal in the frontal cortex. The patient relapsed after neuroleptic withdrawal and glucose utilization returned to the untreated level. These data, along with the data in unmedicated patients presented by Buchsbaum et al. (1982b), indicate that the findings of abnormal frontal lobe metabolism in schizophrenics are not likely the result of neuroleptic treatment.

This does not mean that drug effects are unimportant in perfusion or metabolism studies. For example, Risberg (1980) reported on 20 patients displaying "paranoid symptoms (delusions)" who were studied prior to and after treatment with haloperidol. They found a correlation between reduction of symptoms and rCBF values. Six patients with a greater than 50% decrease in symptoms after two weeks showed normal predrug rCBF that decreased by 15% during treatment. Patients with less improvement had normal pretreatment rCBF and showed only small changes during drug administration. They suggest that antipsychotic drugs might considerably influence rCBF. Thus, medication status and history must be carefully taken into account when interpreting metabolic measurements.

Extensive studies of rCBF in schizophrenic patients have been conducted in our laboratory by dynamic SPECT (Paulman et al., in press; Devous et al. 1985a). Currently, this study examines 40 right-handed, male schizophrenic patients, including 21 paranoid, 17 undifferentiated, and 2 disorganized patients. Subjects were screened for past or present neurologic disease and drug/alcohol abuse, and patients with demonstrable focal lesions on CT, localized abnormalities on routine EEG, or past history of insulin shock or electroconvulsive treatment were excluded. Twenty of the patients were studied following a 7–14-day medication washout period, while an additional 20 were receiving neuroleptic medication at the time of evaluation. These subjects have been contrasted to 31 age-matched, right-handed, male volunteers. The volunteers were also carefully screened for past or present psychiatric illness, neurologic disease, drug/alcohol abuse, or history of psychiatric illness in first-degree relatives.

Twenty-nine of these patients have undergone extensive neuropsychological evaluation including the WCST (a test of abstraction and cognitive flexibility requiring intact frontal lobe function for successful completion), the Luria–Nebraska battery (LNNB, an instrument which provides a comprehensive evaluation of brain function), and the finger-tapping test (FT, a general indicator of frontal lobe function, particularly motor and pre-motor areas). These studies were all administered within one week of rCBF measurements.

rCBF data have been analyzed both by visual inspection and by quantitative analysis of anatomically oriented regions of interest. Interrater reliability assessed among three expert readers yielded agreement on the occurrence of low-flow areas 82% of the time, regardless of which pair of interpreters were cross-interpolated.

Schizophrenic subjects had significantly higher incidence of both left- and right-frontal hypoperfusion ($\chi^2(1,71) = 4.4$, $p < 0.05$; $\chi^2(1,71) = 7.70$, $p < 0.01$; respectively). Although the prevalence of hypofrontality was not statistically different between paranoid and nonparanoid patients, the paranoid subjects did manifest a significantly greater incidence of frontal hypoperfusion relative to controls, while the incidence in nonparanoid subjects was not significantly different from normal controls. Two examples of frontal hypoperfusion in paranoid schizophrenic subjects studied at rest are shown in Figure 20. Several frontal deficits are seen in the study shown on the left, while more moderate frontal hypoperfusion is seen in the study shown on the right.

Our data and those of others suggest that decreased frontal rCBF may be inherent to the subgroup of paranoid schizophrenics. In particular, of those schizophrenics with abnormal left- or right-frontal rCBF, 84% were diagnosed as paranoid. The only other brain areas showing decreased blood flow in schizophrenics were the left and right temporal region (left: $\chi^2(1,71) = 3.99$, $p < 0.05$; right: $\chi^2(1,71) = 9.81$, $p < 0.01$). Right temporal hypoperfusion was the only statistically significant difference

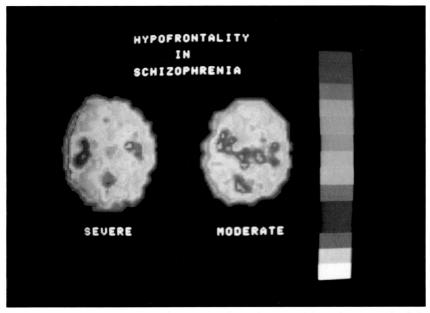

FIGURE 20. Frontal hypoperfusion in schizophrenics. The subject on the left illustrates severe bilateral frontal hypoperfusion coupled with bilateral temporal hypoperfusion. In contrast, the subject on the right shows moderate left frontal hypoperfusion and mild right frontal hypoperfusion, while temporal lobe flow is normal.

between nonparanoid schizophrenics and normals. While we have not yet systematically evaluated regional hypoperfusion in other patient groups, an early comparison between schizophrenics and a small mixed psychiatric sample found hypofrontality in 43% of schizophrenics compared to 11% of psychiatric controls ($\chi^2(1,48)$ = 4.17, p < 0.05; Devous et al. 1985b).

Analysis of hemispheric flow values provided an interesting result. Paranoid schizophrenic patients had significantly higher left- and right-hemispheric rCBF than normal controls (left—70 ± 11 ml/min/100 g, and right—73 ± 12 for patients; left—64 ± 11, and right—65 ± 11 for controls, p < 0.25). Nonparanoid schizophrenics did not differ from controls (left—67 ± 14, right—68 ± 13). These data are illustrated in Figure 21. Our data indicate that paranoid patients have focal frontal rCBF hypoperfusion only within the context of bilaterally elevated hemispheric flow. Similar results have been presented by Buchsbaum et al. (1984) in which a decreased antero–posterior glucose metabolic gradient was found in schizophrenic patients and the decreased gradient was composed primarily of elevated posterior metabolic rates.

Preliminary analyses of Pearson correlations between selected neuropsychological (NP) measures and rCBF measures suggest that left frontal rCBF deficit was related to global NP dysfunction in that it was inversely correlated with an increased number of Luria–Nebraska basic

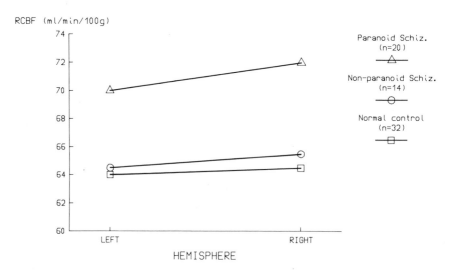

FIGURE 21. Hemispheric cerebral blood flow values in normal controls and nonparanoid and paranoid schizophrenic patients. Note that rCBF is higher in both hemispheres for paranoid schizophrenics than for either normal controls or nonparanoid schizophrenics.

scale elevations (Devous et al. 1985a; Paulman et al., in press). This correlation is striking given that the mean number of Luria–Nebraska elevations for our patient sample was only in the mildly impaired range (3.9 ± 2.7). Left frontal hypoperfusion was also correlated with specific measures of frontal lobe function. For example, subjects with lowered left frontal rCBF committed more WCST errors and made fewer category set shifts than those with normal perfusion. They also had greater difficulty with motor functions of both hands (finger tapping, LNNB motor scale). The correlation between left frontal rCBF and NP measures of frontal function supports the concept that frontal hypoperfusion can affect cognitive function. These findings are especially striking when one realizes that resting rCBF studies and NP assessment normally occurred on separate days. Thus, regional hypoperfusion might be a relatively stable phenomenon in most of our patients.

The relationship of symptomatology to rCBF is very interesting. Preliminary analyses of Pearson correlation coefficients in 15 patients show that the presence of positive or negative symptoms was uncorrelated to frontal blood flow. However, positive symptoms were correlated with left temporal, and mildly correlated with right temporal, rCBF. In contrast, negative symptoms were inversely correlated with right temporal flow.

Medicated and unmedicated subgroups did not differ relative to any rCBF or NP variable. In addition, when neuroleptic dosages of medicated schizophrenics were converted to chlorpromazine equivalents (range 700 to 32,000 mg) and correlated with rCBF ratios and neurological scores, no significant correlations were obtained.

While not all schizophrenics manifest hypofrontality at rest, such an occurrence seems to be more likely in paranoid than in nonparanoid patients. As described earlier, Weinberger and colleagues (Berman et al. 1984, 1986; Weinberger et al. 1986) successfully used the WCST during rCBF measurements as a frontal challenge task to "unmask" latent anterior brain dysfunction. That we found an association between a version of this same task and resting left frontal rCBF (assessed on different days) suggests that regional flow deficits in schizophrenics are relatively stable phenomena with ongoing relationship to NP function.

To further document this finding we have extended our studies to include SPECT rCBF measurements while performing the WCST (Devous et al. 1985a). Initially, we examined 15 chronic schizophrenics. In this group right frontal rCBF declined significantly during the cognitive task (t = − 2.66, p < 0.05). However, when the 11 paranoids in this group were analyzed separately, both left and right frontal rCBF declined during the activating condition (t = − 2.78, p < 0.02). No changes were seen in any other region and all t tests were nonsignificant in the very small nonparanoid sample. An example of the rCBF response to the WCST of two paranoid subjects is shown in Figure 22, and of two nonparanoid patients in Figure 23. A significant decrease in frontal rCBF is seen in the paranoid patient with intact resting flows (Figure 22, top), while the paranoid subject with pre-existing frontal hypoperfusion does not further decrease rCBF during the task (Figure 22, bottom). In contrast, both nonparanoid subjects demonstrated increased frontal rCBF during the WCST (Figure 23).

These data, and the data of others, suggest that anterior brain regions fail to activate in response to learning and effortful problem solving in these patients. We have continued this investigation and visual rCBF determinations are now available in 14 paranoid, 5 nonparanoid, and 11 normal controls performing resting or WCST rCBF examinations. While quantitative analyses are still under way, visual interpretations demonstrate that 10 of 14 paranoids decreased frontal flow during WCST, while only 1 of 5 nonparanoids showed rCBF declines in frontal regions during WCST.

A very curious result is that 5 of 11 normal controls also demonstrated declines in frontal rCBF. The meaning of this latter finding is unknown at

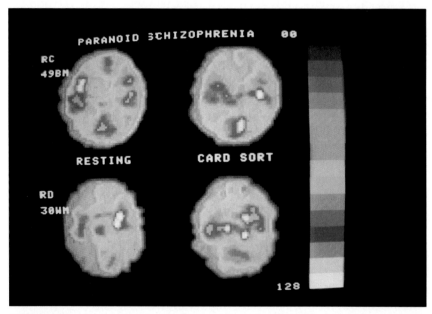

FIGURE 22. Two examples of the response of paranoid schizophrenics to the frontal lobe-activating Wisconsin Card Sort task. The subject at the top shows normal flow at rest and a substantial decrease in frontal rCBF during the Card Sort. The subject at the bottom shows frontal and temporal hypoperfusion with some increase in temporal flows and a very mild decrease in frontal flow during the Card Sort.

this time but is undergoing extensive continuing investigation. Weinberger et al. (1986) have suggested that the separation between schizophrenics and normal controls on the WCST requires a carefully designed control task rather than comparisons to resting states. They indicate that the difference between schizophrenics and controls is not present when WCST-activated flows are compared to resting controls in the patient population. The positive findings are present only when WCST-rCBF values are compared to those obtained while subjects are performing a number-sequencing task.

In a subgroup of schizophrenic patients undergoing resting and WCST-activated SPECT studies, simultaneous topographic EEG data were obtained. This includes six paranoid and five nonparanoid subjects, and eight normal controls. Fourier transforms of artifact-free EEG were averaged for each recording session and compartmentalized into classical bandwidths (Herman et al. 1986). Delta and alpha frequencies decreased in amplitude in normal controls and increased in paranoids during activation. This effect was consistent only at frontal sites, as confirmed by a

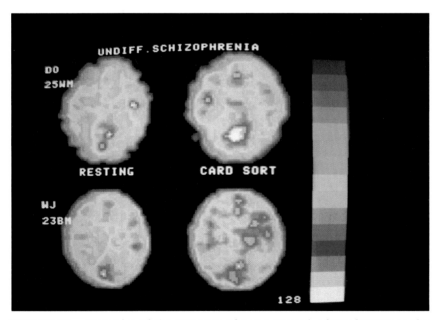

FIGURE 23. Examples of the response of non-paranoid schizophrenics to the frontal lobe-activating Wisconsin Card Sort task. The subject on the top shows frontal hypoperfusion and left temporal hypoperfusion at rest but activates to a normal study during the Card Sort. The subject on the bottom shows normal frontal flow and a left medial temporal defect at rest, but similarly activates to a normal study during the Card Sort.

groups-by-condition-by-sites ANOVA. This data analysis is very preliminary but implies that electrophysiologic function of the cortex is also
altered in schizophrenic patients during WCST.

In summary, there is substantial information from our laboratory and
from others that frontal cortical function is abnormal in schizophrenic
patients, possibly more marked on the left side. This abnormal function
occurs in the context of globally elevated flow and metabolism such that a
decreased antero–posterior gradient characterizes schizophrenic patients.
Buchsbaum et al. (1984) find a similar shift in patients with affective
disorders, while no such evidence is present in our data for depressed
subjects. Correlation between NP function and rCBF indicates that these
metabolic and perfusion findings have strong implications concerning
cognitive function in this patient group. Similar studies from our laboratory relating resting rCBF to NP test results in patients with seizure disorders confirm a correlation between cognitive dysfunction and rCBF deficits (Homan et al. 1984; Homan et al., in press).

Dementia

The most common cerebral illness in middle-aged and elderly people is
dementia. It may be defined as a global deterioration of higher mental
function in its intellectual, cognitive, and emotional aspects (Mayer-Gross
et al. 1969). The National Institute of Neurological and Communicative
Disorders and Stroke estimates that 15% of people over 65 years of age
have varying degrees of dementia, but dementia may also occur in younger
individuals. For example, Alzheimer's disease (AD), which accounts for
more than 50% of the dementias occurring over the age of 65, may occur
in persons in their forties in a form that appears to be genetically transmitted as a dominant trait. Patients with Down's syndrome may also demonstrate an Alzheimer-like dementia at an early age. Dementia may be the
consequence of genetically transmitted disorders such as Huntington's
disease or slow-virus infections such as in the case of Creutzfeldt–Jakob
disease. The onset of dementia associated with generalized neuronal degeneration is typically insidious and slow in it progression (Blessed 1980;
Roth 1978). Developed symptoms may or may not be reversible.

Some dementias have a vascular origin. Individuals suffering from a
series of small cortical strokes can elicit many of the same symptoms of
dementia as individuals suffering from neuronal degeneration. In some
cases the symptoms associated with this latter form of dementia (often
called multi-infarct dementia, MID) can be distinguished by the rather
sudden appearance of emotional instability with well-preserved intelligence and personality, and the later addition of depressive symptoms. The
course with MID has been described as mostly intermittent and fluctuat-
ing (Blessed 1980; Roth 1978).

AD represents 60–70% of the dementias, MID 20–30%, and both disorders are present in 15–20% of demented patients (Tomlinson 1980). AD is often divided into pre-senile and senile forms based solely on the age of onset. However, they are generally regarded as variations of the same degenerative process. AD is characterized by gyral atrophy primarily in frontal and temporal lobes. The anterior parts of middle and superior temporal gyri and hippocampus are most severely affected. A marked loss of cortical neurons is found with an increased number of fibrous astrocytes. Neuritic plaques and neurofibrillary tangles are present throughout the cerebral cortex, but both are particularly common in the anteromedial areas of the temporal lobes (Tomlinson 1980; Terry et al. 1981; Terry 1982). There seems to be a correlation between the abundance of neuritic plaques and the severity of impairment in cognition (Blessed et al. 1968).

Postmortem studies of brain from AD patients demonstrate a selective loss of cholinergic neurons in the temporal lobes and hippocampus (Perry et al. 1978) along with significant reductions in acetylcholine synthesis (Sims et al. 1980). These findings correlated with the number of neuritic plaques and neurofibrillary tangles found. Muscarinic cholinergic receptor binding sites however were found to be unchanged in AD patients (Davies and Verth 1977; Perry et al. 1978). Therefore, the presynaptic cholinergic system seems to be selectively affected in AD patients (White et al. 1977; Rosser et al. 1982). Interestingly, Holman et al. (1985) reported on I-123 QNB (a muscarinic cholinergic antagonist) uptake in a single AD patient. Uptake was reduced relative to a single normal control, but no regional asymmetries in its distribution were found.

Hoyer (1982) has provided an excellent review of global changes in rCBF, oxidative metabolism, and glucose metabolism in abnormal brain aging. He concludes that early in the onset of AD, cerebral blood flow and the cerebral metabolic rate for oxygen ($CMRO_2$) are found to be normal, while the cerebral metabolic rate for glucose (CMRgl) is reduced. In contrast, in MID, rCBF and oxygen metabolism are within the normal range while glucose metabolism is found to be abnormally increased. As the severity of dementia increases in AD rCBF, $CMRO_2$, and CMRgl become tightly coupled. Similarly, advanced MID symptoms are associated with changes in blood flow and metabolism similar to variations seen after ischemic/anoxic insults. Thus, early in the onset of both types of dementia there is a close correlation between rCBF and $CMRO_2$ while they seem to be decoupled from glucose metabolism. As the course of the disorder advances, blood flow, oxygen metabolism, and glucose metabolism follow similar degeneration to reduced levels. Hoyer concludes that in this circumstance global measurements provide no distinction between the dementia types. However, Hoyer does indicate that the severity of dementia is correlated to reductions in perfusion and metabolism.

Dastur (1985) recently reviewed and re-analyzed data from an early NIH study (originally conducted in 1956–1958) of global measures of rCBF and metabolism in normal active elderly men with a mean age of 71 years, relative to normal young subjects with a mean age of 21 years. There was no difference in mean rCBF or CMRO$_2$ values between the two populations. However, there was a significant reduction (approximately 23%) in the metabolic rate for glucose in the aged group relative to the younger group. Dastur also reported on two groups of elderly subjects not considered to be normal and active. In the group with moderate elevations of mean arterial blood pressure and cerebral vascular resistance (asymptomatic but with signs of early atherosclerosis), small but statistically significant reductions in cerebral blood flow were found. In the group with severe atherosclerosis and signs of dementia, cerebral blood flow was significantly reduced as were CMRO$_2$ and CMRgl. The decline in CMRgl was nearly twice the magnitude of that in rCBF or CMRO$_2$.

Shaw et al. (1984) have extensively studied the relationship of cerebral vascular disease to cerebral blood flow changes in aged individuals. They have conducted a cross-sectional analysis of rCBF among 668 volunteers and patients subdivided according to age, gender, and degree of cerebral vascular disease. In addition, a four-year longitudinal analysis was carried out in 230 subjects from this original sample. Patients were subdivided into healthy volunteers, volunteers with risk factors for stroke, subjects with a history of transient ischemic attacks (TIA), patients with completed stroke, and patients with multi-infarct dementia. Decrements in regional cerebral blood flow were evinced by both the cross-sectional and longitudinal analyses in relation to advancing age, progressive cerebral vascular disease, and dementia. In normal individuals they found a progressive decline in gray-matter flow values between the ages of 40 and 100 years with higher flow values in women than in men only for subjects prior to 60 years of age. They also found a heterogeneous, age-related decline in rCBF in normal subjects only in prefrontal, parietal, inferior temporal, motor, and frontal/temporal areas. They suggested that these were related to changes in levels of functional activity within different brain regions. They also found that healthy subjects with risk factors for stroke (i.e., hypertension, heart disease, hyperlipidemia, and/or diabetes mellitus) had lower bihemispheric flow values compared with nonrisk volunteers for subjects in the age range of 40–70 years, independent of gender. The three most significant risk factors associated with these rCBF changes were hypertension, smoking, and alcohol consumption. Of these, hypertension emerged as the single most important predisposing factor for significant rCBF declines.

The interactive effects of advancing age and progressive cerebral vascular disease and/or dementia were established in both their cross-sectional and longitudinal data. This interaction led to decreases in rCBF that were much greater than those seen in the normal aging process. These did not appear to have regional correlates. rCBF distinctions among individuals with progressive cerebral vascular disease, dementia, and just advanced age tended to converge with increasing age. Thus, bihemispheric gray-matter perfusion at rest offered little disease discrimination among the very old.

There have been a number of studies of rCBF in both AD and MID using two-dimensional probe systems and Xe-133. Ingvar et al. (1975) demonstrated reduced flow responses to mental activation as well as abnormal activation patterns in demented patients. Risberg (1980) commented that it is difficult to interpret findings on mental activation due to the influence of aphasia and low motivation in these patients. In two subsequent reports (Gustafson et al. 1984; Risberg 1985), this group extended their studies in dementia to include four subcategories: presenile AD, $N = 28$; senile AD (SDAT), $N = 27$; Pick's disease (PD), $N = 22$; and MID, $N = 4$. They found significant differences by region among the groups. For example, AD and PD groups differed in that AD patients had significant flow reductions in parietal, parieto-occipital and parieto-temporal regions, while PD patients evinced lowest flow values in pre-motor, supplementary motor, and prefrontal regions. In both groups, rCBF reductions were symmetric across hemispheres. AD and SDAT groups were similar in most respects, although AD patients had a more focalized postcentral flow reduction, while SDAT flow reductions were more widespread and appeared to involve the frontal lobes to a greater extent. Both groups evinced preservation of flow to rolandic, occipital, and fronto-temporal structures.

MID patients had evidence of a large variation in mean rCBF. Flow patterns were heterogeneous with no systematic patterns. Patients with early clinical signs with small and/or deep infarcts evinced normal flow levels and a normal regional distribution. However, in the more advanced stages right–left asymmetries were generally observed. They reported that some but not all MID cases could be distinguished from the AD, PD, and SDAT groups as a result of asymmetric and "spotty" flow patterns.

Meyer and colleagues have also published several reports concerning rCBF determinations and dementia (Meyer et al. 1980; Yamaguchi et al. 1980; Tachibana et al. 1984). They compared resting rCBF values to those obtained during the performance of a multiple psychological activation test in 8 MID, 11 AD, 3 Korsakoff's encephalopathy, 2 Parkinson-dementia complex, and 2 Creutzfeldt–Jakob disease patients. All subjects showed failure of normal cortical activation during the task and in most cases regional decreases in gray-matter flow resulted. Others have reported a "paradoxical deactivation" during psychological stimulation in patients with underlying cerebral vascular disease attributing this phenomenon to "steal," whereby blood was redistributed from areas of infarcted brain to normal brain (Hoedt-Rasmussen et al. 1967). However, Meyer et al. suggest that this is an unlikely explanation in patients with dementia since decreased rCBF during activation was found diffusely throughout the brain and little or no evidence of underlying cerebral vascular disease was evident except in the MID subjects. They suggest that in patients with dementia of neuronal origin there is a failure of normal afferent synaptic connections from the brain stem and diencephalic structures to the cortical neurons. Thus, under the stress of enhanced multiple sensory input, there appears to be a decrease rather than an increase of afferent neuronal volleys to the cerebral cortex. This could be due to disordered neurotransmission and/or enhanced synaptic inhibition. In support of this concept (that activation of the cerebral cortex by a brain stem connection is hindered), Meyer et al. found that the normal increase in brain stem–cerebellar flow that occurs during activation was absent or decreased in demented patients.

Their AD and MID patients were distinguished by evidence of bilateral and symmetric rCBF reductions in AD but patchy reductions in MID, although the sensitivity of the discrimination was not reported. In addition, the rCBF vasodilatory increase in response to 5% CO_2 inhalation was reduced in MID patients but was normal in AD patients. They also found a significant correlation between reductions in mean flow values and severity of dementia (Tachibana et al. 1984).

Very recently this same group (Rogers et al. 1986) published the results of a 7-year prospective study among 181 neurologically normal elderly volunteers (mean age, 71 years). In the 7-year duration of the study, 6 volunteers (3.3%) were diagnosed as having senile dementia of the Alzheimer's type (SDAT) and 10 patients (5.5%) were diagnosed as having MID. Only 1 AD patient had a history of risk factors for stroke while all 10 of the MID patients had a least one risk factor (hypertension, heart disease, diabetes mellitus, or hyperlipidemia). Eighty percent of these patients, but only 18% of the original volunteer group, had hypertension and a history of heavy cigarette smoking (one pack per day for at least 10 years).

In addition, the incidence of MID was 11.4% in the subgroup of original volunteers ($N = 88$) with predisposing risk factors for cerebral vascular disease. Of the MID patients, 70% evinced subcortical lacunar lesions predominantly in the distribution of the middle cerebral artery on CT exam, and one-half of the MID patients had transient ischemic attacks before onset of cognitive declines.

More importantly, analyses of variance of mean bihemispheric gray-matter rCBF values (F_1) were conducted for diagnostic criteria that were obtained during yearly examinations over the 7-year time interval with the following results: 1) Two years prior to the onset of symptoms, MID patients had significantly lower F_1 values than subjects who later developed AD, or subjects who remained normal (both those with and without risk factors). In addition, the risk-factored normal volunteers had significantly lower F_1 values than their nonrisk counterparts. No significant difference was observed between AD patients and either of the normal groups. 2) One year prior to the onset of dementia, MID patients had significantly lower F_1 values than any other diagnostic group. 3) At the onset of dementia symptoms, F_1 values for both AD and MID patients were significantly lower than either normal group. At this time, there were no differences in F_1 values between AD and MID patients. 4) One year following the onset of dementia symptoms, mean F_1 values for AD and MID subjects remained lower than for volunteer groups and were not different from each other. Risk-factor volunteers continued to evince lower F_1 values than nonrisk volunteers. None of the differences observed in this study could be related to differences in age or pulmonary function (expired CO_2, expired oxygen levels, and respiration rates) among the groups.

These investigators concluded that patients at risk for MID have patchy reductions of cerebral blood flow levels at least 2 years before the onset of signs or symptoms. In addition, the rCBF pattern in AD differed from MID. In AD, rCBF levels were maintained immediately prior to the onset of symptoms but rCBF decreased rapidly and diffusely as cognition declined. They conclude that, in AD, the rCBF reductions are subsequent to reductions in cerebral oxygen utilization and declining cognition. They point out that this differs from the pattern in normal aging where CBF declines prior to reductions in cerebral metabolism as a consequence of reduced neuronal activity and progressive narrowing and rigidity of cerebral vasculature.

Zemcov et al. (1984) have evaluated the sensitivity and specificity of two-dimensional probe measurements of rCBF in distinguishing among various dementia subtypes. In distinguishing patients with all forms of dementia from age-matched normals they found a sensitivity of 65% (19/29) and specificity of 77% (24/31). Sensitivity was defined as true positives divided by the sum of true positives plus false negatives, and specificity as true negatives divided by the sum of true negatives plus false positives. The sensitivity and specificity values for detecting organic dementia alone were 68% (15/22) and 97% (30/31), respectively. The rCBF criteria used to identify MID were relatively insensitive (57%, 4/7) but reasonably specific (81%, 25/31). These criteria were: for AD, bilateral focal decreases in parieto-temporal and parieto-occipital regions; for SDAT, AD criteria plus decreased flow in frontal regions; for Pick's disease, bilateral frontal and frontotemporal rCBF decreases in combination with preservation of posterior flow levels; for MID, right–left asymmetries of hemispheric flow and regional flow reductions.

Although no known cure exists for Alzheimer's disease, MID is at least theoretically treatable in that further progression of the disease can be limited. The role of rCBF measurements in monitoring such therapy has been minimal, but there are three reports of such efforts. Risberg (1980) studied the effects of piracetam (Notropil) in 9 patients with AD comparing rCBF, psychiatric ratings, and psychometric determinations. No beneficial effects were observed in any of the parameters. However, the patients under study had organic dementia rather than dementia of vascular origin. Hagstadius et al. (1984) in the same laboratory studied the effects of bromvincamine and vincamine on rCBF and mental function in MID patients. Treatment with vincamine led to a significant increase in global flow and a reduction in initial right–left asymmetry of hemispheric means. Performance scores on verbal memory tests increased significantly. No significant effects on rCBF were observed with bromvincamine, although performance on the two memory tests did improve significantly. Hartmann (1985) used a comparative randomized study to examine cerebral blood flow after long-term administration of pentoxifylline and co-dergocrine mesylate in patients with chronic cerebral vascular disease. A statistically significant rCBF increase over baseline was found at 4 and 8 weeks in patients on pentoxifylline. No such findings occurred in controls or co-dergocrine mesylate-treated patients. Symptoms of dizziness, insomnia, and tinnitus improved in the pentoxifylline group but not in others. Cognitive function was not assessed in these groups.

PET studies of rCBF, $rCMRO_2$ and rCMRgl in dementias and normal aging have produced controversial results. For example, Frackowiak et al. (1981) and Kuhl et al. (1982b), studying cerebral metabolism and aging, concluded that $rCMRO_2$, rCBF, and rCMRgl were reduced in the elderly relative to young controls. However, Duara et al. (1983, 1984) examined similar subjects with special attention to screening individuals for any condition that might contribute to cerebral dysfunction and studied subjects with minimal sensory input (eyes covered and ears plugged) to reduce age-related effects of reduced sensory sensitivity. In their examination of right-handed males, ages 21–83, they found that glucose metabolism did not correlate with age, whether raw metabolic data or data normalized to whole-brain levels were used. Subsequently, Frackowiak and Gibbs (1983) re-analyzed their PET data and concluded that blood flow but not oxygen metabolism was age-related, due to increases in the oxygen-extraction ratio. Duara et al. (1984) also reported that psychometric measurements (e.g., WAIS, Benton Visual Retention tests) correlated with regional glucose metabolism when age factors were removed. This is a curious conclusion since they state that their measurements were not age-related.

This same group (Rapoport et al. 1984) examined the relationship between rCMRgl and performance on verbal and full scale WAIS scores, and on the Wechsler Memory Scale in patients with mild to moderate AD. In their study no psychometric measure, nor the severity of the disease, was significantly correlated with rCMRgl. However, they also analyzed their data for asymmetries (examined left minus right for individual lobes and hemispheres divided by the mean metabolic rate) and established a rank order in their 10 patients between language ability (syntax comprehension test) and visual constructive praxis (extended-range drawing test) by establishing a language rank minus visual constructive rank score. Under these conditions, significant correlations between metabolic and psychometric asymmetry indices emerged. They summarized their data as follows: Age differences were not found for rCMRgl in healthy subjects provided metabolism was measured at rest and with reduced sensory stimulation; there was no correlation between parameters of cognitive function and resting glucose metabolism in healthy subjects; rCBF was reduced throughout the brain in relation to the severity of AD with specific declines in temporo-parietal cortex during late stages of the disease; rCMRgl may not be significantly correlated with neuropsychometric deficits in patients with mild to moderate AD due to the high variability of the metabolic measurements; and, right–left asymmetries in cerebral metabolism appeared early in AD and were correlated with asymmetries in language compared with visual constructive abilities.

Foster et al. (1983) and Mazziotta (1985) have pointed out that there is a problem in interpreting PET studies in patients with cerebral atrophy, which problem also applies to two-dimensional probe measurements of rCBF and to SPECT. The problem is twofold. First, the measuring instruments suffer form partial volume effects. That is, the spatial resolution is insufficient to resolve cortical structures. Thus, measurements obtained will include data from cortex, white matter, and cerebrospinal fluid spaces. In addition, it is well known that there is, in Alzheimer's disease, significant cell loss (46% of large neurons in the temporal cortex and 40% of neurons in the frontal cortex in advanced cases; see Terry et al. 1981). It would be unclear whether reduced metabolism or rCBF observed in the cortex reflects neuronal cell death or abnormal function of preserved neurons. In addition, one must cautiously interpret correlations of abnormal NP factors with focal areas of hypometabolism due to the difficulties of applying correlational statistics of multiple comparisons between partially interdependent variables (Foster et al. 1983).

Even in the face of these difficulties, most PET studies have reported a correlation between severity of dementia and reductions in rCMRgl, rCMRO$_2$, or rCBF in whole brain (Foster et al. 1984; Kuhl et al. 1983). For example, in a series of papers, Foster and colleagues (Foster et al. 1983, 1984; Chase et al. 1984) examined patients with AD who had specific predominant symptoms of constructional abnormalities, language abnormalities, or pure memory disorders. In the patients with abnormal spatial and constructional test scores, a 31% decrease in rCMRgl was found in the right parietal cortex relative to the left, while patients with specific language abnormalities had an 18% decrease in left frontoparietal and temporal regions relative to the right side. Patients who predominantly had memory abnormalities had no left–right metabolic asymmetries.

In general, AD patients exhibited reduced glucose metabolism in posterior parietal and contiguous portions of posterior temporal and anterior occipital cortex with relative sparing of the frontal cortex. When they compared patients with early AD to those with more advanced symptoms, a substantial decline in glucose metabolism was noted prior to the observation of significant cognitive impairment. However, small additional metabolic decrements led to marked deterioration in intellectual function. That is, there were relatively small differences in cortical glucose metabolism between patients with mild AD and those with severe cognitive impairments. Foster and colleagues (1984) interpret these data to indicate that the cortex has a considerable margin of safety in regard to neuronal injury since a relatively high threshold of cortical metabolic dysfunction must be exceeded before cognitive dysfunction occurs. They then state that this implies a model for AD in which the disease is viewed as having reduced the safety margin so that relatively minor changes in glucose metabolism led to major changes in mentation. They continue to emphasize the point that metabolic deterioration due to a loss of intrinsic cortical neurons cannot easily be distinguished from hypofunction caused by partial degeneration or deafferentation.

Other groups have confirmed global reductions in metabolic activity in AD patients with maximal focal abnormalities in the parietotemporal regions and relative sparing of the primary sensorimotor cortex and subcortical structures (DeLeon et al. 1983; Friedland et al. 1983; Kuhl et al. 1983). These studies also support the concept that the severity of dementia is directly related to the severity of metabolic impairment, although no specific information has been provided with respect to memory dysfunction, largely due to difficulties in the imaging technology associated with defining mesial temporal structures such as the amygdala and hippocampus, which have been implicated in memory function (Foster et al. 1984).

The question of the role of cerebral atrophy in creating apparent metabolic depression in patients with dementia was addressed in part by Kuhl et al. (1985b) and by DeLeon et al. (1983). Cerebral atrophy was rated from CT scans in these patients and neither group found any correlation between the degree of atrophy and the degree of reduced glucose metabolism. Kuhl et al. found a distinction between MID and AD patients as expected. In MID, the glucose images consisted of random focal deficits in an otherwise normal metabolic distribution. They also noted that the PET glucose image was a more sensitive indicator of stroke sequelae than CT. That is, both CT and PET demonstrated evidence of frank tissue destruction within focal infarcts, but only metabolic images were altered in more distant projection sites. Presumably, disconnection of fiber tracks had resulted in mild hypometabolism within structurally intact tissue due to deafferentation. In contrast, AD patients had the expected pattern of reduced metabolism in cortex, principally parietal and parietotemporal with preservation in caudate, thalamus, anterior cingulate gyrus, pre- and post-central gyrus, and calcarine occipital cortex. These changes did not relate to CT evidence of atrophy, implicating neuronal degeneration without destruction as the primary cause of functional image abnormalities.

More recently, Kuhl et al. (1985a) have studied regional glucose metabolism using PET techniques in patients with basal ganglia disorders, which are a less common source of dementia. In Parkinson's disease, they found a 20% reduction in global glucose metabolism relative to age-matched controls. However, there was no particular regional pattern to these reductions. They concluded that chronic alterations in the striatal dopaminergic system of Parkinson's patients do not have major selective effects on striatal or cortical glucose utilization. By visual interpretation their images could not be distinguished from normal subjects in mildly demented Parkinson's patients. They also studied 13 patients with Huntington's disease with somewhat different results. Global glucose metabolism was not different from normal controls, nor did cortical or thalamic metabolic rates vary from those in a normal population. However, Huntington's patients did have significantly reduced metabolism in the caudate when corrected for age. In fact, metabolic depression in the caudate and putamen were found regardless of disease duration or the presence or absence of caudate atrophy. Thus, caudate hypometabolism appears to precede bulk loss of striatal tissue. Kuhl et al. (1985a) have also examined 15 subjects at risk for Huntington's disease. The subjects at risk had normal structural features, but indices of caudate metabolism differed by more than two standard deviations from the normal mean in 6 of the 15 at-risk subjects. They suggested that striatal glucose utilization may be reduced in asymptomatic carriers of the autosomal dominant Huntington's disorder gene. Indeed, 3 of these 6 individuals subsequently developed symptoms of the disorder.

We have studied patients with dementia due to Alzheimer's disease, MID, Pick's disease, and Creutzfeldt–Jakob disease using SPECT determinations of rCBF (Bonte et al. 1986; Bonte et al. in press). Studies were conducted at rest in 37 patients ranging in age from 50 to 93 years referred with a diagnosis of probable Alzheimer's disease. These patients manifested progressive intellectual decline involving memory, language, and cognitive functions, with relative preservation of social graces, personal hygiene, and normal elementary motor and sensory functions. All patients were ambulatory and did not require custodial care. Evaluations to rule out differential diagnoses of MID, frontal meningioma, subdural hematoma, hydrocephalus, hypothyroidism, vitamin B_{12} deficiency, and depression were conducted. Neither biopsy nor autopsy confirmation of the diagnosis was available in any of these patients.

Six of the 37 patients were unable to cooperate with the inhalation technique in order to obtain satisfactory studies. Five of the remaining patients had normal rCBF results, and another 5 were later rediagnosed to have underlying vascular disease as the cause of dementia. In addition, one patient was subsequently found to have temporal lobe glioblastoma multiforme and one patient was classified as having Pick's disease. Thus, 19 of 24 patients presumed to have Alzheimer's disease had abnormal SPECT rCBF images. These data are summarized in Table 7. The last column of this table includes the results of visual image inspection. The most commonly observed rCBF abnormality was hypoperfusion in the temporal lobes bilaterally (Figure 24a). The region of interest designated temporal lobes in the slice obtained 6 cm above and parallel to the cantho-meatal line contains portions of the superior–posterior temporal lobe and the posterior–inferior parietal lobe. Temporal hypoperfusion was evident in all 19 subjects. In addition, 5 patients had evidence of reduced frontal flow, with a more significant reduction on the left (Figure 24b). Quantitative analyses of rCBF data were compared to results obtained in 13 normal volunteers ranging in age from 50 to 71 years. Hemispheric and whole-slice rCBF were lower in AD patients than in the controls (11%, $p<0.05$). In addition, statistically significant bilateral temporal lobe flow reductions were found in AD patients ($p<0.02$, left; $p<0.05$, right).

When flow values were normalized by constructing region-to-hemispheric flow ratios, the differences between patients and normal controls were more significant. In the controls, the left temporal-to-hemisphere flow ratio was 0.97 ± 0.03 and right was 1.0 ± 0.04. In AD patients the temporal lobe ratio on the left was 0.88 ± 0.04 ($p<0.001$), and on the right 0.92 ± 0.05 ($p<0.001$). In the 5 patients demonstrating decreased frontal lobe flow on visual interpretation, frontal flow ratios did not differ significantly from the control population. Nine of the patients listed in Table 7 have flow ratios for both temporal lobes two standard deviations below the mean value for elderly normals. An additional 4 patients have at least one temporal lobe that is outside the normal range.

These data are preliminary and further analyses are required. For

TABLE 7. Regional Cerebral Blood Flow (rCBF) Abnormalities in Patients with Alzheimer's Disease

Patient No.	Sex	Age	Mean Flow (ml/min/100 g)	LT/LH	RT/RH	Areas of Reduced Flow
1	F	55	50	0.82	0.84	LT, RT
2	M	65	55	0.87	0.89	LF, LT, RT
3	M	74	61	0.90	0.97	LT, RT
4	F	63	54	0.92	1.0	?LT, RT
5	M	70	54	0.81	0.88	LF, LP, LT, RT
6	F	50	60	0.87	0.91	LP, RP, LT, RT, LO, RO
7	F	58	53	0.94	1.0	LT
8	F	93	64	0.80	0.88	LT, RT, LO, RO
9	F	84	45	0.86	0.96	?LT
10	M	65	59	0.93	0.97	LT, LF, RF
11	F	66	73	0.94	1.0	?LT
12	F	67	64	0.87	0.88	LT, RT
13	F	61	74	0.88	0.89	LT, RT
14	M	63	44	0.88	0.89	LT, RT
15	M	67	64	0.92	0.88	LP, RP, LT, RT
16	F	68	66	0.89	0.83	LT, RT, LO, RO
17	M	59	82	1.04	1.0	?LT, RT, LF
18	F	70	77	0.97	0.92	LT, RT, LF
19	M	70	62	0.83	0.98	LF, LT, RT
X ± SD		67 ± 9	61 ± 10	0.89 ± 0.06	0.92 ± 0.05	

F = frontal; P = parietal; T = temporal; O = occipital; H = hemisphere; L = left; Right = right; ? = questionable.
LT/LH = 0.97 ± 0.03 and RT/RH = 1.00 ± 0.04 in age-matched normal controls

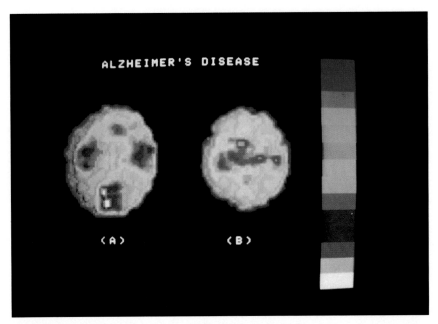

FIGURE 24. rCBF images from a subject with Alzheimer's disease demonstrating the classic finding of bilateral posterior temporal hypoperfusion (a, left). Another rCBF image from a subject with Alzheimer's disease demonstrating bilateral posterior temporal hypoperfusion (b, right). In addition, this subject has bilateral frontal hypoperfusion, a less common finding in these patients.

example, neuropsychological evaluation, duration and age at onset, and medication status have not been related to rCBF findings at this time. However, the general findings in our preliminary studies are in good agreement with findings described above from PET or two-dimensional probe measurements of rCBF, glucose metabolism, or oxygen metabolism.

Only 5 patients studied in our laboratory have had a primary diagnosis of MID. Each of these subjects demonstrated a patchy appearance to the rCBF image while quantitative hemispheric flow values were not different from normal controls (Figure 25, left). This is too small a group to evaluate in a statistically meaningful way. However, none of these patients showed the bilateral temporoparietal flow reductions which are seen so commonly in patients with Alzheimer's disease. In the one patient observed with a primary diagnosis of Pick's disease, significant frontal lobe flow reductions were apparent (Figure 25, right). We also studied a single patient with a diagnosis of Creutzfeldt–Jakob disease. This patient, although young, showed extensive bilateral temporoparietal flow reductions which mimic the findings observed in AD.

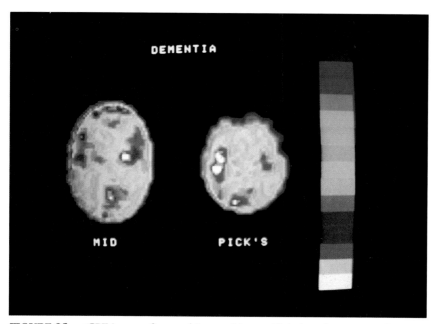

FIGURE 25.   rCBF images from subjects with non-Alzheimer's sources of dementia. A subject with multi-infarct dementia (MID, left) shows severe unilateral left temporal hypoperfusion indicative of stroke, and 2 other small focal underperfused areas typical of the multi-infarct dementia syndrome. Frontal hypoperfusion in a subject with Pick's disease (right) sharply contrasts with the posterior lesions normally seen in Alzheimer's disease.

Clinical Applications

Although SPECT imaging has not yet entered the realm of routine clinical application, recent developments in radiopharmaceuticals and instrumentation should significantly enhance that potential. The various research applications outlined above give some guide to the areas in which anticipated clinical utility might occur. For example, the comparison of resting to Wisconsin Card Sort-activated rCBF responses appears to provide additional differential data in the diagnosis of schizophrenia. Similarly, the distinction between multi-infarct dementia and dementia of nonvascular origin should be enhanced through SPECT rCBF studies. However, the sensitivity and specificity of these techniques in the clinical environment have yet to be established.

One might also imagine that SPECT would be a useful screening tool to rule out traumatic or ischemic causes of psychiatric symptoms. It is already well established that extensive and severe biochemical alterations can be present without clear-cut evidence of structural lesions on either CT or MRI, or in the presence of very small lesions which do not seem to account for extensive symptomatology. The mismatch between structural lesions and functional disturbance is illustrated in Figure 26. A small left frontoparietal lesion is present on CT (top), while a large left-hemispheric rCBF reduction is present in the SPECT image (bottom). The patient's continuing aphasia and hemiparesis three months following a stroke are more easily explained by the SPECT image than by the CT image. Even today, a psychiatrist might wish to obtain a SPECT rCBF study in any patient in which symptoms do not seem to correlate with other laboratory evidence of brain function or structure. There have been a few instances in our experience in which SPECT data have led to subsequent diagnoses not originally envisioned. In some cases, SPECT abnormalities may be so severe or extensive that a CT or MRI study would be requested in a patient for whom it had not previously been considered.

Longitudinal studies for the purpose of diagnosis or to monitor therapy appear promising. Kuhl et al. (1985a) have offered provocative data indicating that PET glucose measurements in subjects at risk for Huntington's disease might be used to distinguish those who will ultimately exhibit symptoms from those who will not. It should be possible to obtain similar data with high-resolution SPECT. Very preliminary data in our laboratory evaluating stroke patients with speech disorders hint that rCBF changes with time and following speech-related task challenges may distinguish those who ultimately develop useful speech patterns from those who do not.

Short-term and long-term responses to therapeutic interventions may also be followed by SPECT rCBF studies. One promising line of research (Risberg 1980) indicates that pre- and post-SPECT rCBF can distinguish between patients who have a successful response without remission and those with a poorer course and a higher probability for remission. However, further research is needed to evaluate the role of SPECT in monitoring therapy, particularly in light of evidence in our own laboratory and in those of others indicating that hypofrontality in schizophrenic patients does not correlate with current levels or previous history of neuroleptic medications.

Monitoring the effects of surgical interventions, particularly those related to cognitive deficits, could easily be an important arena for SPECT evaluations. Devous et al. (1986a) have reported that areas of cerebral steal associated with surgical intervention can be evaluated by SPECT for vascular reactivity using a comparison of resting flow values to those obtained after stimulation with Diamox. Diamox (acetazolamide) is a carbonic anhydrase inhibitor that causes cerebral CO_2 retention. This produces autoregulatory-linked vasodilatation symmetrically throughout

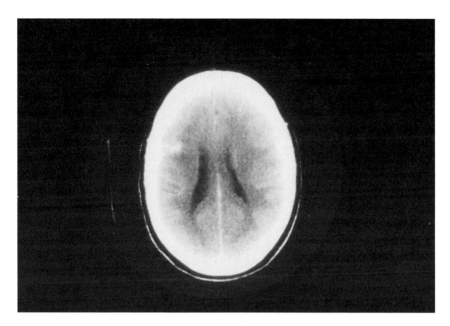

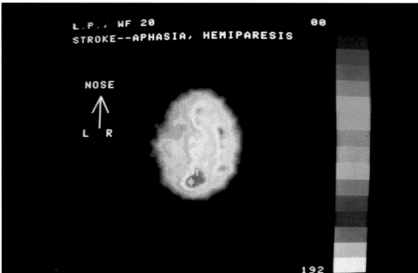

FIGURE 26. CT and rCBF images in a subject suffering from fronto-parietal stroke. The CT (top) shows only a small left fronto-parietal lesion (left is on the left as in the rCBF images). In contrast, the rCBF image (bottom) illustrates hypoperfusion throughout the entire left hemisphere. This mismatch of structural and functional lesions is common and demonstrates the value of obtaining functional measurements even when underlying structural pathology has been identified.

the brain. Hypoperfused regions with normal vascular reserve respond to Diamox by increasing perfusion in a way proportional to or greater than normal tissue, while tissues at risk fail to show significant rCBF increases. Tissues with abnormal vascular responsiveness may not be able to provide normal cognitive function. While our current studies were conducted in patients with arteriovenous malformations, they could be applied to patients undergoing other surgical interventions that might produce either short-term or long-term cognitive deficits. The predictive value of such measurements would be twofold: They might distinguish patients at risk for intra- or postoperative ischemic episodes, and they might distinguish patients who would benefit from postoperative therapeutic efforts.

The strong relationship between cognitive function, assessed by a variety of NP measurements, and resting or stimulated rCBF values suggests a useful future of SPECT measurements in clinical psychiatry (Devous et al. 1986b; Paulman et al. 1985; Homan et al. 1985). Such links should provide the basis for direct interpretation of the relationship between rCBF measurements and clinical syndromes. However, extensive research will be required before this relationship is sufficiently well established to apply it in routine clinical diagnoses. It is our current belief that resting data will be much less informative than data obtained during cognitive or pharmacologic stimulation.

In summary, SPECT is at present primarily a research tool in psychiatry. Research results to date and the development of affordable radiopharmaceuticals and SPECT instrumentation indicate that SPECT may also become a clinical tool in psychiatry. It remains the obligation of both the research community and clinical psychiatrists to apply this technology across a variety of disorders and in sufficiently large patient populations to clearly define its clinical utility.

OVERALL ASSESSMENT

Strengths

SPECT has two major strengths to offer clinical psychiatry. The first of these is its capability to provide three-dimensional measurement of regional cerebral blood flow throughout the entire brain. The resolution of these measurements is adequate for most structural distinctions, and the link between rCBF and cellular metabolism is strong in most circumstances. The second strength that SPECT brings to clinical psychiatry is its availability. Moderate-resolution SPECT instrumentation is available today in almost every nuclear medicine department around the country and certainly in every major city. Availability of high-resolution SPECT instrumentation is limited only by production in the industrial arena; thus, within a few years such instruments should also be widely available. Radiopharmaceuticals for rCBF measurements will soon be available 24 hours per day, 7 days per week. They can be used with both moderate-resolution instruments (rotating gamma cameras) and high-resolution instruments (dedicated SPECT instruments such as PRISM).

It is important to realize that this is not an area of hypothesized clinical availability but in fact very real clinical availability. The only alternate technology is PET. Currently, PET is available on a very restricted basis, and not for routine clinical referral, because of its substantial technological requirements. Some PET researchers believe that it may be possible to obtain tomographs and cyclotrons at lower costs so that it could be made more widely available, but this has not yet come to pass. Given the much more moderate costs of SPECT instrumentation, and the lack of need for on-site production of radiopharmaceuticals, SPECT has many advantages over PET particularly for hospitals not connected with large research-oriented university medical centers.

Limitations

The most striking limitation for SPECT is the lack of research and clinical experience. This reasonably new technology will require time and application to fully appreciate its true utility. Further limitations include modest resolution and a lack of radiopharmaceuticals for measurements other than perfusion. Modest resolution available through rotating gamma camera systems will limit SPECT applications to studies not requiring fine anatomic positioning. Fortunately, recent instrumentation improvements described above have significantly improved SPECT resolution through the use of a dedicated tomograph.

Radiopharmaceutical development has both encouraging and discouraging aspects. Encouraging aspects include the recent development of Tc-99m agents for rCBF determination. These agents permit significant activity to be delivered with minimum radiation exposure so that high-resolution studies can be obtained in short periods of time. Considerable work will be required with these agents, as has been true in the past with PET radiopharmaceuticals, to verify models which permit the radiotracer distribution obtained from images to be converted into quantitative flow values (e.g., ml/min/100 g). It is also encouraging that a receptor ligand labeled with I-123 has been demonstrated to represent the distribution of muscarinic cholinergic receptors in both animal models and in humans. In addition, I-123-labeled receptor ligands for dopaminergic and serotonergic studies have successfully been used in animals, and it is anticipated that they will be available for SPECT studies in humans in the near future. Thus, radiopharmaceuticals for rCBF and receptor distribution measurements seem to be within the grasp of current SPECT technology.

On the discouraging side, very little progress has been made developing either an iodinated or technetium-labeled radiopharmaceutical that distributes in relation to glucose metabolism. The value of regional glucose metabolic rate determinations in brain has been amply demonstrated by PET investigators using F-18 fluorodeoxyglucose. It does not appear that such measurements will be paralleled in SPECT in the near future. Fortunately, rCBF and glucose metabolism are tightly linked in most circumstances. This is not true at some stages during an ischemic insult, in certain tumors, and perhaps in certain conditions with very high flow or metabolism (extreme neuronal discharges).

However, even in these circumstances it has not been clearly established whether rCBF or regional glucose metabolic measurements are preferable. For example, anaerobic glycolysis can lead to normal or elevated glucose uptake in ischemic tissue. Such a result could lead one to believe that the associated tissue was normal, while an rCBF measurement would correctly identify the low-flow area. Conversely, hyperemia (luxury perfusion) is sometimes observed in seriously injured tissue, leading to false conclusions of healthy neuronal populations when a glycolitic measurement might be more informative. As indicated above, in early Alzheimer's disease rCBF and oxygen metabolism are coupled, but glucose metabolism is independent. It is not clear which parameter is most clinically relevant. Nonetheless, a significant spectrum of measurement potentials exists for SPECT today which should be adequate to subserve many, if not all, needs in clinical psychiatry.

Costs

SPECT is the least expensive of all tomographic imaging modalities. CT, MRI, and PET are all characterized by instrumentation costs in the $1–2-million range. The least expensive SPECT tomographs (rotating gamma cameras) can be obtained for approximately $150,000, and the most expensive SPECT tomographs range from $500,000–700,000. Radiopharmaceutical costs are minimal for rCBF agents. Xe-133 has been routinely used for pulmonary imaging in nuclear medicine for several decades. It is widely available and inexpensive. I-123, the agent attached to the rCBF agents IMP and HIPDM, and the first radioisotope bound to receptor imaging ligands, is not as widely available and is significantly more expensive. However, the recent development of Tc-99m-labeled rCBF agents will completely eliminate the need for I-123-labeled rCBF agents, leaving only receptor ligands as those requiring I-123. Thus, the cost of radiopharmaceuticals will range from approximately $25 to $200 per patient. In contrast, PET radiopharmaceuticals generally require on-site production via cyclotrons. Some estimates of these radiopharmaceutical costs are as high as $10,000 per patient, and at present they are certainly no lower than $2,000 per patient. There is some indication that these costs could decrease in the future, but it is unlikely that they will ever be as inexpensive as SPECT agents. One might anticipate that SPECT studies with the most elaborate radiopharmaceuticals and the very best tomographs might eventually be comparable in price to a current CT examination.

Future Directions

The future for SPECT imaging of the brain is very bright. One would anticipate that continued extensive research and initial clinical applications will be the hallmarks for the next five years. During that same time period, receptor imaging with SPECT should evolve. The radiopharmaceuticals for such an effort are too new to have provided a clear indication of their value, but similar imaging efforts with dopamine-receptor ligands in PET have been very provocative (Wagner et al. 1983). Instrumentation development will continue to focus on tomographs dedicated to head imaging and should continue to improve in both resolution and sensitivity.

Applications is psychiatry will be well served by extensive studies of normal cerebral function at rest. Studies during cognitive or pharmacologic activation will also likely play a dominant role in the future. Research should focus on an elucidation of the effects of simple stimuli as building blocks for more complex probes of cognitive function. Similarly, specific probes of biochemical pathways using rCBF as the responding variable and pharmacologic agents as the stimulus should provide useful information concerning underlying causes of psychiatric disorders. Preliminary data from our laboratory concerning the effects of arecoline on cholinergic function indicate that such efforts will be fruitful.

To begin the process of clinical validation of SPECT brain imaging it will be necessary to run sensitivity/specificity studies for diagnosis and monitoring of therapy. This should be feasible since SPECT instruments should be widely available across the nation and thus large numbers of patients should be available for recruitment into such studies. Contrast comparisons with other imaging modalities must be conducted in order to determine when SPECT should be the initial study that serves to recommend further imaging by such modalities as MRI or CT, and when it should be used as end-stage imaging after structural abnormalities have been discovered. One might also anticipate a significant use of SPECT imaging for patients with cognitive dysfunction secondary to nonpsychiatric disorders, including acute head trauma, acute ischemia, drug abuse, and hypertension-related emergencies.

In summary, SPECT has arrived. Tomographs for high-resolution, three-dimensional imaging exist and radiopharmaceuticals for rapid rCBF measurements are now available. Instrumentation and imaging agents have been designed to be applied both in the research setting and in clinical environments. SPECT may eventually permit imaging technologies previously available only in major research institutions to be routinely applied in the diagnosis and therapy of patients with psychiatric disorders.

Acknowledgments

Much of the work described in this book chapter was performed by or supported by my colleagues at the University of Texas Health Science Center at Dallas. These same colleagues have contributed substantially to the writing of this book chapter through their comments and reviews. Most importantly, I wish to acknowledge Frederick J. Bonte, M.D., Director of the Nuclear Medicine Center, and my partner in rCBF imaging. In addition, the significant support and editorial assistance of my colleagues A. John Rush, Jr., M.D., John H. Herman, Ph.D., Ron G. Paulman, Ph.D., and Joachim A. Raese, M.D., in the Department of Psychiatry are greatly appreciated. The assistance of Ms. Juanita M. Hernandez in data analysis, figure preparation, and numerous other tasks is also gratefully acknowledged. Finally, the secretarial and editorial assistance of Ms. Sarah J. Schulz was invaluable in the preparation of this chapter. Only through her ardent assistance did this work come to fruition.

References

Amano T, Meyer JS, Okabe T, et al: Stable xenon CT cerebral blood flow measurements computed by a single compartment-double integration model in normal aging and dementia. J Comput Assist Tomogr 6:923-932, 1982

American Psychiatric Association: Diagnostic and Statistical Manual of Mental Disorders, Third Edition (DSM-III). Washington, DC , American Psychiatric Association, 1980

Anger HO: Scintillation camera. Reviews of Scientific Instruments 29:27-36, 1958

Ariel RN, Golden CJ, Berg RA, et al: Regional cerebral blood flow in schizophrenics: tests using the Xenon-133 inhalation method. Arch Gen Psychiatry 40:258-263, 1983

Baron JC, Steinling M, Tanaka T, et al: Quantitative measurement of CBF, oxygen extraction fraction (OEF) and $CMRO_2$ with the 15-0 continuous inhalation technique and positron emission tomography (PET): experimental evidence and normal values in man. J Cereb Blood Flow Metab 1:S5-S6, 1981

Baxter LR, Phelps ME, Mazziotta JC, et al: Cerebral metabolic rates for glucose in mood disorders. Arch Gen Psychiatry 42:441-447, 1985

Behringer D, Birdsall T, Brown M, et al: A demonstration of ocean accoustic tomography. Nature 299:121-125, 1982

Berman KF, Weinberger DR, Morihisa JM, et al: Regional cerebral blood flow: applications to psychiatry research, in Brain Imaging in Psychiatry. Edited by Morihisa J. Washington, DC, American Psychiatric Press, pp. 41-64, 1984

Berman KF, Zec RF, Weinberger DR: Physiologic dysfunction of dorsolateral prefrontal cortex in schizophrenia, II: role of neuroleptic treatment, attention, and mental effort. Arch Gen Psychiatry 43:126-135, 1986

Blessed G: Clinical aspects of senile dementia, in Biochemistry of Dementia. Edited by Roberts PJ. Chicester, England, Wiley, 1980

Blessed G, Tomlinson BE, Roth M: The association between quantitative measures of dementia and of senile change in the cerebral gray matter of elderly subjects. Br J Psychiatry 114:797-811, 1968

Bonte FJ, Stokely EM: Single-photon tomographic study of regional cerebral blood flow after stroke: concise communication. J Nucl Med 22:1049-1053, 1981

Bonte FJ, Devous MD, Chehabi HH, et al: SPECT study of regional cerebral blood flow in dementia. J Nucl Med 27:732, 1986

Bonte FJ, Devous MD, Chehabi HH, et al: SPECT study of regional cerebral blood flow in Alzheimer disease. J Comput Assist Tomogr 10:579-583, 1986b

Bracewell RN, Riddle AC: Inversion of fan-beam scans in radioastronomy. Astrophysical Journal 150:427-434, 1967

Bruder G, Sutton S, Berger-Gross P, et al: Lateralized auditory processing in depression: dichotic click detection. Psychiatry Res 4:253-266, 1981

Buchsbaum MS, Coppola R, Cappelletti J: Positron emission tomography, EEG and evoked potential topography: new approaches to local function in pharmacoelectroencephalography, in EEG in Drug Research. Edited by Herrmann J. New York, Gustav Fisher, 1982a

Buchsbaum MS, Ingvar DH, Kessler R, et al: Cerebral glucography with positron tomography: use in normal subjects and in patients with schizophrenia. Arch Gen Psychiatry 39:251-259, 1982b

Buchsbaum MS, Holcomb HH, Johnson J, et al: Cerebral metabolic consequences of electrical stimulation in normal individuals. Human Neurobiol 2:35-38, 1983

Buchsbaum MS, DeLisa LE, Holcomb HH, et al: Anteroposterior gradients in cerebral glucose use in schizophrenia and affective disorders. Arch Gen Psychiatry 41:1159-1166, 1984

Budinger TF: Physical attributes of single-photon tomography. J Nucl Med 21:579-592, 1980

Carroll BJ, Feinberg M, Greden JF, et al: A specific laboratory test for the diagnosis of melancholia. Arch Gen Psychiatry 38:15-22, 1981

Celsis P, Goldman T, Henricksen L, et al: A method for calculating regional cerebral blood flow from emission computerized tomography of inert gas concentrations. J Comput Assist Tomogr 5:641-645, 1981

Charles G, Uytdenhoef P, Portlange P, et al: The dexamethasone suppression test and cerebral blood flow in primary major depression. Biol Psychiatry 18:1336-1338, 1983

Charney DS, Menkes DB, Heringer GR: Receptor sensitivity and the mechanism of action of antidepressant treatment: implications for the etiology and therapy of depression. Arch Gen Psychiatry 38:1160-1180, 1981

Chase TN, Foster NL, Fedio P, et al: Regional cortical dysfunction in Alzheimer's disease as determined by positron emission tomography. Ann Neurol 15 (Suppl):S170-S174, 1984

Cormack AM: Representation of a function by its line integrals, with some radiological applications. J Appl Phys 34:2722-2730, 1963

Crawley JCW, Smith T, Zanelli GD, et al: Dopamine receptors in the human brain imaged with a new ligand labelled with 123-I. Clinical Science 70(Suppl 13):53P, 1986

Dastur DK: Cerebral blood flow and metabolism in normal human aging, pathological aging, and senile dementia. J Cereb Blood Flow Metab 5:1-9, 1985

Davies P, Verth AH: Regional distribution of muscarinic acetylcholine receptors in normal and Alzheimer's-type dementia brains. Brain Res 138:385-392, 1977

DeLeon MJ, Ferris SH, George AE, et al: Positron emission tomographic studies of aging and Alzheimer's disease. Am J Neurol 4:568-571, 1983

Devous MD, Rush AJ, Schlesser MA, et al: Single-photon tomographic determination of regional cerebral blood flow in psychiatric disorders. J Nucl Med 25:P57, 1984

Devous MD Sr, Raese JD, Herman JH, et al: Regional cerebral blood flow in schizophrenic patients at rest and during Wisconsin Card Sort tasks. J Cereb Blood Flow Metab 5:S201-S202, 1985a

Devous MD Sr, Stokely EM, Bonte FJ: Quantitative imaging of regional cerebral blood flow in man by dynamic single-photon tomography, in Radionuclide Imaging of the Brain. Edited by Holman BL. London, Churchill-Livingstone, 1985b

Devous MD Sr, Batjer HH, White SR, et al: DSPECT determination of regional cerebral blood flow at rest and following Diamox-induced vasodilatation in patients with arteriovenous malformations. J Nucl Med 27:734, 1986a

Devous MD Sr, Bonte FJ, Stokely EM: The normal distribution of regional cerebral blood flow measured by dynamic single-photon emission tomography. J Cereb Blood Flow Metab 6:95-104, 1986b

Devous MD Sr, Kulkarni PV, Bonte FJ: A comparison of cerebral blood flow measured with radioactive tracer microspheres and the distribution of I-125-labeled diamine or amphetamine. Eur J Nucl Med (in press)

Drayer PP, Wolfson SK, Reinmuth OW, et al: Xenon enhanced CT for analysis of cerebral integrity, perfusion and blood flow. Stroke 9:123-126, 1978

Duara R, Margolin RA, Robertson-Tchabo EA, et al: Cerebral glucose utilization, as measured with positron emission tomography in 21 resting healthy men between the ages of 21 and 83. Brain 106:761-775, 1983

Duara R, Grady C, Haxby J, et al: Human brain glucose utilization and cognitive function in relation to age. Ann Neurol 16:700-713, 1984

Eckelman WC, Reba RC, Rzeszotarski WJ, et al: External imaging of cerebral muscarinic acetylcholine receptors. Science 223:291-293, 1984

Eckelman, WC, Eng R, Rzeszotarski WJ, et al: Use of 3-quinuclidinyl 4-

iodobenzilate as a receptor binding radiotracer. J Nucl Med 26:637-642, 1985

Farkas T, Reivich M, Alavi A, et al: The application of (18F)2-deoxy-2-fluoro-d-glucose and positron emission tomography in the study of psychiatric conditions, in Cerebral Metabolism and Neural Function. Edited by Passonneau JV, Hawkins RA, Lust WD, Welsh FA. Baltimore, Williams & Wilkins, 1980

Farkas T, Wolfe AP, Jaeger J, et al: Regional brain glucose metabolism in chronic schizophrenia: a positron emission transaxial tomographic study. Arch Gen Psychiatry 41:293-300, 1984

Flor-Henry P: On certain aspects of the localization of the cerebral systems regulating and determining emotions. Biol Psychiatry 14:677-698, 1979

Flor-Henry P, Koles ZJ: EEG studies in depression, mania and normals: evidence for partial shifts of laterality in the affective psychoses. Adv Biol Psychiatry 4:21-43, 1980

Foster NL, Chase TN, Fedio P, et al: Alzheimer's disease: focal cortical changes shown by positron emission tomography. Neurology 33:961-965, 1983

Foster NL, Chase TN, Mansi L, et al: Cortical abnormalities in Alzheimer's disease. Ann Neurol 16:649-654, 1984

Fox PT, Perlmutter JS, Raichle ME: A stereotactic method of anatomical localization for positron emission tomography. J Comput Assist Tomogr 9:141-153, 1985

Frackowiak RSJ, Gibbs JM: Cerebral metabolism and blood flow in normal and pathologic aging, in Functional Radionuclide Imaging of the Brain. Edited by Magistretti PL. New York, Raven Press, 1983

Frackowiak RSJ, Lenzi GL, Jones T, et al: Quantitative measurement of regional cerebral blood flow and oxygen metabolism in man using 15-0 and positron emission tomography: theory, procedure, and normal values. J Comput Assist Tomogr 4:727-736, 1980

Frackowiak RSJ, Pozzilli C, Legg NJ, et al: Regional cerebral oxygen supply and utilization in dementia: a clinical and physiological study with oxygen-15 and positron tomography. Brain 104:753-778, 1981

Friedland RP, Budinger TF, Ganz E, et al: Regional cerebral metabolic alterations in dementia of the Alzheimer's type: positron emission tomography with (18F)fluorodeoxyglucose. J Comput Assist Tomogr 7:590-598, 1983

Gibson, RE, Weckstein DJ, Jogoda EM, et al: The characteristic of I–125 4–IQNB and H–3 QNB in vivo and in vitro. J Nucl Med 25:214-222, 1984

Glass HI, Harper AM: Measurement of regional blood flow in cerebral cortex of man through intact skull. Br Med J 1:593, 1963

Greenberg J, Reivich M, Alavi A, et al: Metabolic mapping of functional activity in human subjects with the (18F)-fluorodeoxy-glucose technique. Science 212: 678-680, 1981

Grubb RL Jr, Raichle ME, Eichling JO, et al: The effects of changes in $PaCO_2$ on cerebral blood volume, blood flow, and vascular mean transit time. Stroke 5:630-639, 1974

Gruzelier J, Venables R: Bimodality and lateral asymmetry of skin conductants orienting activity in schizophrenics: replication and evidence of lateral asymmetry in patients with depression and disorders of personality. Biopsychiatry 8:55-73, 1974

Gur RC, Reivich M: Cognitive tasks effects on hemispheric blood flow in humans. Brain and Language 9:78-93, 1980

Gur RC, Gur RE, Obrist WD, et al: Sex and handedness difference in cerebral blood flow during rest and cognitive activity. Science 217:256-261, 1982

Gur RE, Skolnick BE, Gur RC, et al: Brain function in psychiatric disorders, I: regional cerebral blood flow in medicated schizophrenics. Arch Gen Psychiatry 40:1250-1254, 1983

Gur RE, Skolnick BE, Gur RC, et al: Brain function in psychiatric disorders, II: regional cerebral blood flow in medicated unipolar depressives. Arch Gen Psychiatry 41:695-699, 1984

Gustafson L, Risberg J, Johanson M, et al: Evaluation of organic dementia by regional cerebral blood flow measurements and clinical and psychometric methods. Monogr Neural Sci 11:111-117, 1984

Hagstadius S, Gustafson L, Risberg J: The effects of bromvincamine and vincamine on regional cerebral blood flow and mental functions in patients with multi-infarct dementia. Psychopharmacology 83:321-326, 1984

Halsey JH, Blauenstein UW, Wilson EM, et al: The rCBF response to speaking in normal subjects and the time course of alterations in patients recovering from left and right hemisphere stroke. Neurology 27:351-352, 1977

Hartmann A: Comparative randomized study of cerebral blood flow after long-term administration of pentoxifylline and co-dergocrine mesylate in patients with chronic cerebral vascular disease. Curr Med Res Opin 9:475-479, 1985

Hauge A, Nicolaysen G, Thoresen M: Acute effects of acetazolamide on cerebral blood flow in man. Acta Physiol Scand 117:233-239, 1983

Heilman KM, Van Den Abell T: Right hemispheric dominance from mediating cerebral activation. Neuropsychologia 17:315-321, 1979

Herman JH, Raese JD, Devous MD Sr, et al: EEG and cerebral blood flow in schizophrenics during rest and activation. Proceedings of the Society of Biological Psychiatry, Washington, DC, 1986

Heyman A, Patterson JL, Jones RW: Cerebral circulation and metabolism in uremia. Circulation 3:558-564, 1951

Hill TC, Holman BL, Lovitt R, et al: Initial experience with SPECT (single-photon computerized tomography) of the brain using N-isopropyl I-123 p-iodoamphetamine: concise communication. J Nucl Med 23:191-195, 1982

Hoedt-Rasmussen K, Skinhøj E, Paulson O, et al: Regional cerebral blood flow in acute apoplexy: the "luxury perfusion syndrome" of brain tissue. Arch Neurol 17:271-281, 1967

Holm S, Anderson A, Vorstrup S, et al: Cerebral blood flow measured within ten seconds using dynamic SPECT and lipophilic Tc-99m compounds, PnAO and HM-PAO. J Cereb Blood Flow Metab 5:S565-S566, 1985

Holman BL, Zimmerman RE, Schapiro JR, et al: Biodistribution and dosimetry of N-isopropyl-p-123-iodine iodoamphetamine in the primate. J Nucl Med 24:922-931, 1983

Holman BL, Lee RGL, Hill TC, et al: A comparison of two cerebral perfusion tracers, N-isopropyl-I-123 p-iodoamphetamine and I-123 HIPDM, in the human. J Nucl Med 25:25-30, 1984

Holman BL, Gibson RE, Hill TC, et al: Muscarinic acetylcholine receptors in Alzheimer's disease: in vivo imaging with I-123-labeled 3-quinuclidinyl-4-iodobenzilate and emission tomography. JAMA 254:3063-3066, 1985

Homan RW, Paulman RG, Devous MD Sr, et al: Neuropsychological function and regional cerebral blood flow in epilepsy, in Advances in Epileptology: Fifteenth Epilepsy International Symposium. Edited by Porter RJ. New York, Raven Press, 1984

Homan RW, Paulman RG, Devous MD Sr, et al: Cognitive function and regional cerebral blood flow abnormalities in partial seizures. Arch Neurol (in press)

Hommes OR, Panhuysen LH: Depression and cerebral dominance: a study of bilateral intracarotid amytal in 11 depressed patients. Psychiatrie Neurologie Neurochirurgie 74:259-270, 1971

Hounsfield GN: Computerized transverse axial scanning (tomography), I: description of system. Br J Radiology 46:1016-1021, 1973

Hoyer S: The abnormally aged brain: its blood flow and oxidative metabolism: a review—part II. Arch Gerontol Geriatr 1:195-207, 1982

Hoyer S, Oesterreich K: Blood flow and oxidative metabolism of the brain in the course of acute schizophrenia, in Cerebral Function, Metabolism and Circulation. Edited by Ingvar DH, Lassen NA. Copenhagen, Munksgaard, 1977

Ingvar DH: Abnormal distribution of cerebral activity in chronic schizophrenia: a neurophysiological interpretation, in Perspectives in Schizophrenia Research. Edited by Baxter C, Melnechuk T. New York, Raven Press, 1980

Ingvar DH, Franzen G: Abnormalities of cerebral blood flow distribution in patients with chronic schizophrenia. Acta Psychiatr Scand 50:425-462, 1974

Ingvar DH, Risberg J: Increase of regional cerebral blood flow during mental effort in normals and in patients with focal brain disorders. Exp Brain Res 3:195-211, 1967

Ingvar DH, Risberg J, Schwartz MS: Evidence of subnormal function of association cortex in presenile dementia. Neurology 10:964-974, 1975

Ingvar DH, Rosen I, Eriksson M, et al: Activation patterns induced in the dominant hemisphere by skin stimulation, in Sensory Functions of the Skin. Edited by Zotterman Y. London, Pergammon Press, 1976

Ishihara N, Meyer JS, Deshmukh VD, et al: Non-invasive measurement of regional cerebral blood flow (rCBF) in man: normal values, effect of age, cerebral dominance and activation. Neurology 27:401, 1977

Kanno I, Lassen NA: Two methods for calculating regional cerebral blood flow from emission computed tomography of inert gas concentrations. J Comput Assist Tomogr 3:71-76, 1979

Kanno I, Eumura J, Miura S, et al: HEADTOME: A hybrid emission tomograph for single-photon and positron emission imaging of the brain. J Comput Assist Tomogr 5:216-226, 1981

Kety SS, Schmidt CF: The nitrous oxide method for quantitative determination of cerebral blood flow in man: theory, procedure, and normal values. J Clin Invest 27:475-483, 1948

Koslow SH, Maas JW, Bowden CL, et al: CSF and urinary biogenic amines and metabolites in depression and mania. Arch Gen Psychiatry 40:999-1010, 1983

Kuhl DE, Edwards RQ: Image separation radioisotope scanning. Radiology 80:653-662, 1963

Kuhl DE, Edwards RQ, Ricci AR, et al: The Mark IV system for radionuclide computed tomography of the brain. Radiology 121:405-413, 1976

Kuhl DE, Barrio JR, Huang SC, et al: Quantifying local cerebral blood flow by N-isopropyl I-123 p-iodoamphetamine (IMP) tomography. J Nucl Med 23:196-203, 1982a

Kuhl DE, Metter EJ, Riege WH, et al: Effects of human aging on patterns of local cerebral glucose utilization determined by the (18F)fluorodeoxyglucose method. J Cereb Blood Flow Metab 2:163-171, 1982b

Kuhl DE, Metter EJ, Riege WH, et al: Local cerebral glucose utilization in elderly patients with depression, multiple infarct dementia and Alzheimer's disease. J Cereb Blood Flow Metab 3:S494-S495, 1983

Kuhl DE, Markham CH, Metter EJ, et al: Local cerebral glucose utilization in symptomatic and pre-symptomatic Huntington's diease. In Brain Imaging and Brain Function. Edited by Sokoloff L. New York, Raven Press, pp 199-209, 1985a

Kuhl DE, Metter J, Riege WH: Patterns of cerebral glucose utilization in depression, multiple infarct dementia, and Alzheimer's disease, in Brain Imaging and Brain Function. Edited by Sokoloff L. New York, Raven Press, 1985b

Kung HF, Tramposch KM, Blau M: A new brain perfusion imaging agent: (I–123) HIPDM: N,N,N'-trimethyl-N'-(2-hydroxy-3-methyl-5-iodobenzyl)-1,3-propanediamine. J Nucl Med 24:66-72, 1983

Kung HF, Molnar M, Billings J, et al: Synthesis and biodistribution of neutral lipid-soluble Tc-99m complexes that cross the blood-brain barrier. J Nucl Med 25:326-332, 1984

Kushner M, Rosenquist A, Alavi A, et al: Macular and peripheral visual field representation in the striate cortex demonstrated by positron emission tomography. Ann Neurol 12:89, 1982

Lassen NA, Monk O: The cerebral blood flow in man determined by the use of radioactive krypton. Acta Physiol Scand 33:30-49, 1955

Lassen NA, Ingvar DH, Skinhøj E: Brain function in blood flow. Sci Am 239:62-71, 1978

Laux BE, Raichle ME: The effect of acetazolamide on cerebral blood flow and oxygen utilization in the rhesus monkey. J Clin Invest 62:585-592, 1978

Lenzi GL, Frackowiak RSJ, Jones T, et al: $CMRO_2$ and CBF by the oxygen-15 inhalation technique: results in normal volunteers and cerebral vascular patients. Eur Neurol 20:285-290, 1981

Lever SC, Burns HD, Kervitsky TM: The preparation and biodistribution of a Tc-99m triaminodithiol complex designed to reflect regional cerebral blood flow. J Nucl Med 26:18, 1985

Lim C, Gottschalk S, Walker R, et al: Triangular SPECT system for 3-D total organ volume imaging: design concept and preliminary imaging results. IEEE Transactions in Nuclear Science NS32:741-747, 1985

Lucignani L, Nehlig A, Blasberg R, et al: Metabolic and kinetic considerations in the use of 125-I-HIPDM for quantitative measurement of regional cerebral blood flow. J Cereb Blood Flow Metab 5:86-96, 1985

Madsen MT, Hichwa RD, Nickles RD: An investigation of 11-C-methane, 13-N-nitrous oxide and 11-C-acetylene as regional cerebral blood flow agents. Phys Med Biol 26:875-882, 1981

Manuel AA: Construction of the Fermi surface from positron-annihalation measurements. Physiological Reviews 49:1525-1528, 1982

Matsui T, Hirano A: An atlas of the human brain for computerized tomography. Tokyo-New York, IGAKU-SHOIN, pp 147-151, 1978

Matthew RJ, Meyer JS, Semchuk KM, et al: Regional cerebral blood flow in depression: a preliminary report. J Clin Psychiatry 41:12 (Sec. 2, 71-72), 1980

Matthew RJ, Meyer JS, Francis DJ, et al: Regional cerebral blood flow in schizophrenia: a preliminary report. Am J Psychiatry 138:112-113, 1981

Matthew RJ, Duncan GC, Weinman ML, et al: Regional cerebral blood flow in schizophrenia. Arch Gen Psychiatry 39:1121-1124, 1982

Maximilian VA: Cortical blood flow asymmetries during monaural verbal stimulation. Brain and Language 15:1-11, 1982

Mayer-Gross W, Schlader E, Roth M: Clinical Psychiatry, third edition. London, Bailliere, Tindall and Carssell, 1969

Mazziotta JC: Human cerebral metabolism: studies in normal subjects and patients with dementia and amnesia. Ann NY Acad Sci 444:269-286, 1985

Mazziotta JC, Phelps ME, Carson RE, et al: Tomographic mapping of human cerebral metabolism: auditory stimulation. Neurology 32:921-937, 1982

Mazziotta JC, Phelps ME, Carson RE: Tomographic mapping of human cerebral metabolism: subcortical responses to auditory and visual stimulation. Neurology 34:825-828, 1984

McAfee JG, Subramanian M, Esser PD: Appendix: radionuclides used for imaging, in: Clinical Scintillation Imaging, Second Edition. Edited by Freeman LM, Johnson PM. New York, Grune & Stratton, 1975

Melamed E, Lavy S, Portnoy Z: Regional cerebral blood flow response to hypocapnia in the contralateral hemisphere of patients with acute cerebral infarction. Stroke 6:503-508, 1975

Mesulam MM: A cortical network for directed attention and unilateral neglect. Ann Neurol 10:309-325, 1981

Meyer JS: Improved method for non-invasive measurement of regional cerebral blood flow by 133-Xenon inhalation, part II: measurements in health and disease. Stroke 9:205-210, 1978

Meyer JS, Sakai F, Deshmukh V, et al: Testing cerebrovascular functional reserve using 133-Xenon inhalation measurements of rCBF in health and disease, in Cerebral Function Metabolism and Circulation. Edited by Ingvar DH, Lassen NA. Copenhagen, Munksgaard Press, 1977

Meyer JS, Sakai F, Yamaguchi F, et al: Regional changes in cerebral blood flow during standard behavioral activation in patients with disorders of speech and mentation compared to normal volunteers. Brain and Language 9:61-77, 1980

Meyer JS, Hayman L, Amano T, et al: Mapping local blood flow of human brain by CT scanning during stable xenon inhalation. Stroke 12:426-436, 1981

Myslobodsky MS, Horesch N: Bilateral electrodermal activity in depressive patients. Biol Psychiatry 6:111-120, 1978

Obrist WD, Thompson HK Jr, King CH, et al: Determination of regional cerebral blood flow by inhalation of 133-Xenon. Circ Res 20:124-135, 1967

Obrist WD, Thompson HK Jr, Wang HS, et al: Regional cerebral blood flow estimated by 133-Xenon inhalation. Stroke 6:245-256, 1975

Paulman RG, Raese JD, Herman JR, et al: Neuropsychological correlates of structural and metabolic brain abnormalities in schizophrenia. Paper presented at the Annual Meeting of the American Psychological Association, Los Angeles, August 1985

Paulman RG, Devous MD Sr, Gregory RR, et al: Hypofrontality and cognitive impairment in schizophrenia. Dynamic single-photon tomography and neuropsychological assessment of schizophrenic brain function. Arch Gen Psychiatry (in press)

Perry EK, Tomlinson BE, Blessed G, et al: Correlation of cholinergic abnormalities with senile plaques and mental test scores in senile dementia. Br J Med 2:1457-1459, 1978

Phelps ME, Mazziotta JC, Kuhl DE, et al: Tomographic mapping of human cerebral metabolism: visual stimulation and deprivation. Neurology 31:517-529, 1981

Phelps ME, Huang S-C, Hoffman EJ, et al: An analysis of signal amplification using small detectors in positron emission tomography. J Comput Assist Tomogr 6:551-565, 1982

Powers WJ, Raichle ME: PET: the new focus of nuclear medicine? J Nucl Med 26:1499-1500, 1985

Prohovnik I, Hakansson K, Risberg J: Observations on the functional significance of regional blood flow in "resting" normal subjects. Neuropsychologia 18:203-217, 1980

Radon J: On the determination of functions by their integral values along certain manifolds. Leipzig, Saechsische Akadmie der Wissenschaften. Berichte uber die Verhandlungen 69:262-271, 1917

Rapoport SI, Duara R, Haxby JV: The need for the external validation of assessment instruments for evaluating pharmacologically induced change in Alzheimer's disease. Psychopharmacol Bull 20:466-471, 1984

Reivich M, Cobbs W, Rosenquist A, et al: Abnormalities in local cerebral glucose metabolism in patients with visual field defects. J Cereb Blood Flow Metab (Suppl 1)1:471-472, 1981

Reivich M, Alavi A, Gur RC, et al: Determination of local cerebral glucose metabolism in humans: methodology and applications to the study of sensory and cognitive stimuli, in Brain Imaging and Brain Function. Edited by Sokoloff L. New York, Raven Press, 1985

Risberg J: Regional cerebral blood flow measurements by 133-Xenon-inhalation: methodology and applications in neuropsychology and psychiatry. Brain and Language 9:934, 1980

Risberg J: Cerebral blood flow in dementias. Dan Med Bull 32 (Suppl 1):48-51, 1985

Risberg J, Ingvar DH: Patterns of activation in the gray matter of the dominant hemisphere during memorization and reasoning: a study of regional cerebral blood flow changes during psychological testing in a group of neurologically normal subjects. Brain 96:737-756, 1973

Risberg J, Ali Z, Wilson EM, et al: Regional cerebral blood flow by 133-Xenon inhalation: preliminary evaluation of an initial slope index in patients with unstable flow compartments. Stroke 6:142-148, 1975a

Risberg J, Halsey JH, Wills EL, et al: Hemispheric specialization in normal man studied by bilateral measurements of the regional cerebral blood flow: a study with the 133-Xenon inhalation technique. Brain 98:511-524, 1975b

Risberg J, Maximilian AV, Prohovnik I: Changes of cortical activity patterns during habituation to a reasoning test: a study with the 133-Xe inhalation technique for measurement of regional cerebral blood flow. Neuropsychologia 15:793-798, 1977

Rogers RL, Meyer JS, Mortel KF, et al: Decreased cerebral blood flow precedes multi-infarct dementia, but follows senile dementia of Alzheimer type. Neurology 36:1-16, 1986

Ross ED, Rush AJ: Diagnosis and neuroanatomical correlates of depression in brain-damaged patients. Arch Gen Psychiatry 38:1344-1354, 1981

Rosser MN, Emson PC, Mountjoy CQ, et al: Neurotransmitters of the cerebral cortex in senile dementia of the Alzheimer's type, in The Aging Brain: Physiological and Pathophysiological Aspects. Exp Brain Res (Suppl)5:153-157, 1982

Roth M: Diagnoses of senile and related forms of dementia, in Alzheimer's Disease: Senile Dementia and Related Disorders. Edited by Katzman R, Terry RD, Bick KL. New York, Raven Press, 1978

Rush AJ, Schlesser MA, Stokely EM, et al: Cerebral blood flow in depression and mania. Psychopharmacol Bull 18:6-8, 1982

Scheinberg P, Stead EA: The cerebral blood flow in male subjects as measured by the nitrous oxide technique: normal values for blood flow, oxygen utilization, glucose utilization and peripheral resistance, with observations on the effect of tilting and anxiety. J Clin Invest 28:1163-1171, 1949

Shaw TG, Mortel KF, Meyer JS, et al: Cerebral blood flow changes in benign aging and cerebrovascular disease. Neurology 34:855-862, 1984

Sims NR, Bowen DM, Smith CCT, et al: Glucose metabolism and acetylcholine synthesis in relation to neuronal activity in Alzheimer's disease. Lancet 1:333-336, 1980

Smith GT, Stokely EM, Lewis MH, et al: An error analysis of the double-integral method for calculating brain blood perfusion from inert gas clearance data. J Cereb Blood Flow Metab 4:61-67, 1984

Spitzer RL, Endicott J, Robbins E: Research diagnostic criteria: rationale and reliability. Arch Gen Psychiatry 35:773-782, 1978

Stoddart HF, Stoddart HA: A new development in single gamma transaxial tomography: Union Carbide focused collimator scanner. IEEE Transactions in Nuclear Sciences NS26:2710-2712, 1979

Stokely EM, Sveinsdottir E, Lassen NA, et al: A single-photon dynamic computer-assisted tomograph (DCAT) for imaging brain function in mulitple cross-sections. J Comput Assist Tomogr 4:230-240, 1980

Stokely EM, Totah J, Homan RW, et al: Interactive graphics method of regional quantification of tomographic brain blood flow images. Proceedings of MEDCOMP, pp 316-318, 1982

Sumiya H, Matsuda H, Seki H, et al: Quantitative cerebral blood flow measurements using N-isopropyl-p-I-123-iodoamphetamine and single photon emission computed tomography with rotating gamma camera. J Nucl Med 26:106, 1985

Sveinsdottir E, Larsen B, Rommer P, et al: A multidetector scintillation camera with 254 channels. J Nucl Med 18:168-174, 1977

Tachibana H, Meyer JS, Kitagawa Y, et al: Effects of aging on cerebral blood flow in dementia. J Am Geriatr Soc 32:114-120, 1984

Ter-Pogossian MM: PET, SPECT and NMRI: competing or complimentary disciplines? J Nucl Med 26:1487-1498, 1985

Terry RD: Brain disease in aging, especially senile dementia, in Neural Aging and Its Implications in Human Neurological Pathology. Edited by Terry RD, Bolis CL, Toffano G. New York, Raven Press, 1982

Terry RD, Peck A, deTerasa R, et al: Some morphometric aspects of the brain in senile dementia of the Alzheimer's type. Ann Neurol 10:184-192, 1981

Tomlinson BE: The structural and quantitative aspects of the dementias, in Biochemistry of Dementia. Edited by Roberts PJ. Chichester, England, Wiley, 1980

Trevarthen C: Brain bisymmetry and the role of the corpus callosum in behavior and conscious experience, in Cerebral Interhemispheric Relations. Edited by Cernacvek J, Podivisky F. Bratislava, The Publishing House of the Slovak Academy of Science, 1972

Uytdenhoef P, Portlange P, Jacguy J, et al: Regional cerebral blood flow and lateralized and hemispheric dysfunction in depression. Br J Psychiatry 143:128-132, 1983

Volkert WA, Hoffman TJ, Seger RM, et al: 99m Tc-propylene amine oxime (99m Tc-PnAO): a potential brain radiopharmaceutical. Eur J Nucl Med 9:511-516, 1984

Vorstrup S, Henriksen L, Paulson OB: Effect of acetazolamide on cerebral blood flow and cerebral metabolic rate for oxygen. J Clin Invest 74:1634-1639, 1984

Wagner HN Jr: PET: the new focus of nuclear medicine? Reply. J Nucl Med 26:1500-1501, 1985

Wagner HN, Burns HD, Dannals RF, et al: Imaging dopamine receptors in the human brain by positron tomography. Science 22:1264-1266, 1983

Wastek GJ, Yamamura HI: Biochemical characterization of the muscarinic cholinergic receptor in human brain: alteration in Huntington's disease. Mol Pharmacol 14:768-780, 1978

Wehr TA, Wirz-Justice A: Circadian rhythm mechanisms in affective illness and in antidepressant drug action. Pharmacopsychiatria 15:31-39, 1982

Weinberger DR, Berman KF, Zec RF: Physiologic dysfunction of dorsolateral prefrontal cortex in schizophrenia, I: regional cerebral blood flow evidence. Arch Gen Psychiatry 43:114-124, 1986

Wexler BE: Cerebral laterality in psychiatry: a review of the literature. Am J Psychiatry 137:279-291, 1980

White P, Hiley CR, Goodhardt MJ, et al: Neocortical cholinergic neurons in elderly people. Lancet 2:668-671, 1977

Widen L, Bergstrom M, Blomqvist G, et al: Glucose metabolism in patients with schizophrenia: emission computed tomography measurements with 11-C-glucose. J Cereb Blood Flow Metab 1:S455-S456, 1981

Wilkinson IMS, Boll JWD, du Boulay GH, et al: Regional blood flow in the normal cerebral hemispheres. J Neurol Neurosurg Psychiatry 32:367-378, 1969

Winchell HS, Baldwin RM, Lin TH: Development of I-123 iodophenyalkyl amines in rat brain. J Nucl Med 21:940-946, 1980

Yamaguchi F, Meyer JS, Yamamoto M, et al: Noninvasive regional cerebral blood flow measurements in dementia. Arch Neurol 37:410-418, 1980

Yamamoto YL, Thompson CJ, Meyer E, et al: Dynamic positron emission tomography for study of cerebral hemodynamics in a cross-section of the head using positron-emitting 68-Ga-EDTA and 77-Kr. J Comput Assist Tomogr 1:43-56, 1977

Zemcov A, Risberg J, Barclay LL, et al: Diagnosis of Alzheimer's disease and multi-infarct dementia by rCBF compared to clinical classification. Monographs in Neural Psychiatry 11:104-106, 1984

Chapter 5

Positron Emission Tomography: Measuring the Metabolic and Neurochemical Characteristics of the Living Human Nervous System

Henry H. Holcomb, M.D.
Jonathan Links, Ph.D.
Caroline Smith, Ph.D.
Dean Wong, M.D.

History of PET Technology and Its Relation to Biological Psychiatry

In 1965, Schildkraut (Schildkraut 1965) and Bunney (Bunney and Davis 1965) proposed a general hypothesis regarding the roles of catecholamines in affective illness. That hypothesis became the springboard for biological research that continues to this day. Much information regarding monoamine regulation of mood has been obtained from urine, plasma, and cerebrospinal fluid (CSF) measurements. These are, however, biochemically distant measurements with respect to behavior. Most of the nerve cells that contribute to CSF monoamine metabolites cannot be directly implicated as neural substrates for mood regulation. It is, furthermore, not possible to specify to what extent a given group of cells changes its activity in association with behavior when relying on CSF measurements.

235

In 1979, Reivich (Reivich et al. 1979) and Phelps (Phelps et al. 1979) first described a noninvasive method of quantitatively measuring local rates of cerebral glucose utilization (milligrams glucose/100 g brain tissue/minute) in conscious, behaving human beings. By combining a rigorously developed metabolic model for brain glucose metabolism (Sokoloff et al. 1977), positron emission tomography (PET) (Ter-Pogossian et al. 1975, 1978a, 1978b), and radionuclide chemistry (fluorine 18 2-D-deoxyglucose, FDG) (Gallagher et al. 1977; Ido et al. 1978; Tewson et al. 1978), these investigators provided the clinical neuroscience research community with its first glimpse of a biochemically proximal measurement system. With the subsequent development of 'fast' or dynamic cerebral blood flow studies (Herscovitch et al. 1983; Raichle et al. 1983; Raichle 1985) we gained a new opportunity for studying physiobehavioral relationships in normal (Fox and Raichle 1984; Fox et al. 1985a, 1985c, 1986) and abnormal (Baxter et al. 1987; Volkow et al. 1986b; Wong et al. 1986c) diagnostic groups. Finally, quantitative PET determinations of neuroreceptor density and occupancy states are providing direct windows into the complex subcellular interactions that regulate abnormal behavior, drug responsiveness, and pharmacobehavioral relationships (Bice et al. 1986; Brodie et al. 1986; Frost et al. 1985, 1986; Persson et al. 1985; Sedvall et al. 1986).

From the early 1960s to the present, clinical neurobiologists have been frustrated by their inability to use biochemical measurements of body fluid monoamine metabolites to assess specific behaviors and pathological states more sensitively, reliably, and physiologically. PET offers the promise of localization in multiple domains (metabolic, receptor, neurotransmitter, and enzymatic). That promise has been long in coming.

What Is PET? What Does It Do?

In an effort to better understand how the brain's myriad cells interact with one another, investigators have created methods of measuring the metabolic activities and neurochemical properties of brain regions in conscious, behaving human beings and animals. These methods broadly fall under the label of emission computed tomography. Both single photon emission computed tomography (SPECT) and positron emission tomography (PET) provide the clinical neurobiologist with quantitative, physiologically relevant information. The regional chemical composition and metabolic activity of the brain in the context of complex behavioral and pharmacological conditions can be elucidated with the aid of these technologies. Psychiatrists, neurologists, psychologists, neurosurgeons, and others are now able to systematically study a subject multiple times with a variety of radiotracers. From these studies we can generate metabolic activity maps of the brain in association with sensory, cognitive, motor, and pharmacologic interventions. Similarly, we can measure and characterize a variety of neuroreceptor systems, with and without agonist/antagonist blockade; these include dopamine (DA), serotonin, acetylcholine, benzodiazepine, and opiate binding sites.

Clinical brain imaging is the product of a highly productive marriage between the technologies of digital image acquisition, nuclear chemistry, metabolic modeling, biochemistry, physiology, and neuroscience. This chapter describes how some of these component parts support the generation and interpretation of useful information regarding regional brain function as determined by PET and quantitative autoradiography.

Advantages and Applications

What Do We Want to Know About the Nervous System and How Can We Learn It?

Information regarding the central nervous system is usefully divided into four general categories: 1) anatomic—fiber pathway topology, morphology, growth patterns, differentiation, and synaptic specificity; 2) biochemical—structural and metabolic characteristics of subcellular neuronal systems including enzymes (e.g., hexokinase) and neurotransmitters; 3) physiological—hemodynamic and electrochemical; and 4) behavioral—sensory, motor, cognitive, affective, and appetitive. Ideally, we would like to know the static and dynamic characteristics of all subsystems supporting a given behavior. That goal requires us to make appropriate measurements in our subject at the time he or she is performing or experiencing the task/condition/state of interest.

For example, when a person takes a dose of amphetamine several things happen in the nervous system to cause feelings of euphoria/dysphoria, anxiety, restlessness, or hyperactivity. The clinical investigator presiding over a study of amphetamine neuropharmacology would like to measure the firing rate of various neurons in multiple brain regions, the release and metabolism of multiple neurotransmitters, regional second by second changes in glucose/oxygen utilization, local changes in tissue pH, and focal modifications in blood flow. All measurements should be made in real time, in association with constant monitoring of CNS/peripheral amphetamine distribution. The subject's task performance could also be quantitatively tracked, measured, stored, displayed, and analyzed. Most components of this experiment are now operational (Brodie et al. 1986).

How Can We Noninvasively Measure Significant Neurophysiological Processes?

In 1948, Kety and Schmidt produced in vivo cerebral energy metabolism measurements using the nitrous oxide technique. This method, however, measures the average rates of energy metabolism in the brain as a whole and does not provide regional information. The imaginary experiment described above can now, when performed with PET technology, provide detailed, high-resolution, biochemically and metabolically useful information about specific brain regions.

Consider the experiment in pieces. First, the subject's dopamine system can be probed with L-dopa tagged with the positron-emitting radionuclide fluorine-18 (Garnett et al. 1983). This radiotracer provides estimations of dopamine synthesis and release in the rapid turnover pools located in the striatum and frontal cortex. Dopamine-receptor occupancy by the endogenous neurotransmitter can be estimated by subsequently administering raclopride (Farde et al. 1986) labeled with positron-emitting carbon-11 (^{11}C). Quantitative estimates of neurotransmitter synthesis and release and of receptor occupancy are not established at this time. In contrast, measurements of cerebral oxygen metabolism, cerebral blood flow and blood volume (using oxygen-15-labeled water) are standard and routine operations at several PET centers (Raichle 1983). Brain-tissue pH determination is also available using ^{11}C-labeled dimethyloxazolidinedione. This agent is especially useful in assessing pathological processes that chronically alter tissue metabolism, such as brain tumor, infection, or infarction. Chronic amphetamine abuse may or may not produce focal abnormalities in brain pH, but degenerative disorders (multiple sclerosis) and neoplastic processes appear to characteristically modify tissue pH by reducing local oxygen-extraction fraction (OEF) (Buxton et al. 1985).

Regional (local) measurements of cerebral blood flow (rCBF) and cerebral glucose utilization (rCMRgl) constitute the day-to-day workhorses of cerebral metabolic research. Though there is no method at present for measuring electrical activity of discrete neurons in man noninvasively, rCMRgl is an excellent representation of local synaptic activity. The measurement of local glucose metabolism provides an accurate representation of neuronal activity and as such "captures" the functional metabolic profile of the CNS as it exists in the 10–15-minute period after administration of radiolabeled 2-deoxy-D-glucose (2DG). ^{11}C and ^{18}F are both used to label 2DG (Huang et al. 1980b; Reivich et al. 1979, 1982, 1985).

The principal advantage of using oxygen-15 (^{15}O)- labeled water is that one can perform multiple blood-flow studies in rapid back-to-back fashion in a short period of time owing to the short half-life of oxygen-15

(2.07 min) and the model used to calculate blood flow; a dynamic scanner is necessary. The radioactive decay characteristics of carbon-11 (half-life, 20.4 minutes) and fluorine-18 (half-life, 109.7 minutes) preclude more than three CDG or two FDG studies per day (Brooks et al. 1987). When measuring the cerebral metabolic rate for glucose one is constrained by the Sokoloff model regarding the frequency of tracer infusions. One could legitimately start an additional study 45 minutes after a previous 2DG administration if appropriate steps are taken to correct for residual tracer retention. When using ^{11}C-2DG, one can follow one study with another, five half-lives of time after the first infusion (that is, about 100 minutes), without consideration of previous tracer infusions.

Returning to the imaginary subject in the amphetamine experiment, we can appreciate the practicality of performing multiple rCBF studies over a two-hour period of time, before and after drug administration. By coupling the scan to a variety of other measures, including blood amphetamine levels, task performance, and subjective mood scales, we could reasonably expect to obtain an informative repeated measures analysis of the drug's influence on brain metabolism and behavior. From such data one might learn which blood flow profiles were associated with various mood and performance changes. In this way, clinical research questions previously addressed only in animal studies are now given a more complete examination.

How Is PET Most Useful?

Investigators learn the most about the things they know the most about. That is to say, it is often more fruitful to ask a focused and highly constrained question than to enter new and uncharted territory, where the landscape is new and difficult to understand. This methodological strategy also applies to PET research. PET metabolic studies are most useful in diagnosing central nervous system illnesses and treatment strategies that are complicated by overlapping clinical features and by similar clinical profiles.

Two examples illustrate this point. First, if a 60-year-old patient exhibits forgetfulness and an acute personality change the consulting physician may reasonably wonder whether depression or Alzheimer's disease is the underlying pathologic process. PET measurements of rCMRgl in this patient will most likely reveal hypometabolism in the temporal, frontal, and parietal regions if the patient is afflicted with Alzheimer's disease (McGeer et al. 1986a) (also see Figures 1, 2, and 3). Depression is not likely to be associated with multiple hypometabolic foci, but rather with a right temporal hypometabolic pattern (Post et al. 1987).

Second, radiation treatment of brain tumors often generates tissue

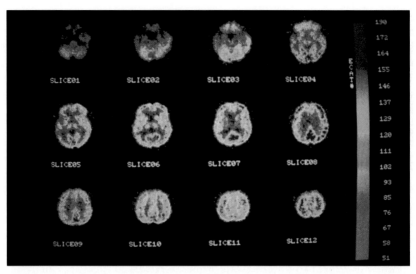

FIGURE 1. 62-year-old man with a two-year history of progressively worsening memory: the presumptive diagnosis is Alzheimer's disease. His primary symptom is word-finding difficulty. Note the marked left temporal lobe hypometabolic asymmetry in the top two rows of images. (Courtesy of Dr. Barry Gordon, Neurology Department, Johns Hopkins Medical Institutes, Baltimore, Maryland)

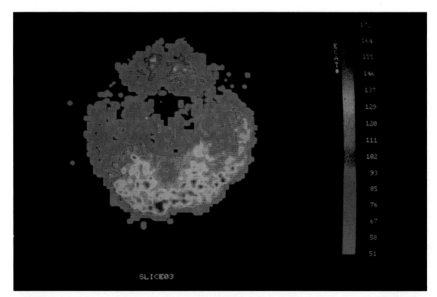

FIGURE 2. Same patient described in Figure 1; PET scan 32 mm above and parallel to the canthomeatal axis. (Courtesy of Dr. Barry Gordon, Neurology Department, Johns Hopkins Medical Institutes, Baltimore, Maryland)

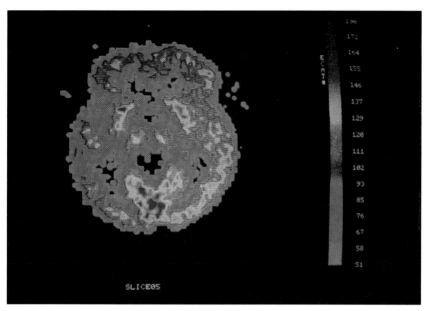

FIGURE 3. Same patient described in Figure 1; PET scan 64 mm above and parallel to the canthomeatal axis.(Courtesy of Dr. Barry Gordon, Neurology Department, Johns Hopkins Medical Institutes, Baltimore, Maryland)

necrosis. X-ray computed tomography (XCT) scans do not readily distinguish necrotic from tumor tissue. PET studies of [^{11}C]-methionine uptake, with and without oral phenylalanine pretreatment, indicate a sharp distinction between tumor and necrotic tissue (Figure 4). The former will not retain [^{11}C]-methionine in phenylalanine-pretreated patients, whereas tissue damaged by radiation necrosis will sequester the radiotracer; this is presumably due to loss of blood–brain barrier integrity (Bergstrom et al. 1987; O'Tuama et al. 1987; Wagner 1986). Brain-tumor studies are further improved by using rCMRgl to grade the neoplasm (DiChiro et al. 1985).

These two clinical examples suggest that PET is most useful as a functional diagnostic probe. Unlike MRI or CT, PET provides local functional information. If we know what to look for and how to interpret it, then we can ask highly sophisticated questions about neural activity networks and cellular function with this new methodology.

Basic Principles

A radiotracer is only useful if we know its *metabolic fate*. This fundamental principle has several pieces. First we need to know the physiologi-

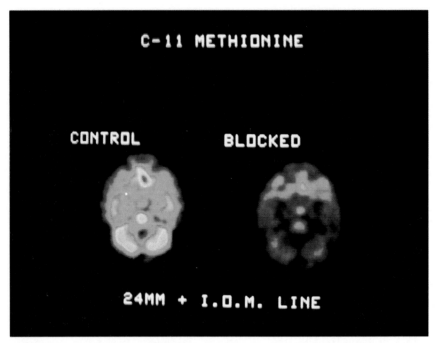

FIGURE 4.   Glioblastoma PET image acquired with [^{11}C]methionine in the *(left)* unblocked (no oral phenylalanine pretreatment) and *(right)* radiotracer uptake blocked (20 milligrams/kilogram) conditions. (Courtesy of Dr. L. O'Tuama, Nuclear Medicine Division, Johns Hopkins Medical Institutes, Baltimore, Maryland)

cal disposition of the biologically active substance and its metabolites. For example, spiroperidol and raclopride bind to D2 dopamine receptors; carfentanil binds to mu opiate receptors; glucose (deoxyglucose) is used primarily by nerve terminals in maintaining ionic gradients through the generation of adenosine triphosphate; oxygen-15-labeled water reflects the dynamic properties of blood and oxygen; leucine is used primarily in protein synthesis whereas methionine is used in both protein synthesis and as a methyl group donor. A tracer's metabolic fate is defined in terms of tissue/cellular specificity and its dynamic properties. We need to know where it goes, how fast it gets there, how long it stays there, what happens to it while it resides there, how fast it leaves, what form it takes when it leaves (is it carrying the radioactive label), and where it goes in its various modified states when it does leave (water or fat, excreted or stored).

Initially, these questions are answered by rodent and primate studies. Rodent studies rely heavily on *autoradiographic* analysis of tracer concentrations in tissues and continue to contribute fundamental information for the quantitative 2DG model (Sokoloff et al. 1977). Primate studies have been used heavily for neuroreceptor modeling (Arnett et al. 1986; Perlmutter et al. 1986) and are usually performed with PET to determine tissue tracer concentration.

This section describes the two primary technical foundations of metabolic modeling: 1) PET tracer and detector physics instrumentation and 2) physiological/biochemical modeling of tracer dynamics. It is important to appreciate that PET detection/imaging systems only provide numbers, which in turn become pictures of how many radioactive particles are located in a given brain region. An image is only useful if the user can *interpret* the numbers that generate the image he or she is looking at, and interpretation is entirely dependent on the model that is applied to the tracer being used. The model is simply our best effort to describe what a cell, or group of cells, is doing with the molecules we are trying to understand.

The Physics and Instrumentation of PET

The Physics of Positron Decay

The power of PET comes from the physics, chemistry, and biochemistry inherent in positron decay and the positron-emitters of interest. Unstable nuclides with an excess of protons in the nucleus can undergo radioactive decay via positron emission. A positron is an antimatter electron; it has the same rest mass as an electron, but a +1 charge. Nuclides undergoing positron decay increase their neutron-to-proton ratio. A given radionuclide which undergoes positron decay gives off positrons with a range of energies up to some maximum determined by the radionuclide. The average positron energy is about one-third of the maximum.

Once emitted, the positron travels several millimeters in tissue, depositing its kinetic energy in the process of ionization of atoms in the tissue. When the positron expends all of its kinetic energy and is at rest, it meets up with a "free" (i.e., unbound) electron in the tissue. Since the positron is an antimatter electron, mutual annihilation occurs. In order to obey the law of conservation of energy, two 511 KeV gamma ray photons appear in the place of the positron and electron. (From $E=mc^2$, 511 KeV is the energy equivalent to the rest mass of a positron or electron.) In order to obey the law of conservation of momentum (equal to mass $\times$ velocity), which is zero at the point of annihilation, the two 511 KeV photons are emitted exactly 180 degrees back-to-back. It is these two photons which are detected in PET (Figure 5).

The detection of the "annihilation photons," rather than the positron itself, fundamentally limits the achievable spatial resolution in PET by two processes (Figure 6). First, the positron travels some distance in tissue

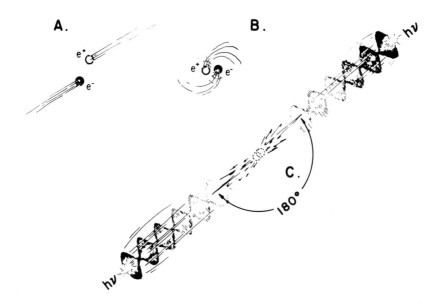

FIGURE 5.   A: A positron approaches an electron; B: The two particles interact; C: A pair of photons is created, each having about 511 keV energy and traveling colinearily. (Courtesy of Dr. M.M. Ter-Pogossian, Washington University School of Medicine, St. Louis, Missouri; "PET Instrumentation," in Positron Emission Tomography, M. Reivich and A. Alavi [eds], New York, Alan R. Liss Inc., pp. 48-49, 1986)

before depositing all its kinetic energy, but the PET scanner only detects the site of annihilation; spatial resolution cannot be better than this "positron range." (Radionuclides with lower maximum positron energies permit better resolution than those with higher positron energies; higher energies correspond to longer distances traveled in tissue.) Second, the positron is not always at rest at the time of annihilation; this net momentum is reflected in noncolinearity. The angular deviation from 180 degrees is determined by the net momentum of the positron and electron. The larger the diameter of the PET scanner, the greater this effect on spatial resolution. There is general agreement that these two processes limit the achievable spatial resolution to about 2 to 3 mm. Figures 7, 8, and 9 illustrate the resolution available with present 5-mm within-plane FWHM resolution (supplied as a courtesy of CTI, Knoxville, Tennessee).

PET Scanners: How Do They Work?

A PET scanner can be conceptually reduced to a ring of radiation

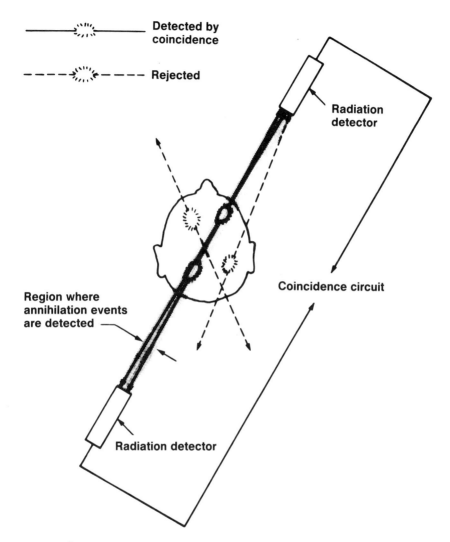

FIGURE 6. PET uses this form of electronic coincidence collimation; without a coincidence circuit a pair of photons is not detected. (Courtesy of Dr. M.M. Ter-Pogossian, Washington University School of Medicine, St. Louis, Missouri; "PET Instrumentation," in Positron Emission Tomography, M. Reivich and A. Alavi [eds], New York, Alan R. Liss Inc., pp. 48-49, 1986)

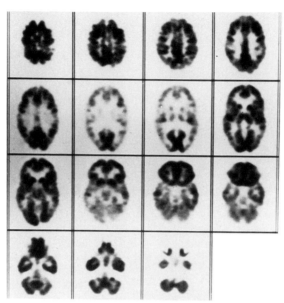

FIGURE 7. High resolution PET FDG brain images from a normal human subject, 5 mm FWHM within plane resolution, transverse. (Courtesy of CTI, Knoxville, Tennessee; and UCLA PET Facility, Los Angeles, California)

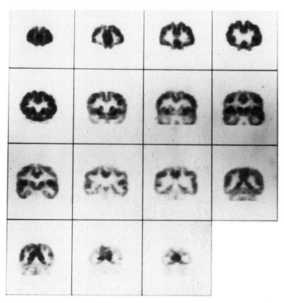

FIGURE 8. High resolution PET FDG brain images from a normal human subject, 5 mm FWHM within plane resolution, coronal. (Courtesy of CTI, Knoxville, Tennessee; and UCLA PET Facility, Los Angeles, California)

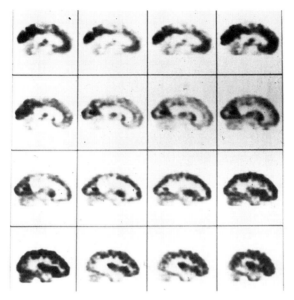

FIGURE 9. High resolution PET FDG brain images from a normal human subject, 5 mm FWHM within plane resolution, sagittal. (Courtesy of CTI, Knoxville, Tennessee; and UCLA PET Facility, Los Angeles, California)

detectors surrounding a patient. These detectors count the number of emitted 511 KeV photons from a large number of angles around the patient, and use these data to reconstruct a cross-sectional image of the distribution of the positron-emitting radiopharmaceutical in the patient (Ter-Pogossian et al. 1975, 1978a, 1978b, 1981, 1982).

The most commonly used detectors are crystals which scintillate (give off light) when energy is deposited in them via interactions between the 511 KeV photons and molecules in the crystal lattice. Early PET scanners used sodium iodide crystals, which are the crystals of choice in conventional nuclear medicine instrumentation. Newer PET scanners have switched to bismuth germinate crystals. These crystals are denser than sodium iodide, and are thus more efficient at detecting the 511 KeV photons, which are of higher energy than generally encountered in conventional nuclear medicine. Some of the newest PET scanners use cesium fluoride (Ter-Pogossian et al. 1982) or barium fluoride crystals, in conjunction with a technique called "time of flight," to be described below (Figure 10).

While it would be possible to construct the PET scanner so that each detector worked alone to count individual photons, it is more efficient to simultaneously detect both of the annihilation photons in opposing detec-

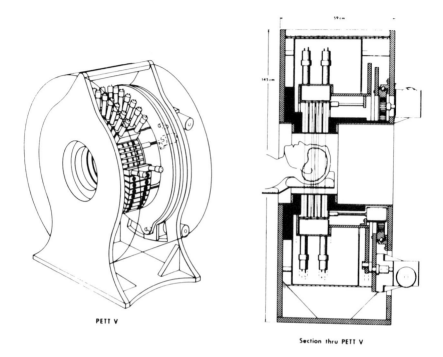

PETT V

Section thru PETT V

FIGURE 10.   *Left:* a simplified drawing of PETT V scanner. *Right:* a section through PETT V. (Courtesy of M.M. Ter-Pogossian, Journal of Computer Assisted Tomography 2:539-544, 1978)

tors. This requires the presence of a *coincidence circuit.* Opposing detectors in the ring are electronically coupled "in coincidence." When two opposing crystals simultaneously detect 511 KeV photons, an annihilation event is assumed to have occurred along the line joining the two detectors. A PET scan consists, in essence, of the acquisition of a large number of these *coincidence lines* (Figure 11).

In theory, the cross-sectional image could be reconstructed by simply retracing all of the acquired coincidence lines. Wherever they are superimposed in the image and reinforced, a significant amount of radioactivity would be presumed to be present at that site. In practice, the data are reoriented so as to appear to have come from a CT scanner; the image is then reconstructed with a standard filtered back-projection algorithm. As with other cross-sectional reconstruction techniques, perhaps the most important consideration is the choice of reconstruction filter. A "sharp" filter will preserve spatial resolution in the reconstructed image, but will amplify the random noise in the image. (This noise is the result of the statistical nature of radioactive decay.) Conversely, a "softer" filter will

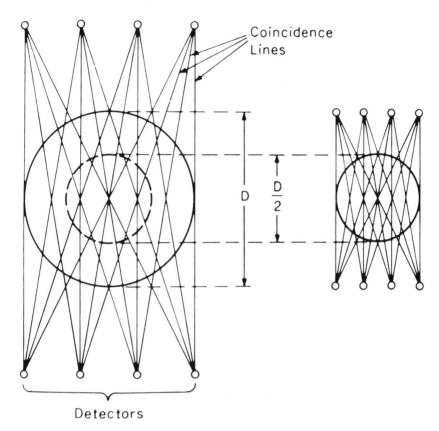

Detectors

FIGURE 11. Coincidence lines are more efficiently measured if the maximum field size of the system is matched to the size of the region imaged. (Courtesy of M.M. Ter-Pogossian, Journal of Computer Assisted Tomography 2:539-544, 1978)

reduce both spatial resolution and statistical noise. This is because both statistical noise and the edges of objects are rich in high spatial frequencies. A filter which attenuates high frequencies in the data will simultaneously reduce noise and smear object edges. This inevitably results in resolution degradation. The choice of an appropriate filter is dependent on the required spatial resolution and statistical precision of the study (Hoffman et al. 1983, 1984) (Figure 12).

A major refinement of the reconstruction algorithm is the use of *time-of-flight* information (Ter-Pogossian et al. 1981). The two annihilation photons differ in their arrival times at the two opposing detectors, depending on the proximity of the two detectors to the annihilation site. This difference in photon arrival time can be used to position the annihilation event along the coincidence line. Since the photons are traveling at

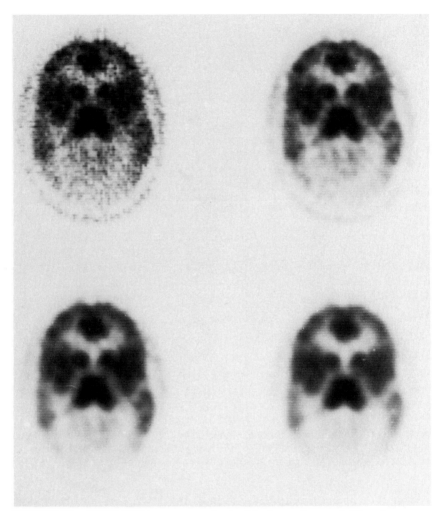

FIGURE 12. NMSP PET images acquired with sharp *(upper left)* and progressively softer *(lower left, upper right,* and *lower right)* filters. (Courtesy of Dr. J. Links, Johns Hopkins Medical Institutes, Nuclear Medicine Division, Baltimore, Maryland)

the speed of light, very fast scintillation crystals and electronics are required. ("Fast" scintillators, such as cesium fluoride and barium fluoride, give off a large fraction of their light in a very short time after energy has been deposited in them.) Available PET scanners have arrival time resolution on the order of several hundred picoseconds, which limits spatial resolution to several centimeters. Thus, time-of-flight information is used

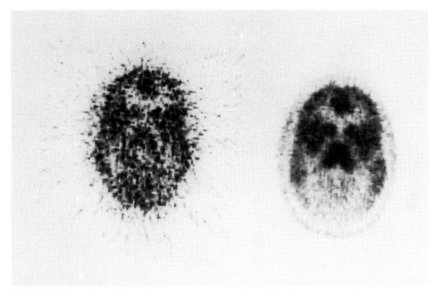

FIGURE 13. Signal level alters image quality. The left and right images have equal resolution but the left image was produced with one minute of counts and the right images with 30 minutes of counts. Brief measurement schedules produce images with high noise due to poor statistical accuracy. (Courtesy of Dr. J. Links, Johns Hopkins Medical Institutes, Nuclear Medicine Division, Baltimore, Maryland)

in conjunction with filtered back-projection in the reconstruction process, as it does not provide adequate spatial resolution by itself.

The scanner design factor which has the major influence on achievable spatial resolution is the crystal's cross-sectional dimensions. A new technique called *signal amplification* uses extremely small crystals (Phelps et al. 1982). This produces an increase in the signal levels of the higher spatial frequencies. This increased signal level can be used to either increase the spatial resolution in the reconstructed image with no increase in noise, or to decrease the noise with no deterioration in spatial resolution (Figure 13).

Factors Affecting Quantification

The principal aim of PET research is not the production of an image per se, but the measurement of physiologic and biochemical processes. The conversion of an image into physiologically meaningful quantities is a complex, multistep function. The first step is to convert observed "count rate" into true radioactivity. A metabolic model (Huang and Phelps 1986) is then invoked to describe the biological fate of the radioactive tracer in space and time. From this model, the physiologic variables of interest are computed.

From a physics point of view, there are many factors which affect the quantification of absolute radioactivity. These include: 1) attenuation of photons by tissue, 2) transaxial spatial resolution and effective slice thickness of the PET scanner, 3) detection of scattered photons, 4) accidental counting of "random" (nonpaired) photons in coincidence, and 5) "noise" resulting from the statistical nature of radioactive decay.

Attenuation.   Introductory discussions of this and other technical aspects of PET instrumentation are available in the review chapter by Hoffman and Phelps (1986).

The annihilation photons are electromagnetic radiation. As such, they undergo two significant interactions in tissue. First, in the photoelectric effect the photon interacts with the Coulomb field of the nucleus of an atom in tissue. The photon disappears, and an electron is ejected from the atom with kinetic energy equal to the photon's energy, minus the binding energy of the electron in the atom. This type of interaction reduces the available number of paired annihilation photons which emerge from the patient. It also increases the radiation dose to the patient. Second, in Compton scattering, the photon collides with an unbound or "free" electron in the tissue. The photon transfers some of its energy to the electron, which becomes the electron's kinetic energy, and the photon and electron go off at different angles. If the photon is scattered "out of the slice" of the PET scanner, one of the pair of annihilation photons is missing, and that annihilation event will not be detected. If the photon is scattered "within the slice," the detected coincidence line does not pass through the true annihilation site. This detection of scattered photons reduces the contrast in the image (Figure 14).

The average attenuation is greatest at the center of an object. Attenuation produces a gradual, increasing underestimation of radioactivity from the edge to the center of the head, by about a factor of five. Thus, it is extremely important to correct for its effects. There are two main approaches to attenuation correction. In the first, attenuation is measured before the PET scan begins by placing a ring of positron-emitting activity around the patient's head, and measuring the fractional transmission of the annihilation photons from the ring through the patient, point-by-point within a given slice.

The second approach to attenuation correction does not require any additional measurements (Bergstrom et al. 1982; Huang et al. 1981a). After the uncorrected image is reconstructed, the PET operator outlines the scalp, usually with an ellipse. An average value for attenuation is then

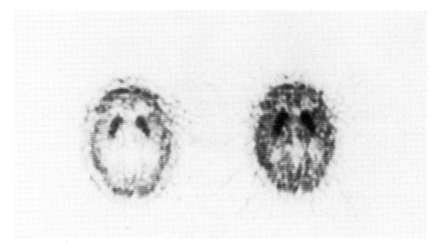

FIGURE 14. Average attenuation is greatest at the center of an object. The left image has not been corrected for attenuation, whereas the right image (otherwise identical) has been corrected using the calculated correction approach. (Courtesy of Dr. J. Links, Johns Hopkins Medical Institutes, Nuclear Medicine Division, Baltimore, Maryland)

assumed for each point within this outline of the head. (This average value depends on both the tissues involved and the characteristics of the particular PET scanner.) The use of a "measured" attenuation correction may be more accurate, but results in propagation of statistical noise from the transmission study into the emission image. It also requires the additional transmission scan. Because of these considerations, most investigators use the "calculated" correction approach, with an ellipse and an assumed attenuation value (Huang et al. 1979).

Finite Spatial Resolution. All PET scanners have a finite ability to resolve small objects. The spatial resolution of a PET scanner can be thought of as that distance by which two small point sources of radioactivity must be separated to be distinguished as separate in the reconstructed image. Finite spatial resolution results in two important effects. First, the image is blurred, with the degree of blurring dependent on the spatial resolution. This blurring prevents the delineation of edges of larger structures in the brain, and may not allow the visualization of smaller ones as distinct objects. Furthermore, in the cortex, the gray and white matter are smeared and averaged together, reducing the measured value in the areas with greater radioactivity (usually gray matter), and increasing it in the areas with lesser radioactivity (usually white matter) (Hoffman et al. 1982).

The second effect is more subtle. Finite spatial resolution produces an underestimation of radioactivity in small structures, with progressive underestimation as the structures get smaller. The effect is not eliminated until the object is approximately three times the resolution of the scanner. This underestimation effect is conceptually separate from the blurring effect, though they both arise from finite spatial resolution. Indeed, blurring from surrounding larger structures can partially compensate for the underestimation in a small structure, by smearing counts into the small structure. Thus, the underestimation is greatest for isolated structures, such as the heads of the caudate nuclei.

This effect can be corrected if the size and shape of the structure is known, and if the physical characteristics of the PET scanner have been quantified with the use of calibrated objects such as hollow spheres filled with known concentrations of radioactivity. The *recovery coefficient* describes the ratio between measured and true radioactivity, and can be used to multiplicatively boost the observed values to compensate for the underestimation (Hoffman and Phelps 1986). In practice, it is difficult to assess accurately the size and shape of each patient's brain regions of interest, and recovery coefficient techniques are only applied in those situations where the effects are significant (for example, in comparison of receptor-binding in the head of the caudate in normal persons and patients with Huntington's chorea, where the head of the caudate shrinks considerably).

Partial Volume Effects.   Partial volume effects are related to finite spatial resolution effects, but apply to the so-called z axis, along the long axis of the patient (Hoffman et al. 1984). If the object is smaller than about three times the slice thickness, the averaging and underestimation effects described above will occur. The underestimation can be corrected with a recovery coefficient. Orthogonal one-dimensional x, y, and z recovery coefficients could be sequentially applied, or an "effective" three-dimensional coefficient can be used. It is important to note that the term *slice thickness* is really a misnomer, as the profile of the slice is not a square wave with a uniform width, but rather more like a bell-shaped curve. Slice thickness is usually given as the "full-width-at-half-maximum" of this Gaussian function. Thus, radioactivity lying outside the "slice thickness" still contributes to the slice (though much less so), and not all the activity "within" the slice is detected with equal sensitivity.

Scattered Photons.   As described above, annihilation photons can undergo Compton scattering in the patient. Detection of these photons, which is unavoidable to a certain extent, is determined by the physical geometry of the scanner and any electronic scatter-rejection circuit settings, produces a "background" haze in the image, which reduces contrast. This background results in an overestimation of the radioactivity in structures, especially those structures containing less activity than their surroundings. Some PET scanners implement scatter correction by estimating its contribution. This estimate is usually based on both the characteristics of the scanner, and the actual distribution of radioactivity in the slice, as given by the (uncorrected) reconstruction.

Accidental Coincidences. The basis of PET scanning is coincidence detection of the annihilation photons. In the real world, *coincidence* or *simultaneity* must have a finite definition (Hoffman et al. 1981). In most PET scanners, the *coincidence time window*, which defines these terms, is 5–20 nanoseconds (10^{-9}) wide. It is possible for two photons from different annihilation events to be detected as though they were from the same event. A false coincidence line will thus be generated. The probability of detecting these accidental or random coincidences increases as the coincidence time window is widened, and as the radioactivity in the PET scanner increases. In fact, since the true coincidences increase linearly with increasing radioactivity, while random coincidences increase with the square of activity, the fraction of total coincidences detected which are random increases with increasing activity.

Accidental coincidences are usually subtracted from the detected total by separately measuring their contribution during scan acquisition. This can be done, for example, by using a second coincidence time window that is purposely offset in time so that all coincidences which fall within this window must be random.

Statistical Noise. All of the above effects result in reductions in the accuracy of quantification. There is one fundamental factor which limits the precision of measurements made with PET. The statistical nature of radioactive decay, described by the Poisson distribution, produces noise in the measurements. This noise is visible in reconstructed images as a mottled or salt and pepper appearance. Since the relative noise decreases as the observed counts increase, longer scanning times result in less noise. Additionally, most PET scanners offer two or more resolution/sensitivity options. As sensitivity is increased, to increase count rate, resolution deteriorates.

Finally, spatial resolution and noise can be traded off in the reconstruction process. The filter used in filtered backprojection boosts the high spatial frequencies at which noise resides. If the filter is rolled off at high frequencies, the noise will not be accentuated as much. However, the true high frequencies will also not be boosted as much, resulting in poorer resolution in the image. This tradeoff is dependent on the particular application at hand; most PET scanners offer a range of filters from which to choose.

Imaging Protocols

As the above discussion should make obvious, there are a lot of compromises necessary in real-world PET scanning. The choice of an imaging protocol is dependent on many factors, including the required spatial and temporal resolution, the amount of radioactivity in the patient (which determines available count rate), and the characteristics of the scanner. It is extremely important to define these requirements a priori, as certain decisions cannot be altered after acquisition.

Metabolic and Neuroreceptor Models

Local Cerebral Glucose Utilization: The Quantitative Model

Measuring Biochemical Processes in Vivo

With positron emission tomography, clinical neurobiologists can measure the rates of biochemical reactions in human tissues. Other analogous tools used in animal research are liquid scintillation counting and quantitative autoradiography. Measurements of biochemical reaction rates follow similar principles when used in the context of various techniques. Chemical and enzyme kinetics and tracer theory are used in PET research in the same way they are used in animal autoradiography. Because of the constraints inherent in emission tomography, the traps and pitfalls are even greater with PET than with the more conventional biochemical techniques.

A chemical reaction is the conversion of one species of molecule to another. The rate of the reaction can be measured by the determination of the rate of formation of product or the disappearance of reactant(s). Generally, it is preferable to measure the rate of product accumulation because the percentage change in the amount of product accumulation is much greater than the percentage change in the amount of reactant or precursor. The addition of a radiolabel to one of the reactants in molecular concentrations too small to alter the kinetics of the overall reaction can facilitate the measurement of either the reactant or product but it also introduces complications. The rate of chemical transformation of the labeled species is not the rate of the reaction of the nonradioactive species which is the reaction to be measured. To derive the rate of the total reaction from the measurement of the rate of the labeled species, it is necessary to know the specific activity of the precursor pool (i.e., the ratio of the concentrations of labeled to total precursor molecules). The rate of the overall reaction can be calculated from the rate of radioactive product formation as follows:

$$\text{rate of reaction} = \frac{\text{labeled product formed in interval, 0 to } T}{\text{integrated specific activity of precursor}}$$

Occasionally the labeled species exhibits a kinetic difference from the natural compound, the so-called isotope effect; this isotope effect can be evaluated and appropriate correction made for it. The assay of biochemical reactions in vivo usually involves the use of specialized separation techniques to isolate and identify the labeled product and therefore confine the measurement of the radioactivity to the specific chemical product of the reaction. The specific activity of the precursor molecule in in vitro experiments is constant over the time course of the interval and is predetermined by the investigator.

Quantitative autoradiography and positron emission tomography make it possible to measure the concentration of radioisotopes in tissue regions. These techniques coupled with in vivo administration of the radiotracer provide a method for measuring the rate of a reaction in local regions of a tissue in vivo. The requirements for such a technique are considerable. The labeled chemical compound must be judiciously selected and the procedure must be carefully designed such that the mathematical function can be solved in this complex situation. Because the precursor pool in the tissue region cannot be sampled directly over the time course of the experiment, it is necessary to develop a model for the behavior of the labeled molecule in the tissue and the blood. The model must be based on known biochemistry. If the method requires the use of a poorly characterized tracer molecule, it will be necessary to determine the biochemical behavior of the molecule before formulating a model. The method will only be as accurate as the model is reliable. Fits do not define a model. From a kinetic analysis of the model an equation can be derived which expresses the rate of the reaction in terms of measurable variables (i.e., in terms of concentrations of the labeled and the unlabeled species in the blood and the amount of label in the tissue). Autoradiography and emission tomography measure only the total concentration of the isotope and cannot distinguish among the various chemical species which may be labeled. Methods must ensure that the radioactivity is contained exclusively in the precursor and/or in one or more of the products specific to the chemical reaction to be assayed. The labeled precursor should be selected so that the radioactive label is confined only to the specific pathway under study.

In Vivo Measurement of Energy Metabolism

These general principles have been more or less successfully applied in two currently operational methods for the measurement of energy metabolism in the nervous system of animals and man. One method is the steady state cerebral O_2-consumption technique (Frackowiak et al. 1980a, 1980b; Frackowiak and Lammertsma 1985; Jones et al. 1976, 1982b). Blood flow, blood volume, and oxygen metabolism measurements are discussed in a subsequent section. The other method is the radioactive deoxyglucose technique for the measurement of local cerebral rates of glucose consumption (Sokoloff et al. 1977; Sokoloff 1982). Figure 15 illustrates metabolic pathways utilizing glucose and deoxyglucose. It has been used primarily in association with autoradiography in animals but has been adapted to study human regional cerebral metabolism as indicated above (Reivich et al. 1979; Phelps et al. 1979). The deoxyglucose method is based on the measurement of product accumulation. Because it encompasses almost all the principles to be considered in the measurement of biochemical processes in vivo, it will serve as an informative example of their application. A comparable method, but one designed to measure local cerebral rates of protein synthesis, has also been developed (Smith et al. 1980) and it serves to illustrate additional problems in the assay of biochemical processes in vivo.

Deoxyglucose Method: Theoretical Basis

The deoxyglucose method was developed to measure rates of glucose utilization simultaneously in all structural and functional components of the central nervous system in conscious animals. Although the purpose was to measure the local rates of glucose utilization, the analog of glucose, 2-deoxy-D-glucose (DG), rather than glucose itself, was selected as the labeled precursor because its biochemical properties make it easier to adhere to the essential biochemical principles for the measurement of a biochemical process in vivo by autoradiography or other emission tomographic techniques. If radioactive glucose is used as the precursor, some of the labeled products of glucose metabolism, particularly CO_2 and water, are lost too rapidly from the tissue, and many other labeled products dependent on additional chemical reactions other than glucose metabolism are retained. With radioactive deoxyglucose as precursor, the label is retained in the tissues in either of two chemical species, the unmetabolized precursor molecule or the immediate product of its metabolism. The use of deoxyglucose serves to isolate the chemical process under study to a well-defined reaction, the hexokinase-catalyzed

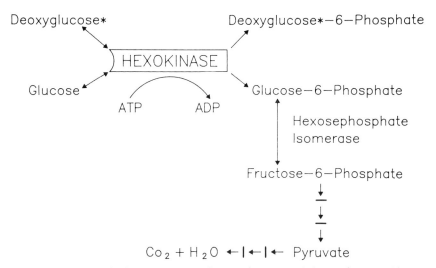

FIGURE 15. Metabolic pathways utilizing glucose and deoxyglucose. Glucose utilization commences with the hexokinase-catalyzed phosphorylation of glucose by ATP, but the product of this reaction, glucose-6-phosphate, is not retained in the tissues. Instead, it is metabolized further to products like CO_2 and H_2O, which leave the tissue. Deoxyglucose, an analog and competitive substrate with glucose in the hexokinase reaction, leads to a product, deoxyglucose-6-phosphate, that does accumulate in the tissue quantitatively for a reasonable length of time. By putting a label on the deoxyglucose, it is possible to measure the rate of labeled deoxyglucose-6-phosphate formation. From a knowledge of the time course of the relative concentrations of labeled deoxyglucose and glucose in the tissue at the enzyme site and the relative Michaelis-Menten constants of hexokinase for the two substrates, it is possible to calculate how much glucose must have also been phosphorylated during the production of the measured amount of deoxyglucose-6-phosphate. The integrated relative concentrations of labeled deoxyglucose and glucose in the tissue are calculated from the measured time courses of the two compounds in the arterial plasma by subtracting from the integrated plasma specific activity a term that corrects for the lag of the tissue behind the plasma. (Courtesy of Drs. L. Sokoloff and C. Smith, Laboratory of Cerebral Metabolism, National Institutes of Mental Health, Bethesda, Maryland)

phosphorylation of the hexose, the first step in the biochemical pathway of glucose metabolism.

The method was derived by analysis of a two-compartment model based on the biochemical properties of 2-deoxyglucose and glucose in brain. 2-Deoxyglucose is transported bidirectionally between blood and brain by the same carrier that transports glucose across the blood–brain barrier. In the cerebral tissues it is phosphorylated, like glucose, by hexokinase to produce 2-deoxyglucose-6-phosphate (DG-6-P). DG and glucose are, therefore, competitive substrates for both blood–brain transport and hexokinase-catalyzed phosphorylation. Unlike glucose-6-phosphate, however, which is metabolized further, eventually to CO_2 and water (Figure 16), DG-6-P cannot be converted to fructose-6-phosphate, and it is also a poor substrate for glucose-6-phosphate dehydrogenase. A small amount (about 2%) of DG-6-P is incorporated into brain glycogen (Nelson et al. 1984) during the 45 minutes following a pulse injection of DG. Radiolabel in the tissue in the form of glycogen, glycolipids, or glycoproteins is trapped in the tissue at least as well as the label in DG-6-P and it is returned to the form of DG-6-P by glycogenolysis. There is relatively little glucose-6-phosphatase activity in brain and even less deoxyglucose-6-phosphatase activity. Deoxyglucose-6-phosphate, once formed, remains, therefore, essentially trapped in the cerebral tissues, at least for 45 min (Sokoloff 1982).

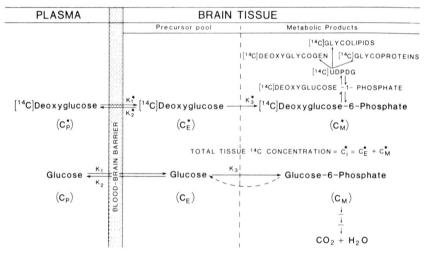

FIGURE 16.   Diagrammatic representation of the theoretical model. C_i^* represents the total ^{14}C concentration in a single homogeneous tissue of the brain. C_P^* and C_P represent the concentrations of $[^{14}C]$deoxyglucose and glucose in the arterial plasma, respectively; C_E^* and C_E represent their respective concentrations in the tissue pools that serve as substrates for hexokinase. C_M^* represents the concentration of $[^{14}C]$deoxyglucose-6-phosphate in the tissue. The constants k_1^*, k_2^*, and k_3^* represent the rate constants for carrier-mediated transport of $[^{14}C]$deoxyglucose from plasma to tissue, for carrier-mediated transport back from tissue to plasma, and for phosphorylation by hexokinase, respectively; the constants k_1, k_2, and k_3 are the equivalent rate constants for glucose. $[^{14}C]$Deoxyglucose and glucose share and compete for the carrier that transports both between plasma and tissue and for hexokinase which phosphorylates them to their respective hexose-6-phosphates. The dashed arrow represents the possibility of glucose-6-phosphate hydrolysis by glucose-6-phosphatase activity, if any. (Courtesy of Drs. L. Sokoloff and C. Smith, Laboratory of Cerebral Metabolism, National Institute of Mental Health, Bethesda, Maryland)

It is critical that the product of 2DG phosphorylation, DG-6-P, be trapped in cerebral tissue for the 45-minute duration of the experiment. Methodological validity turns on this point. Although glucose-6-phosphatase activity in brain is low, it is not zero (Sokoloff 1982). This enzyme is capable of hydrolyzing the product, DG-6-P, to free DG; that action leads to product loss. Fortunately, the product and enzyme are in separate cellular compartments. The DG-6-P is formed in the cytosol and must be transported into the cisterns of the endoplasmic reticulum, where the DG-6-phosphatase resides, before the hydrolysis can occur. In liver this transport process is mediated by a specific carrier. In brain, however, the carrier is absent (Fishman and Karnovsky 1986). The kinetics of this process, namely, a lag with zero phosphatase activity followed by progressively increasing activity, are expected as a consequence of enzyme/substrate separation and a rate-limiting transport of the substrate across the membrane to the enzyme. Although the evidence clearly indicates that phosphatase activity is of no significance to the deoxyglucose method if the experimental period is limited to 45 minutes, a few reports have appeared alleging that phosphatase activity is a major source of error (Hawkins and Miller 1978; Huang and Veech 1982; Sacks et al. 1983). Each of these reports has been shown to be flawed either as a result of the misinterpretation of experimental findings or faulty conduct of biochemical procedures (Nelson et al. 1985, 1986a; Dienel et al. 1986), and therefore have no bearing upon this issue.

If the interval of time following introduction of labeled DG into the tissue is kept short enough to ensure negligible loss of labeled product (DG-6-P), then the quantity of DG-6-P accumulated in any cerebral tissue is a function of the rate of flux of glucose through the hexokinase-catalyzed reaction, the first step in glycolysis. In a steady state, the net rate through any step in a pathway equals the net rate through the overall pathway. Therefore, measurement of the net rate of glucose phosphorylation in a steady state is a determination of the net rate of the entire glycolytic pathway.

In order to determine the rate of glucose phosphorylation it is necessary to measure the amount of labeled product, DG-6-P, formed and the integrated specific activity of the precursor (i.e., the ratio of the concentrations of DG to glucose integrated over time, T). In addition, a correction factor for the *isotope effect* must also be introduced into the expression to correct for the fact that DG rather than glucose is used as the labeled substrate. These relationships can be mathematically defined by mathematical analysis of the model, provided that the following requirements are met:

1. Steady states for glucose (i.e., constant plasma glucose concentration

and constant rate of glucose consumption throughout the experimental period);

2. Homogeneous tissue compartments within which the concentrations of DG and glucose are uniform and exchange directly with the plasma; and

3. Tracer concentrations of DG (i.e., molecular concentrations of free DG that are insignificant compared with the concentration of glucose).

The operational equation which defined R_i, the rate of glucose utilization per unit mass of tissues, i, in terms of measurable variables is as shown in Figure 17, where $C_i^*(T)$ is the concentration of label in the tissue at time T; C_p^* and C_p are the arterial plasma concentrations of DG and glucose, respectively; k_1^*, k_2^*, and k_3^* are the rate constants for the carrier-mediated transport of DG from plasma to the tissue precursor pool, for the carrier-mediated transport of DG back from the tissue to the plasma, and

FUNCTIONAL ANATOMY OF THE OPERATIONAL EQUATION OF THE [^{14}C] DEOXYGLUCOSE METHOD

General Equation for Measurement of Reaction Rates with Tracers:

$$\text{Rate of Reaction} = \frac{\text{Labeled Product Formed in Interval of Time, 0 to T}}{\begin{bmatrix}\text{Isotope Effect}\\\text{Correction Factor}\end{bmatrix}\begin{bmatrix}\text{Integrated Specific Activity}\\\text{of Precursor}\end{bmatrix}}$$

Operational Equation of [^{14}C] Deoxyglucose Method:

$$R_i = \frac{C_i^*(T) - K_1^* e^{-(k_2^*+k_3^*)T}\int_0^T C_p^* \, e^{(k_2^*+k_3^*)t}\, dt}{\left[\dfrac{\lambda \cdot V_m^* \cdot K_m}{\Phi \cdot V_m \cdot K_m^*}\right]\left[\int_0^T \left(\dfrac{C_p^*}{C_p}\right)dt - e^{-(k_2^*+k_3^*)T}\int_0^T \left(\dfrac{C_p^*}{C_p}\right)e^{(k_2^*+k_3^*)t}\, dt\right]} \qquad [\text{Equation 1}]$$

Labeled Product Formed in Interval of Time, 0 to T

Total ^{14}C in Tissue at time, T

^{14}C in Precursor Remaining in Tissue at Time, T

Isotope Effect Correction Factor

Integrated Plasma Specific Activity

Correction for Lag in Tissue Equilibration with Plasma

Integrated Precursor Specific Activity in Tissue

FIGURE 17. Operational equation of the radioactive deoxyglucose method and its functional anatomy. T represents the time of termination of the experimental period; λ equals the ratio of the distribution space of deoxyglucose in the tissue to that of glucose; Φ equals the fraction of glucose which once phosphorylated continues down the glycolytic pathway; and K_m^* and V_m^* and K_m and V_m represent the familiar Michaelis-Menten kinetic constants of hexokinase for deoxyglucose and glucose, respectively. The other symbols are the same as those defined in Figure 16. (Courtesy of Drs. L. Sokoloff and C. Smith, Laboratory of Cerebral Metabolism, National Institute of Mental Health, Bethesda, Maryland)

for the phosphorylation of DG in the tissue, respectively. *T* represents the time of termination of the experiment. L.C., or the lumped constant, is a composite of six constants

$$\frac{\lambda \cdot V_{max}^{\bullet} \cdot K_m}{\Phi \cdot V_{max} \cdot K_m^{\bullet}}$$

which as a whole represents the correction for the kinetic difference between deoxyglucose and glucose; λ is the ratio of the distribution space in the tissue of deoxyglucose and glucose, Φ is the fraction of glucose which once phosphorylated continues down the glycolytic pathway, and $K_m^{\bullet}$, $V_{max}^{\bullet}$, K_m, and V_{max} represent the Michaelis–Menten kinetic constants of hexokinase for DG and glucose, respectively.

The rate constants $k_1^{\bullet}$, $k_2^{\bullet}$, and $k_3^{\bullet}$ are determined in a separate group of subjects by a nonlinear, iterative process which provides the least squares best-fit of an equation which defines the time course of tissue radiolabel concentration in terms of the time, the history of the plasma DG concentration, and the rate constants to the experimentally determined time courses of tissue and plasma concentrations of radiolabel. The Φ and enzyme kinetic constants are grouped together to constitute a single, "lumped constant" (see Figure 17). It can be shown mathematically that this lumped constant is equal to the asymptotic value of the product of the ratio of the cerebral extraction ratios of DG and glucose and the ratio of the arterial blood to plasma specific activities when the arterial plasma DG concentration is maintained constant (Sokoloff et al. 1977). The lumped constant is also determined in a separate group of subjects from arterial and cerebral venous blood samples drawn during a programmed intravenous infusion which produces and maintains a constant arterial plasma DG concentration (Sokoloff et al. 1977).

Despite its complex appearance, the operational equation is really nothing more than a general statement of the standard relationship by which rates of enzyme-catalyzed reactions are determined from measurements made with radioactive tracers. The numerator of the equation represents the amount of radioactive product formed in a given interval of time; it is equal to $C_i^{\bullet}$, the combined concentrations of DG and DG-6-P in the tissue at time *T* measured by the quantitative autoradiographic technique or emission tomography, minus a term that represents the free unmetabolized DG still remaining in the tissue. The denominator represents the integrated specific activity of the precursor pool times a factor, the lumped constant, which is equivalent to a correction factor for an isotope effect. The term with the exponential factor in the denominator takes into account the lag in the equilibration of the tissue precursor pool with that of the plasma.

Procedure

The specific procedure employed has been designed to evaluate the variables and to minimize potential errors that might occur in the actual application of the method. If the rate constants k_1^*, k_2^*, and k_3^* are precisely known, then the equation is generally applicable with any mode of administration of DG and over any time interval. The rate constants have been determined in the conscious rat and in humans for both DG (Sokoloff et al. 1977) and FDG (Reivich et al. 1985), respectively. These rate constants can be expected to vary with the condition of the subject and for most accurate results should be redetermined for each condition studied. The structure of the operational equation suggests a more practical alternative. All the terms in the equation that contain the rate constants approach zero with increasing time if the DG is so administered that the plasma DG concentration also approaches zero. From the values of the rate constants determined in normal animals and the usual time course of the clearance of DG from the arterial plasma following a single intravenous pulse at zero time, it has been determined that an interval of 30 to 45 minutes after a pulse is adequate for these terms to become sufficiently small that considerable inaccuracies in the rate constants are permissible without appreciable error in the estimates of local cerebral glucose consumption (Sokoloff et al. 1977). An additional advantage derived from the use of a single pulse of DG followed by a relatively long interval before measurement of local tissue DG radioactivity level is that, by then, most of the free DG in the tissues has been either converted to DG-6-P or transported back to the plasma. The radioactivity in the tissues then represents mainly the concentration of the product, DG-6-P, and, therefore, reflects directly the relative rates of glucose utilization in the various cerebral tissues.

In animal work, either ^{3}H- or ^{14}C-labeled DG can be used as the tracer and the tissue concentration of label C_i^* can be determined by quantitative autoradiography (Hand 1981). For studies in humans with PET, the DG must be labeled with a positron-emitting isotope. This has been accomplished with the use of either [^{18}F]-fluorodeoxyglucose (Reivich et al. 1979) or [^{11}C]-deoxyglucose (Reivich et al. 1982). It is a common experience that the substitution of the very small F atom in place of a hydrogen at a judicious site in the molecule does not alter the basic biochemical behavior of metabolic substrates. It has been shown that this is the case in animal studies with [^{14}C]-fluorodeoxyglucose (Reivich et al. 1979). In these studies with PET it is often necessary to extend the experimental period to intervals longer than 45 minutes. In this case it is necessary to account for the effects of glucose-6-phosphatase activity. This has been done by modifying the original model to include a k_4^*, the rate constant for DG-6-P hydrolysis by the phosphatase; a new operational equation has been derived that incorporates this variation (Sokoloff 1982).

Local Protein-Synthesis Rates: The Quantitative Model

The basic biochemical principles for the measurement of metabolic rates in vivo, which were so effectively applied in the deoxyglucose technique, also apply to other metabolic processes. A metabolic activity of broad interest is protein synthesis. This biochemical activity is not likely to reflect functional activity directly, at least not accurately, but it may well be involved in slower, more gradual processes in the nervous system, such as growth and development, plasticity, regeneration and repair, response to drugs and hormones, and possibly learning and memory. Protein synthesis may also be altered in pathological states, such as brain tumors, mental retardation due to metabolic errors, aging (Ingvar et al. 1985) and senility, Alzheimer's disease, Huntington's disease, and endocrine diseases.

A method for the measurement of local rates of protein synthesis in the nervous system is under development (Smith et al. 1980). Like the deoxyglucose method it is designed to achieve localization by quantitative autoradiography; recent reports indicate that it is now being adapted to positron emission tomography (Phelps et al. 1985; Bustany et al. 1985). Like the deoxyglucose method it is based on the same biochemical principles described above, but their application to the measurement of local cerebral protein synthesis may be far more complex because of still undefined properties and kinetics of the equilibration of the precursor amino acid pool in the tissue with the circulating amino acid pool in the plasma.

The two essential variables which must be determined in any quantitative radioactive assay of the rate of a reaction are the amount of product formed and the integrated precursor specific activity over a measured interval of time. Because autoradiographic or emission tomographic techniques measure the concentration only of the radioisotope and not that of the radioactive product itself, it is essential that the label in the tissue be confined only to the product molecule itself or, at least, in well-defined chemical species which can be quantified separately. This problem is mitigated by the use of carboxyl-labeled L-leucine, an essential amino acid which is prevalent in most proteins and which, other than incorporation into protein, has a single simple pathway of metabolic degradation.

In the pathway of degradation, the amino acid is first transaminated and then rapidly decarboxylated. The label is then lost as radioactive CO_2, which, because of dilution by the large pool of unlabeled CO_2 constantly generated by carbohydrate metabolism, the relatively slow rate of CO_2 fixation, and the rapid removal of CO_2 from brain tissue by the blood flow, is removed from the tissues. The label is then retained only in the product of the reaction, labeled protein, and the residual unincorporated amino acid. The concentration of free labeled amino acid can be calculated from the history of the plasma concentration and the kinetic constants for the equilibration of the tissue free amino acid pools and the plasma. The concentration of free labeled amino acid in the tissue can be minimized by its intravenous administration as a pulse at zero time and then waiting a sufficiently long time for the plasma and tissue to be cleared of labeled amino acid. One hour after the pulse the fraction of total radioactivity in the tissue that is in the free amino acid pool is small (about 10%) in the rat. In adult monkey and probably in humans, however, it is large (30–50%) because of the relatively slow rates of protein synthesis and of clearance of the free amino acid pools. The error in subtracting a poorly defined free amino acid pool concentration from a total concentration that is not a great deal larger may, of course, be enormous.

An even more difficult problem is the determination of the integrated precursor pool specific activity in the tissue from measurements in the plasma. To accomplish this, it is necessary to know the kinetics of the equilibration of the precursor pool in the cells with that of the plasma. What makes this problem particularly perplexing is that there is evidence that amino acids in the cells are compartmentalized with only a fraction of the total intracellular amino acid content representative of the pool that serves as precursor for protein synthesis. Therefore, although it is relatively simple to measure the rate constants for the equilibration of the total amino acid pool with that of the plasma, there is little assurance that this pool reflects the kinetic behavior of the fraction of it that is the precursor for protein synthesis. A further complication is the possibility of significant dilution of the intracellular precursor amino acid pool by unlabeled amino acid derived from the slow but continuous turnover of the protein components of the cell. The magnitude of this potential dilution is even more difficult to evaluate. Nevertheless, studies in progress (e.g., at NIMH, Laboratory of Cerebral Metabolism) are designed to resolve these problems. If successful, they will not only determine the rate constants for the turnover of the true precursor pool but also the degree of admixture of unlabeled amino acids from protein breakdown with amino acids in the precursor pool.

Although the method is not yet fully developed, experiments with our first and most primitive model already indicate the usefulness for this quantitative local protein synthesis technique. Model I is essentially the same as that for the deoxyglucose method. It assumes a single tissue pool of free amino acid, all of which equilibrates uniformly with the plasma and serves as the precursor pool for protein synthesis with no dilution by unlabeled amino acids derived from protein degradation (Smith et al. 1980). Although the quantitative values obtained with this version of the method are probably not accurate and may be underestimates of the true rates of L-leucine incorporation into protein, the results demonstrate that the rates of protein synthesis do change in specific regions of the brain in response to altered function. For example, in the rat, section of one hypoglossal nerve is followed by increased protein synthesis in the ipsilateral hypoglossal nucleus after a lag of close to 4 days (Agranoff et al. 1980; Smith et al. 1984). The increase reaches a maximum between 20–30%, and protein synthesis does not return to normal until regeneration and restoration of functional activity in the hypoglossal nerve is complete (Smith et al. 1984).

The method has also been used to study plasticity in the binocular visual system of the newborn rhesus monkey (Kennedy et al. 1981). The outputs from the retinae of the two eyes are crossed approximately 50%, and the optic tracts terminate in the lateral geniculate ganglia in six discrete laminae: 1, 4, and 6, the sites of termination of the pathways from the contralateral retina; and 2, 3, and 5, the laminae supplied by the ipsilateral eye. The cells in these laminae project via the geniculocalcarine tracts to the ipsilateral striate cortex in such a way that the two retinal outputs for each point in the visual field converge to two adjacent cortical columns, one for each eye, for the same spot in the visual field. These are the ocular dominance columns, first described by Hubel and Wiesel (Hubel and Wiesel 1968; Hubel et al. 1977) and demonstrated autoradiographically by the [^{14}C]-deoxyglucose method (Kennedy et al. 1976).

The visual system of the newborn monkey exhibits plasticity. Chronic occlusion of one eye in a newborn monkey leads to widening of the ocular dominance columns for the functioning eye at the expense of the columns for the deprived eye until eventually the columns disappear, and the entire striate cortex is taken over to subserve the function of the undeprived eye (Hubel et al. 1977; Des Rosiers et al. 1978). Presumably the axonal terminals of the geniculocalcarine pathway for the functioning eye grow into, and take over, the synaptic connections in the adjacent column normally reserved for the deprived eye. If so, changes in protein synthesis required for axonal growth and sprouting could be involved, and the protein synthesis used for this process occurs in the cell bodies of origin of the pathway (i.e., in the lateral geniculate ganglia).

Figure 18 shows the results of the local protein synthesis method applied to this question. The laminae in the geniculate bodies are clearly visible and relatively uniform in the autoradiographs of the 25-day-old normal monkey. Acute monocular deprivation for 3 h does not alter the rates of protein synthesis in any of the laminae, including those for the deprived eye. Chronic monocular deprivation from 2 days to 25 days of age results in marked reductions in protein synthesis in the laminae normally served by the deprived eye. Apparently chronic reduction in functional activity, in contrast to the acute state, results in a lowering of protein synthesis in the affected pathway. These results suggest that the loss of ocular dominance columns in the striate cortex for the chronically deprived eye is the result of depressed protein synthesis and deficient axonal growth in the geniculocalcarine pathways for the deprived eye.

In conclusion, measurements of local protein synthesis rates in the nervous system will be useful for studying normal and abnormal processes that may not be accessible to other autoradiographic and tomographic procedures, processes such as growth, maturation, plasticity, and actions of hormones. The full potential of this approach must, however, await the development of an accurate and reliable method.

Cerebral Blood Flow and Oxygen Consumption: The Steady State Approach

Frackowiak and Lammertsma (1985) provide a lucid account of the steady

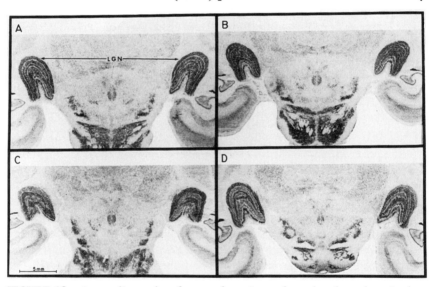

FIGURE 18. Autoradiographs of coronal sections of monkey lateral geniculate nuclei (LGN) obtained with the [^{14}C]leucine method. The left side of the brain is on the left side of the autoradiographs. A: 25-day-old monkey with intact binocular vision. B: 25-day-old monkey with acute occlusion of the left eye. C: 25-day-old monkey with chronic occlusion of right eye initiated on second day of life. D: 25-day-old monkey with chronic occlusion of left eye initiated on second day of life. Note the decreased labeling and therefore, rate of protein synthesis in laminae 1, 4, and 6 of the lateral geniculate ganglion contralateral to the deprived eye, and in laminae 2, 3, and 5 of the ganglion ipsilateral to the deprived eye. (Courtesy of Dr. C. Smith, Laboratory of Cerebral Metabolism, National Institute of Mental Health, Bethesda, Maryland)

state cerebral blood flow (CBF) and metabolism (CMRoxy) methods. Their mathematical analyses of the derivations and limitations of this method are carefully and simply presented in their work which is partially summarized here.

Classical steady state methods of measuring physiological and biochemical processes involve administration of inert, diffusible, and soluble tracers until saturation of the tissue occurs. The rate at which saturation (or desaturation) is achieved provides dynamic information about the metabolic fate of a substance of fluid. In vivo saturation of a tissue by a radioactively labeled tracer is, however, not a realistic goal. Short-lived isotopes permit one to measure the activity at steady state without reaching saturation. That is, the short half-life tracers have a decay constant that is comparable to the transit time of the tracer through cerebral tissue. The steady state is not at saturation when arterial and tissue concentrations are equal; instead, the steady state is at an intermediate level dependent on the rate of delivery (Figures 19 and 20).

If the physiological variables and delivery of short-lived tracer are both constant, the steady state can be maintained. The steady state is dependent on delivery, washout, *and* radioactive decay. The shorter the half-life of the tracer, the more rapidly will the tracer reach equilibrium.

Clinical Measurement of Cerebral Blood Flow

Jones et al. (1976, 1982b) developed the concept of using ^{15}O to label circulating water as a tracer of cerebral perfusion. By using short half-life tracers, he and his colleagues reasoned, one could "freeze" the distribution of tracer in time by continuous tracer administration.

The continuous-inhalation method of CBF measurement depends on the in vivo labeling of water (H_2O) in the pulmonary circulation by the inhalation of trace quantities of ^{15}O-labeled carbon dioxide ($C^{15}O_2$). This occurs quickly and completely in the lungs. The labeled water is then distributed throughout the arterial circulation proportionally to blood flow. Water is an especially good flow marker because it is freely diffusible at physiological flow rates and there is rapid equilibration between tissue and blood. The continuous delivery of $H_2^{15}O$ to the tissue is equaled by its removal into the venous circulation by washout and radioactive decay. Consequently, the tissue activity due to labeled water accumulates until the input to the tissue is balanced by loss and the steady state is established. Understandably, it is important that the physiological status of the tissue not alter during the buildup and time required for activity measurements. The steady state tissue activity is directly proportional to the constant input activity as a function of flow.

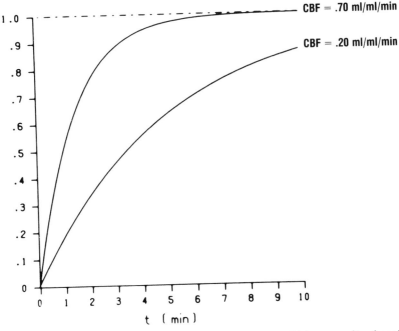

FIGURE 19. Build-up of regional tissue concentration (Tc), normalized against arterial concentration (Ac), in the case of continuous inhalation of a long-lived isotope ($\lambda = 0$). Note that flow information is contained in the time interval it takes to reach equilibrium. In the steady state, however, the tissue signal reflects volume. (Courtesy of Dr. R.S.J. Frackowiak, National Hospital for Nervous Disease, Queen Square, London, England; Positron Emission Tomography, M. Reivich and A. Alavi [eds], Alan R. Liss, New York, p. 156, 1985)

Measurement of Oxygen Metabolism, the Steady State ^{15}O Model

Oxygen-15 is distributed to the cerebral tissue at a rate dependent on CBF. Only 30–40% of the delivered oxygen is extracted for the generation of phosphate bonds and water. Hence, some of the labeled oxygen is transformed to water by virtue of its role as an electron acceptor; some of it traverses the capillaries and arrives in the venous compartment where it is redistributed throughout the circulation. The washout of metabolic water from brain and other tissues accounts for the fact that the venous effluent contains circulating $H_2^{15}O$ as well as hemoglobin-bound $^{15}O_2$. This recirculating labeled water generated in metabolically active tissues during $^{15}O_2$ inhalation provides a contaminating signal that is not dependent on tissue extraction, but rather on blood flow. The tissue signal will then reach a steady state when the accumulation of metabolic and recircu-

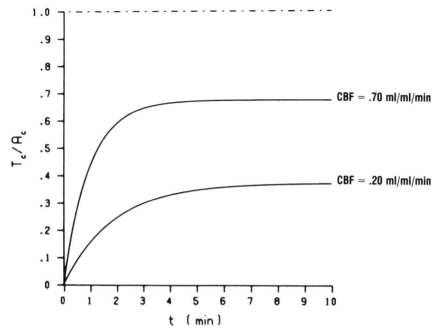

FIGURE 20. As in Figure 19, but now for a short-lived isotope ($\lambda = 0.335$ min -1). Note the steady state is reached much faster than in Figure 19. The steady state level is now dependent on flow. (Courtesy of Dr. R.S.J. Frackowiak, National Hospital for Nervous Disease, Queen Square, London, England; Positron Emission Tomography, M. Reivich and A. Alavi [eds], Alan R. Liss, New York, p. 156, 1985)

lating water is counterbalanced by the water washout and radioactive decay of the short-lived tracer.

If the physiological state remains constant during $C^{15}O_2$ and subsequent $^{15}O_2$ inhalations, then the distribution of the contaminating recirculating $H_2^{15}O$ tissue signal during the oxygen inhalation will be equal to the circulating water signal from the labeled CO_2 inhalation. By normalizing the CO_2 tracer study to the O_2 generated $H_2^{15}O$ signal, one obtains, by simple subtraction, a metabolically generated $H_2^{15}O$ signal that is linearly proportional to oxygen extraction. It is important to note that the recirculating labeled-water signal constitutes 20–30% of the total $^{15}O_2$ cerebral tissue activity and that it appears within 30–40 seconds after bolus tracer administration. Accurate assessments of the blood-recirculating water component are clearly necessary for a dynamic time-activity measurement of oxygen-extraction rate.

CBF and Oxygen Use, Using a Rapid Dynamic-Imaging Approach

In 1983, two papers by the Washington University PET research group described the clinical application of Kety's autoradiographic CBF method (Herscovitch et al. 1983; Raichle et al. 1983). Using $H_2^{15}O$ as the freely diffusible tracer, this group provides detailed analyses of a protocol dependent on a 40-second scan time. This is an accurate replication of the method originally described by Kety (1951, 1960, 1985). Because PET scanners do not have temporal resolution adequate to measure tissue radioactivity instantaneously, a modification was made in the operational equation to provide for integration over the time of the scan. Using that equation, the investigator can use the local radioactivity over the duration of the scan, and the arterial tracer concentration to determine the product of

$$(f) \ (m) \ (\lambda^{-1}),$$

where f is the flow per unit weight of tissue, m is a constant between 0 and 1 that represents the extent to which diffusion equilibrium between blood and tissue is achieved, and λ is the tissue:blood partition coefficient. By strictly limiting the duration of the scan to under 40 seconds, an accurate estimate can be made of CBF.

Cerebral Oxygen Utilization Measured by Dynamic Scanning

As described above for the equilibrium method, it is necessary to measure recirculating metabolic water in order to calculate oxygen metabolism. This is done by measuring blood volume (CBV) and blood flow (CBF) in all regions of interest, and the arterial total oxygen content at the time of the scan. CMRoxy is computed as the product of the local extraction of oxygen, the local CBF, and arterial oxygen content. CBV is determined with $C^{15}O$; this measurement is necessary in order to calculate the $O^{15}O$ in the vascular compartment. Calculations and corrections for metabolic water are similar to those described above.

Dopamine Receptor Measurement in Vivo Using Positron-Emitting Radiotracers

Receptors are membrane-embedded, globular proteins. In vitro binding assays provide reliable estimates of drug and neurotransmitter binding site number. These sites are putative receptors, biologically essential, molecular transducers of neurotransmitter and pharmacological signals. Kinetic and equilibrium studies are both used to determine receptor number and binding affinity. The former consists of adding labeled drug to the tissue membranes and following the time course of association. Equilibrium studies routinely provide quantitative estimates of ligand binding density. This method consists of incubating a radioactive drug and appropriate tissue membranes with progressively increasing doses of unlabeled drug. Unlabeled ligand is added to differentiate between specific and nonspecific binding sites. Excess nonradioactive drug reduces the specific activity of the radioactive drug and increases the amount of nonspecifically bound drug. The amount of activity detected on the filters used to trap these homogenate membranes is the total binding, the sum of specific and nonspecific binding. Filters which contain the membrane with a large amount of unlabeled drug added represents the nonspecifically bound. The specific binding is the difference between these values. By plotting the ratios of bound/free tracer against bound, in the equilibrium condition, one obtains the B_{max} (density of specific binding sites) and K_d (the dissociation constant) characteristics of the tracer–receptor interaction.

In these binding experiments several criteria must be met: 1) saturability of the receptor site with unlabeled ligand; 2) ligand distribution commensurate with in vitro receptor mapping studies; and 3) pharmacologic characterization using appropriate stereospecific isomers and agonist–antagonist combinations.

These techniques can be used to determine both the absolute receptor density (B_{max}) and the dissociation constant (K_d). This technique requires the investigator to identify particular areas of interest and prepare tissue homogenates. Receptor autoradiography is another method which exceeds the sensitivity of the in vitro homogenate technique and shows regional receptor distribution. Quantitative autoradiography can be performed in vitro, whereby a tissue is incubated with labeled ligand and various unlabeled compounds or by an in vivo procedure. The latter depends on the administration of radioactive drug prior to sacrifice. The brain is sectioned and the slices are exposed to x-ray film. Both methods provide cellular receptor distribution maps. The recent development of computer-assisted image analysis permits accurate receptor quantification and three-dimensional representation of neurochemical patterns (Lear 1986). Optical densities in the exposed x-ray film reflect the distribution of tissue-retained radioactivity.

Closely linked to the in vivo procedure of autoradiography is the study of potential new ligands by their in vivo administration to animals. Animals are sacrificed at various times to follow the time course tracer accumulation in the absence or presence of various competing unlabeled ligand concentrations. Counts obtained in specific binding regions are compared to nonreceptor regions such as dopamine D2 and D1 receptors in the caudate and cerebellum, respectively. In vivo binding studies measure the labeling of the receptors in the presence of an intact blood–brain barrier. Many drugs which will specifically bind in vitro will not do so in vivo because of low blood–brain barrier penetration.

Comar et al. (1979) first attempted to measure radiolabeled dopamine receptor binding in living human subjects when he and his coworkers used PET to assess the distribution of [^{11}C]-chlorpromazine in patients with schizophrenia. They concluded that this drug was not appropriate for in vivo dopamine (DA) receptor measurements because specific and nonspecific radiotracer binding could not be distinguished.

More specific and higher-affinity ligands, especially those of the butyrophenone class, were subsequently developed for measuring DA receptors. Because spiperone is such a potent DA antagonist, several groups made an effort to label it with either ^{18}F or ^{11}C. In 1983, a method using a [^{11}C]-methyliodide-labeling procedure to produce [^{11}C]-3N-methylspiperone (NMSP) was established (Burns et al. 1984; Dannals et al. 1986). This approach generated a product with very high specific activity, 1 to 2 Curies/millimole.

In initial studies approximating the rate of NMSP binding to the dopamine receptor, time versus activity curves were based on the ratio of activity in the caudate–putamen divided by the activity in the cerebellum. This is a measure of total binding (specific and nonspecific binding) to that of nonspecific binding. This index had previously been used to compare various pharmacologic relationships between competing drugs (Kuhar et al. 1978). In order to understand radiotracer retention, investigators must clarify multiple pharmacodynamic associations. These include the relationship of this ratio to blood flow, partial volume effects, and the mass of the injected radioligand.

Following the initial imaging of D2 dopamine receptors in human brain (Wagner et al. 1983; Wong et al. 1984) investigators suggested that the caudate–cerebellar ratio and its apparent linearity over the PET scan time of 90 minutes was a process which could be used as an index related to receptor binding and/or affinity under a certain reasonable range of receptor conditions. In these conditions, the slope could be used to estimate the rate of binding to the receptor (k_3). They also presented a preliminary mathematical derivation to explain why the caudate–cerebellar ratio versus time might be linear during the 90-minute time period.

Mintun and colleagues at Washington University (1984a) expanded the standard three-compartment model and supported his recommendations with preliminary results in baboon studies using [^{18}F]-spiperone. This method proposed the necessity of independent measurements of blood flow and blood volume for the receptor density measurements. They suggested a single receptor–ligand scan, as well as one for blood flow and volume to estimate the binding potential (receptor density/ affinity). This was an important initial study but did not include an accounting of plasma metabolites as did a later study by Perlmutter et al. (1986). Other investigators have suggested that it is not necessary to measure independent blood flow, only the transfer constant k_1 (Wong et al. 1984). The three-compartment model is shown in shown in Figure 21.

In an effort to better model the metabolic fate of labeled spiperone and other butyrophenones, the Brookhaven group has emphasized the usefulness of ^{18}F-N-methylspiroperidol (Arnett et al. 1986). Their studies in human subjects extend over several hours and have helped to improve the estimated equilibrium binding characteristics of this tracer.

The Karolinska PET research group (Farde et al. 1985) has recently published a report describing the synthesis of a substituted benzamide, [^{11}C]-raclopride. This compound appears to reach equilibrium during the PET-scan study time. Because of this characteristic, binding data are analyzed with saturation kinetics modeling, an approach similar to that used in 2DG research.

Quantitative Receptor Measurement and Mathematical Modeling of Absolute Receptor Density

In this section D2 radiotracers are discussed in two groups. Full equilibrium tracers (raclopride) achieve an effective equilibrium or constant ratio between at least three compartments: plasma, brain tissue nonspecific binding, and brain tissue specific binding (Sedvall et al. 1986; Farde et al. 1986). A second class consists of tracers which do not reach full equilibrium (NMSP) during the PET scan time but do achieve a steady state between the plasma and the brain tissue nonspecific binding compartments.

D2 Receptor Measurement by Saturation Analysis in Humans. Explanations by Farde (Farde et al. 1986) and Sedvall (Sedvall et al. 1986) are restated in order to clarify the application of saturation kinetics to PET neuroreceptor measurement.

Figures 22 and 23 graphically depict the quantitative relationship between a population of binding sites and a reversibly binding ligand. When a ligand is in equilibrium with its receptor, increasing ligand doses, or concentrations, will generate a rectangular hyperbolic curve characteristic of a progressively falling binding potential. As the ligand concentration increases, the number of potential binding sites falls; the slope of this curve directly reflects the dynamic tendency for the ligand to dissociate. "Tight" ligand–receptor interactions are characterized by a steep slope; a shallow slope indicates binding with a greater probability of

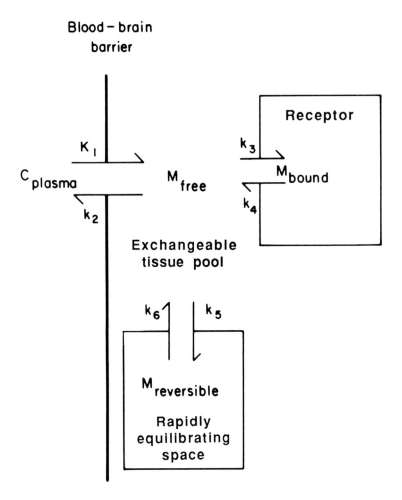

FIGURE 21. Schematic representation of the three compartment model. The accumulation of [^{11}C]NMSP in the brain occurs in two steps. The ligand first crosses the blood-brain barrier, then binds to the receptors. C_{plasma}, concentration of the ligand in arterial plasma; M_{free}, quantity of drug in the exchangeable pool of the tissue; M_{bound}, quantity of ligand bound to the D_2 dopamine receptors; $M_{reversible}$, quantity of drug bound to the secondary or "non-D_2" receptors assumed to be in rapid equilibrium with the free ligand in brain; k_1, clearance from plasma; k_2, rate constant (fractional rate of escape from brain tissue); k_3 and k_4, the rate constants for the association and dissociation of the ligand to and from the D_2 receptors, respectively; k_5 and k_6, rate constants for the lower affinity or secondary, rapidly reversible binding present in the caudate but not the cerebellum. (Courtesy of Dr. D. Wong, Johns Hopkins Medical Institutes, Nuclear Medicine Division, Baltimore, Maryland; Science 234:1559, 1986)

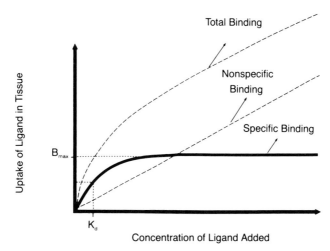

FIGURE 22. Theoretical curve principle of ligand binding to receptors in tissue. Graph demonstrates total binding, nonspecific binding, and specific binding in relation to increasing concentrations of ligand added to tissue specimen during equilibrium. B_{max} indicates maximum binding; K_d, equilibrium dissociation constant. (Courtesy of Dr. G. Sedvall, Karolinska Institute, Stockholm, Sweden; Arch Gen Psychiatry 43:996, 1001, 1986. Copyright 1986 American Medical Association)

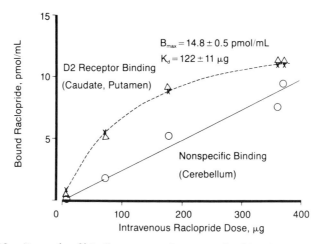

FIGURE 23. Example of binding curve using saturation kinetics. Saturation analysis of carbon 11-labeled raclopride binding to D2 receptors in brain of healthy volunteer. [^{11}C]Raclopride (100 megabecquerels) was injected intravenously on five different occasions, on which different amounts of nonlabeled raclopride were added to tracer dose. B_{max} indicates maximum binding; K_d, equilibrium dissociation constant. (Courtesy of Dr. G. Sedvall, Karolinska Institute, Stockholm, Sweden; Arch Gen Psychiatry 43:996, 1001, 1986. Copyright 1986 American Medical Association)

dissociation. As larger amounts of tracer are added to a system, and fewer sites become available for occupation, the curve bends; it reflects population saturation. It is only by measuring the dynamic shape of the receptor–ligand interaction over a *range* of tracer concentrations that one can independently determine the number of sites available (B_{max}) and the tendency of the tracer to dissociate from the binding site (K_d). *A tracer's retention by a receptor population is the product of its tendency to dissociate from its binding sites and the number of sites available.* It is for this reason that investigators often use the term *binding potential* to indicate the product of K_d and B_{max}.

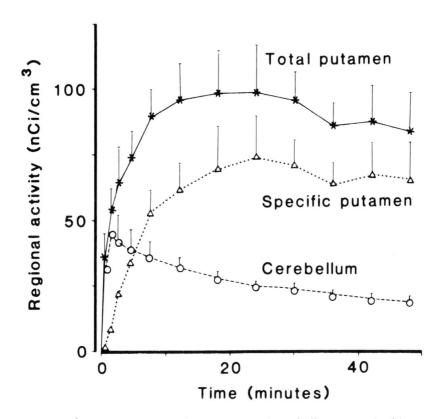

FIGURE 24. Radioactivity in the putamen and cerebellum in six healthy men after intravenous injection of [^{11}C]raclopride (2.7 mCi). The radioactivity was observed sequentially for 1- to 6-minute periods during 50 minutes after the injection. The radioactivity in the cerebellum was assumed to reflect free and nonspecific binding. Specific binding in the putamen was calculated as the difference between radioactivity in the putamen and that in the cerebellum. Values are means ± standard deviations. (Courtesy of Dr. L. Farde, Karolinska Institute, Stockholm, Sweden; Science 231:258, 1986)

By measuring receptor occupancy in association with graduated doses of ligand, determinations of K_d and B_{max} are made independently. This is not, however, an easy task when measurements are made in vivo, with PET or autoradiography. Estimations of free and specifically bound tracer concentration are indirect. Figures 24 and 25 illustrate the use of tracer activity in the caudate–putamen (total activity) versus the cerebellum (free tracer activity) as a means of estimating free and specifically bound (total minus free) ligand. The second set of curves (Figure 25) demonstrates data from four different studies. The saturation curves presented in Figure 25 provided data for Scatchard Plot analyses. This plot of bound/free (*y* axis) versus bound (*x* axis) will produce a straight line

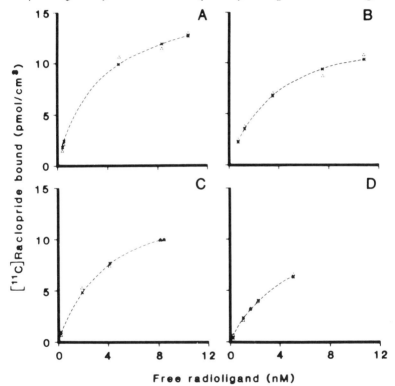

FIGURE 25. Saturation curves for specific [^{11}C]raclopride binding to the putamen in four healthy men (A to D). The curves were obtained by nonlinear regression analysis with five experimental data points, each obtained with different doses (7.5 to 432 μg) of [^{11}C]raclopride (2.7 mCi). Specific binding was calculated as the difference between radioactivity in the putamen and that in the cerebellum. Binding in the cerebellum was assumed to reflect the free radioligand concentration. Triangles represent the experimental data and dashed lines the fitted curves which were determined with an iterative program, BMDP. (Courtesy of Dr. L. Farde, Karolinska Institute, Stockholm, Sweden; Science 231:258, 1986)

with two intercepts, the one on the x axis giving the number of binding sites per molecule of ligand and y intercept providing $1/K_d$. Figure 26 illustrates the good agreement between subjects for these measurements. These data were also used to determine whether raclopride binds to more than one site. Hill plots with coefficients of unity indicate that bound/B_{max} is proportional to the fraction of total sites occupied, strongly arguing that raclopride binds to a single class of sites (Figure 27).

The raclopride method of measuring D2 receptors is valid only insofar as the following assumptions are correct (Sedvall et al. 1986):

1. Total radioactivity in the brain during the experiment represents unchanged [^{11}C]-raclopride; brain metabolism of the tracer must be negligible.

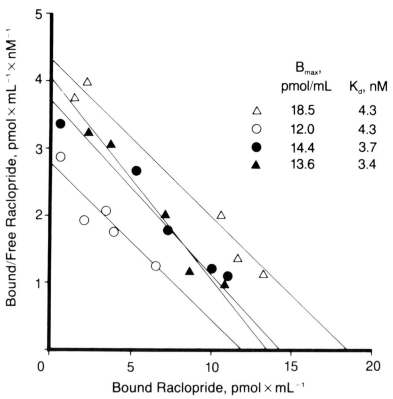

FIGURE 26.   Scatchard plots of [^{11}C]raclopride binding in putamens of four healthy men. B_{max} indicates maximum binding; K_d indicates equilibrium dissociation constant. (Courtesy of Dr. G. Sedvall, Karolinska Institute, Stockholm, Sweden; Arch Gen Psychiatry 43:1001, 1986. Copyright 1986 American Medical Association)

2. Equilibrium is reached within 42 minutes; measurements are taken at that time. K_d values are similar between 36 and 42 minutes. This indicates the presence of equilibrium.
3. Cerebellum radioactivity reflects the free concentration of [^{11}C]-raclopride throughout the brain. This is nonspecifically bound drug, free radioligand, and ligand within the local vasculature.
4. Endogenous dopamine does not influence [^{11}C]-raclopride binding to D2 receptors to any appreciable degree.

From this model the authors were able to determine that clinically effective doses of antipsychotic medication resulted in 84–90% receptor occupancy by medication. It is not known to what extent receptors must be occupied (percentage), and for how long, in order for a medication to have its maximal therapeutic effect.

D2 Receptor Measurement Using N-Methylspiperone. Wong et al. (1986a, 1986b) have presented a model that estimates absolute recep-

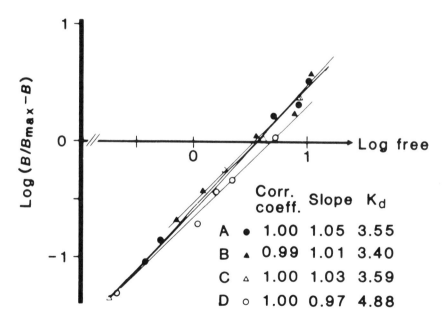

FIGURE 27. Hill plots of the four normative studies presented in figure 25. To calculate the hill plot parameters the B_{max} value from the nonlinear regression analysis of the data for each individual was used. K_d values were determined from the intersection with the abscissa. Coefficients of unity indicate a single species of receptor. (Courtesy of Dr. L. Farde, Karolinska Institute, Stockholm, Sweden; Science 231:259, 1986)

tor density; it requires the onset of a steady state between plasma and nonspecific binding in brain tissue following the [^{11}C]-NMSP injection. This method relies on the measured reduction in available D2 binding sites following unlabeled haloperidol administration. It is assumed that haloperidol equilibrates during the PET scan. The available number of receptors will remain constant during the scan. Taken from a study of normal volunteers, schizophrenic patients previously treated with neuroleptics, and schizophrenics not previously treated with neuroleptics, the following figure illustrates the relationship between the reciprocal of the absolute rate of binding ($1/k_3$) and the haloperidol concentration in the serum. Using this procedure young normal volunteers have demonstrated receptor densities in the order of 10 to 14 pmole/g (Figure 28).

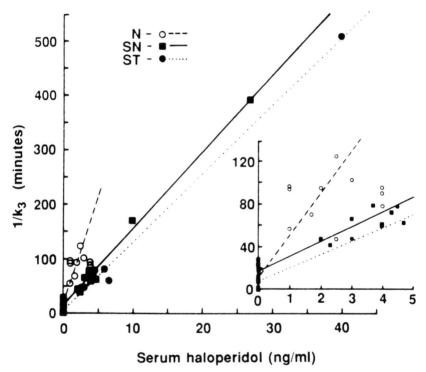

FIGURE 28. Binding rate reciprocal is proportional to plasma haloperidol concentration. This relationship is plotted for normal volunteers (N), neuroleptic treated schizophrenic patients (ST), and neuroleptic naive patients with schizophrenia (SN). The slope of $1/k_3$, plotted against serum haloperidol concentration, for each subject, provides an average slope that is proportional to the reciprocal of [k'off$\times$ B$_{max}$]. The values of the average slopes for all normal (N), drug-naive (SN), and drug-treated (ST) subjects were 39.0 ± 7.2, 13.3 ± 1.4, and 12.0 ± 1.6 min/ng/ml, respectively. (Courtesy of Dr. D. Wong, Nuclear Medicine, Johns Hopkins Medical Institutes, Baltimore, Maryland; Science 234:1560, 1986)

Nonequilibrating tracers such as [^{11}C]-NMSP have been successfully used as a measure of D2 dopamine receptor binding. There are certain advantages to tracers which are effectively "irreversibly bound" over the PET scan period; because the rate of dissociation from the receptor (k_4) is very small or negligible, a high signal-to-noise ratio is achieved. Limitations to the nonequilibrium study of receptors are also evident. When the free-ligand concentration in brain tissue is so small that it becomes insensitive to changes in receptor density, one must reduce the number of available binding sites by pretreating the subject with a neuroleptic. Wong et al. (1984) have found that in normal older subjects it is possible to use the kinetic model previously described to specifically calculate an absolute rate of binding to the receptor (k_3). In patients with schizophrenia or normal young subjects, the high caudate D2 receptor density prevents accurate estimation of k_3 without performing multiple studies with known plasma levels of haloperidol. In the absence of inhibiting or unlabeled competing ligands (e.g., haloperidol), the binding of [^{11}C]-NMSP may be sufficiently high that k_3 estimates become inaccurate. In this situation the steady state slope becomes more like k_1 when k_2 is much less than k_3. *In extremely high receptor concentrations the caudate–cerebellar ratio slope is diffusion limited.* This can be determined kinetically and this limitation on the measurement of k_3 can be removed with prior reduction of the available number of receptors by unlabeled competitors. The caudate–cerebellar ratio reflects the absolute rate of binding to the receptor when the number of receptors is small; it is more a reflection of diffusion limitation in young normals and patients with schizophrenia, who exhibit high receptor concentrations and low free-ligand concentrations. Examples of NMSP time/activity curves are shown in Figures 29 and 30.

Another related point is the effect of an increase in the tracer mass. Increasing the tracer mass (which correspondingly decreases the specific activity of the [^{11}C]-NMSP) enables the caudate–cerebellar-ratio-versus-time and the volume-versus-theta plot to measure the rate of binding if the curves demonstrate equilibrium. With an irreversibly binding ligand the unlabeled NMSP and hence the number of available receptors will change over time. One way to measure the rate of binding to the receptor accurately with such nonequilibrium conditions is to lower the available number of receptors by administering a blocker (Figure 31).

Alternatively, even with a slowly or irreversibly binding ligand it may be possible to estimate B_{max} and association-rate constants using two different specific activities in the same sitting as suggested by Huang et al. (1986a). In their definition of k_3 (different from Wong et al. 1986) there is a time dependence since k_3 depends on the ratio of specifically bound tracer to specific activity. Under the assumption of a "constant k_3" for

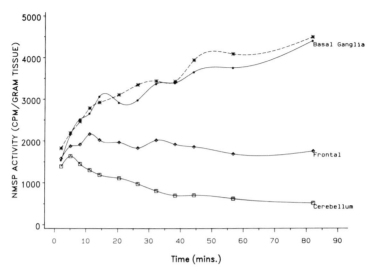

FIGURE 29. NMSP time/activity curves in a 30-year-old depressed man given 1 mg of fluphenazine 4 hours prior to ^{11}C-NMSP administration. Unlike the time/activity curve in Figure 30, these data suggest equilibrium is being approached during the 60–90 minute interval. (Courtesy of Drs. C.A. Tamminga, D. Wong, and H. Holcomb, University of Maryland Psychiatric Research Center, Baltimore, Maryland; and Johns Hopkins Medical Institutes, Baltimore, Maryland)

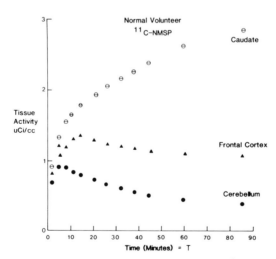

FIGURE 30. NMSP time/activity curves in a 22-year-old normal volunteer without D2 receptor blockade (no neuroleptic). Unlike the cerebellum or frontal cortex (both reach equilibrium early), caudate NMSP binding continues to rise during the 60–90 minute interval. (Courtesy of Dr. D. Wong, Johns Hopkins Medical Institutes, Baltimore, Maryland; Journal of Cerebral Blood Flow and Metabolism 6:141, 1986)

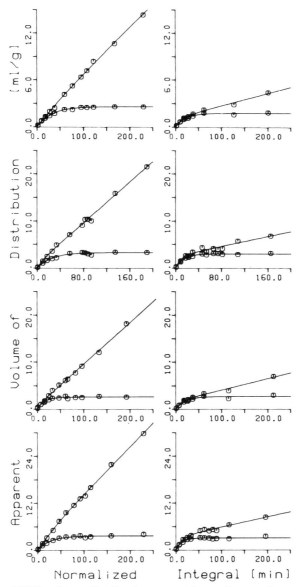

FIGURE 31. NMSP volume distribution curves in caudate nucleus and cerebellum, and the normalized time integral of NMSP in plasma, in four normal volunteers: *(upper curves)* caudate nucleus, *(lower curves)* cerebellum. *Left:* uninhibited uptake of NMSP. *Right:* Haloperidol-inhibited uptake. Abscissas indicate normalized time integral of plasma radioactivities; ordinates indicate apparent volumes of distribution (ml/g). (Courtesy of Dr. D. Wong, Johns Hopkins Medical Institutes, Baltimore, Maryland; Journal of Cerebral Blood Flow and Metabolism 6:150, 1986)

different specific activities, this double injection method can yield receptor estimates. Huang et al. (1986a) also reviewed the two dynamic methods proposed by Wong et al. (1986a, 1986b) and Perlmutter et al. (1986). Both employ an estimate of k_3 without the assumption of Huang et al. (1986a). Perlmutter et al. (1986) proposed an exact solution of the same basic differential equations employed by Wong and Huang et al., but applied them to a baboon study. Wong et al. employed in human studies an analysis algorithm and a normalized integral plot (Patlak et al. 1983) to estimate the k_3. This latter method may be more useful since the exact solution is impractical except for PET scanners with high temporal resolution. Furthermore, Wong et al. (1986b) have employed blocking studies with haloperidol to estimate B_{max}. This avoids the problem of injecting high doses of potent radioligands that have regulatory and safety restrictions. Huang and colleagues (1986a) point out that the equilibrium method proposed by Farde et al. (1986) may not require such rapid temporal sampling.

Opiate and Benzodiazepine Receptor Measurements in Vivo Using Positron Emission Tomography

Reports authored by Persson et al. (1985) and Samson et al. (1985) have recently described the distribution of RO 15-1788, benzodiazepine, binding sites in human brain (Figure 32). By labeling the tracer with ^{11}C, the investigators were able to use PET measurements to determine the highly specific, competitively displaced (with unlabeled RO 15-1788) binding of this potent benzodiazepine antagonist. In Figure 23 (1985), the sensitivity to competitive displacement is clearly shown. The rapid displaceability of [^{11}C]-RO 15-1788 by unlabeled compound, low nonspecific binding characteristics, potent pharmacological properties, and physiologically appropriate binding pattern make this ligand especially promising as a new probe for studying in vivo benzodiazepine pharmacology and related behaviors. The modeling and pharmacology of other benzodiazepine ligands labeled for PET research are in progress (Frost et al. 1986), and should complement the work initiated by Persson et al. (1985) and Samson et al. (1985).

Two studies (Pert et al. 1984; Frost et al. 1985) indicate the feasibility of labeling an opiate antagonist, acetylcyclofoxy (Pert et al. 1984), and agonist, carfentanil (Dannals et al. 1985; Frost et al. 1985), with positron-emitting isotopes ^{18}F and ^{11}C, respectively. The displacement of carfentanil, a potent synthetic agonist, from opiate-rich regions in the human brain by multiple doses of naloxone is shown in Figure 33. The distribution of labeled carfentanil in various brain structures is shown in Figure 34. The high degree of tissue specificity is consistent with animal

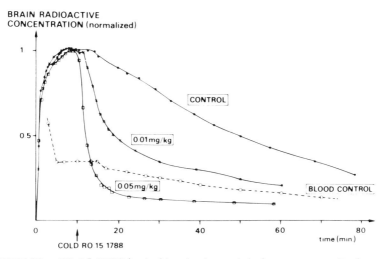

FIGURE 32. RO 15-1788 brain kinetics in occipital cortex: two displacement studies (0.01 mg/kg and 0.05 mg/kg unlabeled tracer) and one control study are shown. Curves are expressed in arbitrary units; the individual activity values are normalized to that obtained at T = 9.5 min. The time course of plasma radioactivity concentration is also shown (dotted line). (Courtesy of Dr. Y. Samson; European Journal of Pharmacology 110:249, 1985)

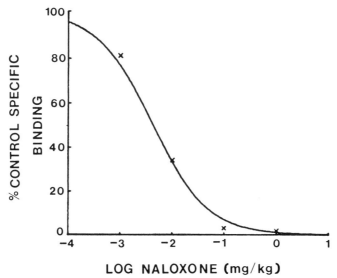

FIGURE 33. Competition curve generated by administering four different doses of naloxone to a subject receiving the same dose of [¹¹C]carfentanil in each study. Measurements were made of the basal ganglia and thalamus. (Courtesy of Dr. J.J. Frost, Nuclear Medicine Division, Johns Hopkins Medical Institutes, Baltimore, Maryland)

studies using other opiate receptor ligands (Kuhar et al. 1973; Herkenham and Pert 1980).

The principal strength of the benzodiazepine and opiate receptor ligand studies briefly presented above lies in their use of compounds which bind reversibly and reach equilibrium conditions within the time frame appropriate for PET measurements using ^{11}C.

Neuropsychiatric Research Using PET: A Review

Common Methodological Problems Encountered in PET Research

Three general groups of technical problems are inevitably encountered in PET research: 1) anatomic identification of regions being measured, 2) the statistical analysis of numerous measurements (many of which are highly intercorrelated) in a small number of subjects, and 3) the physiobehavioral interpretation of complex statistical relationships between regions that share complex physiological connections with one another.

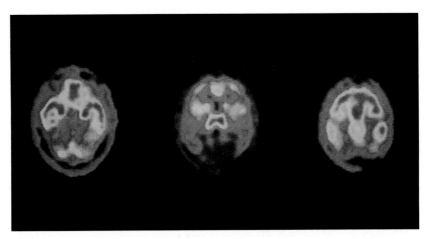

FIGURE 34.   Carfentanil binding at three different brain levels, *(left)* 24 mm, *(center)* 56 mm, and *(right)* 88 mm above the canthomeatal axis. High activity areas in the 24 mm plane include the amygdala, superior temporal lobe, and rectus gyrus. The 56 mm plane reveals high binding activity in the basal ganglia, cingulate cortex, and thalamus. At 88 mm, the regions of highest activity include the cingulate and prefrontal cortical regions; parietal cortex also exhibits substantially higher binding than the occipital region. (Courtesy of Dr. J.J. Frost, Nuclear Medicine Division, Johns Hopkins Medical Institutes, Baltimore, Maryland)

Anatomical Localization for Positron Emission Tomography

PET provides functional metabolic or neurochemical maps of the brain. As a consequence, the anatomical landmarks conventionally used to define the various regions are blurred and difficult to identify accurately. From clinical and experimental viewpoints this is an exceptionally important point. First, one needs to know with certainty what structures, and what part of those structures, are being analyzed. Second, in one's analysis the same structures must be identified reliably among individuals and among groups. Third, correction for tissue atrophy (Alzheimer's and Huntington's diseases) must be included to avoid spurious inflated comparisons. At this time most groups rely either on brain atlas approximations of regional identifications or on structural images (XCT or MRI) using a standardized comparable head position.

Fox and colleagues (1985b) emphasize three criticisms of using closely matched structural images from brain atlases in association with PET images. This group suggests that accurate regional comparisons between PET images of different subjects is not possible with a method based on making comparisons of each subject's PET image with his or her own structural image. First, localization depends on the presence of gross anatomical boundaries evident on the structural image. And second, the identity, or registration, of the scanning planes of the physiological and structural images must be assured. Unless great care is taken to standardize head position, moving a subject from the PET area to the CT or MRI cannot assure perfect image registration. Fox (1985b) and the Washington University School of Medicine PET research group (Herscovitch et al. 1986; Perlmutter et al. 1985b) have published three exceptionally useful papers that describe their efforts to solve this important technical dilemma. Multiple reports from this group (Fox and Raichle 1984, 1985, 1986; Fox et al. 1985a, 1985b, 1985c, 1986) provide a history of physiological research which describes their methods.

A Stereotaxic Method for Standardizing Individual Brain Region Locations

Theory. In the service of providing a three-dimensional coordinate system for neurosurgeons, a line passing through the anterior and posterior commisures (AC–PC line, see Figure 35) has been adopted (Schaltenbrand and Wahren 1977; Talairach et al. 1967) as a common reference axis. The location of any point in this stereotactic coordinate system is defined by its distance from the center of the AC–PC line, a reference established by anatomical–geometrical correlation with skull landmarks (glabella and inion).

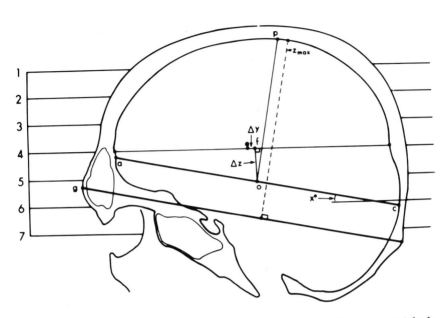

FIGURE 35.   Stereotaxic coordinate generation from sagittal and transaxial planar images. The glabella-inion (GI) line is placed on the radiograph, connecting the most anterior point of the glabella (point g) to the midpoint of the base of the inion (point 1). The line between the anterior and posterior commissures (ac–pc line; line aoc) is drawn parallel to and above the GI line. The GI to ac–pc distance is best estimated as 0.21 times the greatest perpendicular distance from the GI line to the vertex (Z_{max}). Once the ac–pc line (line aoc) is constructed, the measurements defining the relation between the tomographic planes and the stereotactic coordinate system are made. The center (o) of the ac–pc line (aoc) is the origin of the stereotactic coordinate system. The center (e) of the middle tomographic slice (slice 4) is the origin of the tomographic coordinate system. The vertical and anteroposterior distances between the origins are measured from the radiograph. The angle between the xy planes of the two coordinate systems is measured as the angle between the ac–pc line and any wire line. The system of proportionate measurements defines region location by the distance from the center of the ac–pc line relative to the total brain dimensions in each axis. Brain size in the anteroposterior and vertical directions are measured from the radiograph as the length of the ac–pc line and the perpendicular distance from the center of the ac–pc line to the vertex. By combining MR sagittal images showing horizontal plane placement, and horizontal images showing sagittal plane placement, the investigator increases his confidence in knowing where each coordinate is found. (Courtesy of Dr. P.T. Fox, Washington University School of Medicine, St. Louis, Missouri; Journal of Computer Assisted Tomography 9:144, 1985)

Brain orientation and dimensions.   In order to translate the tomographic images into standardized atlas coordinates, the precise relation between the two systems must be defined. This is accomplished by using a lateral skull film taken in conjunction with a calibrated, radiopaque marker or tubing. The marker's calibrations indicate the planes of the PET tomograph. Subsequent alignment of the skull with XCT would also be possible using this lateral film, a necessary step in the correction for cerebral atrophy. The skull radiograph records the positions of the PET 'slices' relative to the skull (a wall-mounted x-ray tube with a fixed focal-film distance facilitates this step).

After the lateral skull film is taken, the subject is placed in the scanner and a multislice transmission scan is taken. (This is commonly accomplished using a positron-emitting ring source, Germanium 68/Gallium 68.) The transmission image provides the transverse dimension of the tomograph. It will also be used to regionally correct all subsequent emission images for the effects of photon absorption (an important complication in basal brain regions). XCT images of the head also provide transaxial transmission scans and lateral topograms.

Transformation of regional coordinates.   The origin of the stereotaxic coordinate system is the center of the AC–PC line, lying in the midsagittal plane. The measurements defining the relationship between the tomographic and stereotactic coordinate systems are made from the skull radiograph and the transmission scan.

Assumptions.   Stereotaxic localization assumes that normal brains are similar in their anatomical relations and overall configuration. By using proportionate measurements the effect of subject-to-subject variation in brain size and shape is minimized. Four additional assumptions are made. First, the location of the glabella–inion (GI) line can be accurately and reproducibly determined from a lateral skull radiograph. Second, the GI line is assumed to be parallel to the AC–PC line. Third, the distance between the GI and AC–PC lines is assumed to be a fixed proportion of the vertical dimension of the brain, measured with a perpendicular to the GI line. Four, the center of the estimated AC–PC line is assumed coincident with the midcommissural point, the center of the atlas coordinate system. The accuracy and reproducibility of this system have been rigorously tested. Ultimately, it is highly desirable to have a standardized format for PET images; automated analysis programs are severely hampered by nonuniform data structures. Because most investigators measure different brain regions in every subject, and rarely provide objective stereotaxic identification of the imaged regions, they cannot specify to what extent measurements of similar regions are accurate. This variability, or heterogeneity, in data structures inevitably reduces the power of statistical analysis and further complicates the task of elucidating physiobehavioral relationships.

The method given above is "described and validated for use in the structurally normal brain. The application of this method to structurally abnormal brains is therefore subject to certain limitations" (Fox et al. 1985b, p. 151). Those groups studying patients with schizophrenia and other psychiatric/neurologic illnesses associated with morphological variations must integrate XCT or MRI scans of the same brain structures measured with PET, using a standardized reference system. Rigid, tightly fitting head-holders and face masks (Greitz et al. 1980) permit reliable *functional* activity measurements in a set of brain planes, specified by fiducial lines drawn on the head-holder; MRI or XCT structural images of those same brain planes may then be acquired. Commercially available image-analysis software will register morphologic and functional images on a pixel-by-pixel basis (Loats Associates, Inc., Westminster, Maryland). Image registration is followed by 'redirected' sampling, measurement of functional image activity from a region specified on the registered structural scan. Accurate assignment of a region's stereotaxic coordinates can be made if the XCT/MRI provides a lateral topogram (or scout film) with superimposed lines indicating the brain-scan planes.

Standard stereotaxic atlases (Schaltenbrand and Wahren 1977; Talairach et al. 1967) generate their x, y, z coordinates from the midline anterior commissure–posterior commissure (AC–PC) axis. MRI scans can locate that internal boundary, as well as the glabella–inion axis. XCT topograms delineate the glabella and inion. The GI line is parallel to the AC–PC axis and the GI-to-AC–PC distance is best estimated as 0.21 times the greatest perpendicular distance from the GI line to the vertex. These measurements made, one can then compute the three-dimensional coordinates of the individual patient's brain and describe regions of interest in standard atlas format. Techniques that rely on identifying specific brain regions from each individual's MRI have the advantage of relative certainty that one actually is measuring activity in that individual's specific brain region, even if individual differences in shape or structure are present. This is especially important for schizophrenia, the dementias, and other illnesses associated with structural abnormalities.

Face Mask Alignment: A Reference for Registering MRI, XCT, and Positron Emission Tomography Head Scans

The relationship of the PET scan plane must be determined with respect to its putative morphological counterpart. An alternative approach to that described above has been developed by one of the authors

(Holcomb et al. 1988). Borrowing from the method developed by Greitz et al. (1980), this method uses a modified face mask; thin (1–3-millimeter) plastic tubes are taped to the mask surface. They are filled with a liquid that is clearly visible in MRI or XCT, vegetable oil or diatrizoate meglumine (containing iodine), respectively. Figure 36 shows such a modification. Because the tubing is applied to the mask in a vertical zigzag pattern, each image plane that intersects the mask will reveal a unique geometric set of tube cross sections; each plane will have its own characteristic interpoint geometry. By measuring the point-to-point distances on the XCT or MRI console and matching those distances with measurements made directly on the mask, the investigator creates a one-to-one correspondence in point geometry between the image plane and the mask's tube configuration. Having obtained a set of morphological images that include these unique point sets, the clinician can then locate, and mark,

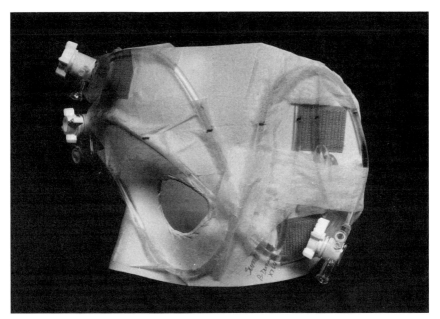

FIGURE 36. Face mask with image reference system. Plastic tubes are attached to the surface of an individually fitted, skin-tight mask. Because of the tube configuration, all image planes passing through the mask–tube assembly (and head inside the mask) will capture a set of tube cross-sectional points unique to that plane. By measuring the interpoint distances, which reflect the tube's distances from one another, on the XCT or MRI console, the investigator identifies the plane's intersection with the mask. That intersection is then reproduced directly on the mask and used for subsequent image alignment. This permits precise inter-image modality registration. (Courtesy of Dr. H.H. Holcomb, University of Maryland Psychiatric Research Center, and Johns Hopkins Medical Institutes, Baltimore, Maryland)

that plane's intersection with the mask and align the PET scanner's detectors with the morphological plane of interest. This permits (within 2–3 millimeters) good interimage matching. Validation of that match can be obtained by emptying the vegetable oil from the tubes and filling them with [¹⁸F]-water (1–5 microCuries/ml). The same point geometry seen in the morphology images should now be found in the PET scan if alignment has been successful.

Accurate Regional Sampling Requires Morphologic Guidance

Perlmutter et al. (1985b) emphasizes that the best way to calculate global values for PET measurements utilizes data from the same anatomical regions for each subject, includes all of the brain, avoids data from nonbrain regions, and is easily implemented. Perlmutter and colleagues (1985b) compare metabolic measurements made on regions corrected for nonbrain tissue versus whole slice metabolism. This emphasizes the point of correcting for nonneuronal tissue and CSF. Redirected sampling from morphologic images circumvents this problem entirely (Figure 37).

Herscovitch and colleagues (1986) further elaborate on this point by comparing elderly normals against age-matched elderly patients with dementia. Inspection of his data strongly argues for this measure in comparing normal groups against patients with degenerative nervous ailments. Oxygen metabolism appears to be significantly higher in normal young subjects than in SDAT subjects prior to correction for atrophy, but not

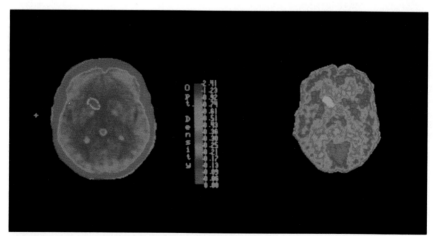

FIGURE 37. Redirected sampling from a registered XCT image (caudate nucleus) to the corresponding PET plane. (Courtesy of H.L. Loats, Loats Associates, Westminster, Maryland)

after correction. Oxygen metabolism, it appears, is a less robust indicator of physiological differences than CBF.

Statistical Analysis of Clinical PET Data

Table 1 provides the interested reader with a list of papers which use and discuss the general problem of analyzing experiments characterized by many highly intercorrelated measurements in a small number of cases. This problem is further complicated by the dearth of test–retest reliability studies (Brooks et al. 1987; Reivich et al. 1982) and the use of different test conditions by the various PET groups. It is, therefore, difficult to assess how much change in how much of the brain is 'real.' It is also difficult to compare one patient group with another due to the differing test conditions (Buchsbaum et al. 1984; Volkow et al. 1986a, 1986b; Gur RE et al. 1987a, 1987b). In each of these schizophrenia studies, FDG was given to patients in different physiobehavioral conditions.

FDG and CDG ([^{11}C]-labeled 2DG) studies carry an inherent limitation not found in dynamic blood flow studies. The former studies use isotopes with relatively long half-lives (109.7 min = FDG, 20.4 min = CDG), whereas blood flow studies use oxygen-15, which has a half-life of 2.07 minutes. If one waits for five half-lives between studies, then one may perform only one FDG, or two CDG, studies per day. In marked contrast, one may easily perform a new blood flow, oxygen-15 study every 10 minutes. If the investigator is able to determine the measurement error in all brain regions in association with each test condition,

TABLE 1. PET Data Analysis: Alternative Statistical Methods Data Papers

Papers	
Univariate ANOVA	Buchsbaum et al. 1984
Multivariate ANOVA	RE Gur et al. 1987a, 1987b
Correlation matrix	Clark et al. 1984
	Metter et al. 1984a, 1984b
	Horwitz et al. 1984, 1986
Regression model	Clark et al. 1986
Principal component analysis	Volkow et al. 1986b
Signal detection through noise subtraction	Fox et al. 1986

Methodological Papers and Editorials

Multiple comparisons	Ford 1983
	Oken and Chiappa 1986
Correlation matrices	Ford 1986
	Clark and Stoessl 1986
	Kennedy 1985
Q-component analysis	Clark et al. 1985

he or she can then determine how much change is necessary for statistical significance. The greater flexibility afforded by using oxygen-15 also facilitates mixing the order of behavioral states, though it has not been demonstrated that order effects play an important role in PET research completed thus far.

Concerning the statistical methods used in the papers listed above, it is important to emphasize two additional complications of PET/DG studies. First, they are expensive, time-consuming, and labor intensive (about 10 people usually participate in each). As a consequence, most studies use relatively small samples of clinically heterogeneous patients. Second, though one may, by carefully controlling the amount of radionuclide given in each study (less than 5 mCi of FDG/injection), perform as many as four metabolic PET experiments in each subject (over a period of days to weeks), significant amounts of time elapse between studies (a minimum of 100 minutes for [^{11}C]-2DG PET) and it is difficult to assure that the anatomic structures subsequently sampled match those of the initial scan. This makes it difficult to assure accuracy in the test–retest design. This problem is reasonably solved by using XCT coimaging and a tightly fitting face-mask or head-holder system. Increasing time intervals between studies will promote greater variance in metabolic measurements. It is important to determine, for any given diagnostic group, the variance associated with each region of interest and each test condition. Ideally, each member of each group should be studied four times, twice in each of two different conditions. That time-consuming and expensive approach would permit error measurement assessment for each region of interest, each subject, and each test condition. That in turn would allow one to determine accurately how much change between conditions, for a given ROI, was due to normal variance and how much to the task in question, for the group being studied.

By way of further emphasizing the power of using multiple studies on single individuals, in combination with a standardized measurement system, Fox and colleagues (1987b) recently mapped functional zones of visual cortex separated by less than 3 millimeters. This was possible by virtue of using a highly sensitive physiological marker (CBF), a powerful stimulus (visual activation), and an imaging strategy that emphasized a signal-to-noise-detection approach to cortical function analysis. *It is for these reasons that dynamic blood flow studies have strong advantages over 2DG studies.* Only by subtracting previous, control-condition scans from test activated-condition images were the investigators reliably able to identify optimal response fields to macular, perimacular, and peripheral stimuli. Conceptually, this method depends on the assumption that zones of brain activity separated by less than one FWHM can be distinguished from one another by sequential activation even though they would not be seen as distinct (not resolved) if activated simultaneously. This signal-detection strategy is identical to that employed by radar detection of moving objects; the field detected in the first moment is subtracted from that detected in a second moment. Only by comparing the same brain region in two or more conditions and performing appropriate subtraction or ratio manipulations can this be accomplished. Visual cortex metabolic mapping is illustrated in Figures 38, 39, and 40. Retinotopy by stimulus eccentricity is shown in Table 2.

Within-Subject Multiple-Test Design

By using each individual as his or her own control in carefully monitored behavioral designs, we may be able to avoid the principal detractor of PET measurements, our inability to know what is, and what is not,

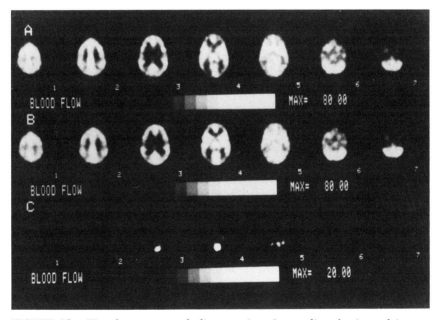

FIGURE 38. Visual cortex metabolic mapping. Seven-slice, horizontal images from a single subject's scanning session. A: Resting state image of cerebral blood flow (CBF). B: CBF image acquired while viewing the peripheral annulus. C: Image of the absolute change in CBF induced by peripheral visual stimulation, determined by subtracting image A from image B. Response location was identified using interslice interpolation and a computerized search routine. This identified the brain volume having the greatest increase in CBF during the stimulus. (Courtesy of Dr. P.T. Fox, Washington University School of Medicine, St. Louis, Missouri; Journal of Neuroscience 7:913-922, 1987)

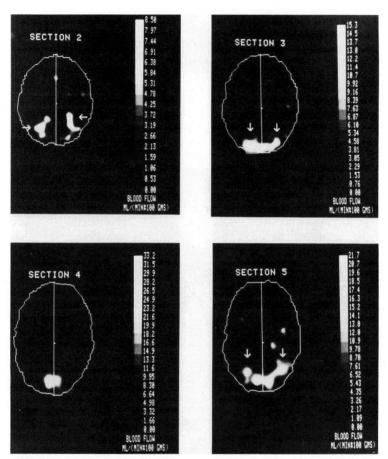

FIGURE 39.   Visual cortex metabolic mapping. Extrastriate visual area responses were elicited in many stimulus trials.

relevant in an individual's brain metabolism. Because each subject has a unique baseline metabolic-activity profile, many subjects must be measured in order to determine the feature most closely related to a given behavior. The problem changes dramatically when one studies a subject twice. By subtracting the complex background patterns (like radar) present in the first and second study, the investigator can determine directly which regions are associated with a given behavior and how much metabolic change is associated with a given behavioral change. When measuring metabolic patterns in patient groups with particularly high levels of variance (e.g., patients with schizophrenia) it is especially im-

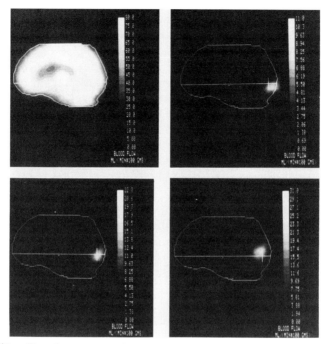

FIGURE 40. Visual cortex metabolic mapping. Macular response focus in a subtraction image format.

TABLE 2. Retinotopy by Stimulus Eccentricity Expressed in Stereotactic Coordinates

	Macula	Perimacula	Periphery
Degrees	0.1–1.5	1.5–5.5	5.5–15.5
n	5	6	6
Anteroposterior axis (cm)			
Mean (SD)	− 6.86 (0.13)	− 6.29 (0.09)	− 5.96 (0.07)
Statistical	ANOVA: $F = 42$, $p < 0.00001$		
Analysis	Newman-Keuls: macula < perimacula < periphery; $p < 0.01$ for all inequalities		
Vertical axis (cm)			
Mean (SD)	− 0.50 (0.36)	− 0.12 (0.32)	0.64 (0.42)
Statistical	ANOVA: $F = 90$, $p < 0.00001$		
Analysis	Newman-Keuls: macula < perimacula < periphery; $p < 0.01$ for all inequalities		

(Courtesy of Dr. P.T. Fox, Washington University School of Medicine, St. Louis, Missouri; Journal of Neuroscience 7:913-922, 1987)

portant to use the within-subject multiple-test design to circumvent the "noisy" data characteristic of heterogeneous groups. Patients suffering from disorders of attention, vigilance, memory, and cognition (e.g., visuospatial relationships, word choice, psychophysical relationships, etc.) are likely to provide the most interpretable test results when studied twice (or more) and compared with a large normative data base. Such a data base should provide the clinician and research neurobiologist with a three-dimensional model relating behavioral performance to two primary brain metabolism measurements: where and how much.

For example, a normal 30-year-old woman with an IQ of 125 may be expected to show high levels of metabolic activation (determined by subtracting her resting, background scans) in the right parietal and left superior frontal region when discriminating between various intensities of brightness presented on a video terminal. Her accuracy in making those determinations may be directly proportional to metabolic activity in one region and inversely proportional to metabolism in another area. Were one to find a task-performance deficit in association with loss of activation in one of these regions, in a particular patient matched for age, gender, IQ, and socioeconomic status, then one might seriously begin to use the PET scan data to 'understand' functional neuropathological syndromes. If depression, for example, were associated with a decrement in right-hemispheric frontoparietal activation, in specific discrimination tasks, the clinician would be able to better diagnose/prognose cognitive deficits commonly seen by psychiatrists and neurologists.

The brain is dynamically and regionally interactive; during any given moment, within any given task session, many regions will be highly intercorrelated. Regional interrelationships are probably stable for a given task (hypothetically) in a given diagnostic group. *It has not been established how best to interpret interrelational changes in association with various tasks in various groups.* Does one predict a higher degree of correlation between motor cortex and basal ganglia in an animal at rest or in an animal actively using its motor system to move? Unilateral nigral stimulation is associated with a significant reduction in ipsilateral corticostriate correlational strength compared with the same regions in animals at rest (0.90 versus 0.78; Holcomb et al., unpublished data). Other studies using PET raise complex and important issues regarding interregional correlational analysis. What, for example, do we make of a different frontoparietal interregional correlation matrix in healthy young normals versus healthy elderly control groups (Horwitz et al. 1986; Kennedy 1985). Only by analyzing the brain's principal components' structure in the same subjects under multiple, controlled, measured conditions can we interpret correlation matrices in a comprehensive and useful physiobehavioral context.

The Physiobehavioral Interpretation of PET Research

Clinical PET studies have recently addressed sensory (Fox and Raichle 1984, 1985; Fox et al. 1987a, 1987b); cognitive (Gur RC and Reivich 1980; Gur RC et al. 1983); and motor function (Fox et al. 1985d) in normal subjects. Quantitative studies relating behavioral performance and pattern/magnitude of CMR have been sparse. Fox and colleagues (1984a, b), measuring cerebral blood flow, have demonstrated a strong linear relationship between rate of visual stimulus and the magnitude of CBF in the human striate cortex (Figure 41). This paper is a striking exception to most PET studies which make no effort to meaningfully correlate performance or stimulus measurements with patterns of metabolic activity. An important opportunity to assess brain–behavior relationships is lost when subjects are studied with either an unmonitored task/stimulus or no task/ stimulus at all. When subjects are given somatosensory, visual, or auditory stimuli it is important to monitor the magnitude of the stimuli electro- physiologically (evoked potentials) or psychophysically (signal detec- tion). When subjects perform psychophysical, motoric, or cognitive tasks it is important to assess, preferably on a trial-by-trial basis, their perfor- mance throughout the study. Finally, when CMR is measured subsequent to drug administration it is important to make serial plasma measurements of both the drug and its active metabolites (Brodie et al. 1986). Ideally, investigators will also acquire independent biological measures of drug action. For example, diazepam's effects on the central nervous system can be monitored by EEG spectral analysis before and during the CMR mea- surements. By assessing behavior and relevant biological variables that coincide with CMR measurements, clinical neurobiologists can better account for the variability in metabolic rate patterns.

A Review of PET Metabolic Research in
Normative and Pathological Conditions

In the following sections numerous topics are considered from the psychi- atric and neurological medical specialties. Many of these studies are pre- sented in a brief, abstracted form. It is beyond the scope of this chapter to consider each topic in the detail an interested reader may want to encoun- ter. An extensive reference list is provided.

Metabolic Studies: Normative Functions

Movement

The only carefully controlled PET study of normal human movement in the literature to date was that conducted by Fox and colleagues

(1985a) (Figure 42, Table 3). The use of five different conditions and dynamic CBF measurements made in normal volunteers makes this a model study. The generation of voluntary saccadic eye movements (SEM) was studied in nine normal, paid volunteers (seven men and two women). The paradigm included three SEM conditions, one finger-movement condition and two control conditions (initial and final). The three SEM condi-

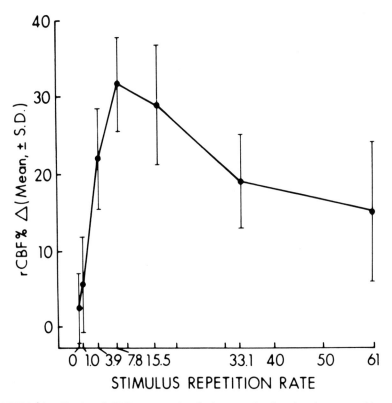

FIGURE 41. Regional CBF versus stimulation rate in the visual cortex of human subjects receiving variable frequency photic stimuli. Increasing the frequency of patterned-flash photic stimulation caused a selective regional CBF increase in striate cortex up to a maximum response at 7.8 Hz. Regional CBF declined with frequency increases beyond 7.8 Hz but remained above the unstimulated state. Each point and error bar represent the mean ± SD at each stimulus frequency. For 1.0 and 61 Hz, N = 8; for all other rates, N = 9. CBF response is expressed as the percent change from the initial unstimulated scan, rCBF% change. All CBF values were obtained from a standard region (5 pixels × 10 pixels × slice width) placed to enclose the area of greatest rCBF% change. For an individual subject, all measurements were taken from identical region coordinates. (Courtesy of Dr. P.T. Fox, Washington University School of Medicine, St. Louis, Missouri; Journal of Neurophysiology 51:1115, 1984)

tions included 1) targeted versus untargeted SEMs; 2) auditorily cued versus visually cued SEMs; and 3) stochastic versus rhythmic SEMs. Saccadic eye movements were associated with rCBF increases within the frontal eye fields, the supplementary motor area, and the cerebellum. Finger movements were associated with rCBF changes within the sensorimotor hand areas, the supplementary motor area, and the cerebellum. The

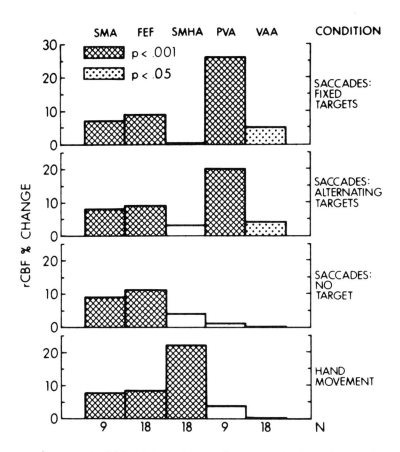

FIGURE 42. Cerebral blood flow changes for various brain regions and motor tasks. This figure illustrates for each brain region and task condition, the magnitude of the induced change in regional cerebral blood flow, expressed as the percentage increase over the mean of the control measurements. The significance levels given are for each region in comparison to control, as determined by the post hoc multiple rank testing described. The brain regions are the supplementary motor area (SMA), frontal eye fields (FEF), sensorimotor hand area (SMHA), primary visual area (PVA), and lateral visual association area (VAA). (Courtesy of Dr. P.T. Fox, Washington University School of Medicine, St. Louis, Missouri; Journal of Neurophysiology 54:348–369, 1985)

TABLE 3. Mean Blood Flow by Brain Region and Condition for Physiologically Defined Regions

	n	Cond. 1 Saccades: Fixed Targets	Cond. 2 Saccades: Alternating Targets	Cond. 3 Saccades: No Targets	Cond. 4 Hand Movement	Cond. 5 Control	Analysis
Supplementary motor area	9	67	67	68	68	62	3 = 4 = 2 = 1 > 5*
Frontal eye fields	18	56	56	57	56	51	3 = 2 = 1 = 4 > 5*
Sensorimotor hand area	18	52	54	54	64	52	4 > 3 = 2 = 5 = 1*
Primary visual area	9	70	67	57	58	56	1 = 2 > 3 = 4 = 5*

The statistical hierarchy shown is from post hoc multiple-range testing (Newman-Keuls procedure). For each region, post hoc analysis was performed only if ANOVA indicated significant variation ($p < 0.01$ after Bonferroni correction) between test conditions. All equalities are for $p < 0.1$; * indicates $p < 0.001$.

(Courtesy of Dr. P.T. Fox, Washington University School of Medicine, St. Louis, Missouri; Journal of Neurophysiology 54:348-369, 1985)

frontal eye fields were consistently active during the generation of voluntary SEMs and uninfluenced by target presence, type of cue, or task complexity. The supplementary motor area (SMA) was consistently active during all motor tasks and was uninfluenced by the degree of task complexity or stochasticity. Lateral occipital visual association cortex activation was present only during targeted saccadic conditions; this was apparently secondary to the presence of a target and not due to occulomotor activity. Interestingly, the caudate nucleus, through which the occulomotor circuit passes, was not activated by any of these procedures.

The primate study conducted by Schwartzman and colleagues (1981) uses the 2DG autoradiographic method to compare the visual, motor, and auditory regions of five *Macacca mulatta* monkeys. Three animals were injected with 2DG while at rest and two were studied while repetitively pulling a 1-pound weight. Working monkeys, operantly conditioned, revealed marked asymmetric patterns of CMRgl in various motor-related brain regions, including motor cortex, caudate nucleus, putamen, globus pallidus, ventroanterior nucleus of the thalamus, ventrolateral nucleus of the thalamus, and subthalamic nucleus. A detailed somatotopic analysis of the precentral gyrus indicates that the regions of greatest increase were the arm and shoulder regions.

The early primate study by Kennedy and coworkers (1980) used four trained monkeys taught to respond to illuminated symbols to obtain a water reward by reaching forward and pressing a plastic key with the left hand. Control studies were completed in four untrained monkeys who were inactive except for sporadic spontaneous movements. In the activated hemisphere the following regions exhibited marked asymmetry: primary motor cortex, primary sensory cortex, the superior parietal lobule (area 5), ventral posterior lateral nucleus of the thalamus, the globus pallidus, and the ipsilateral cerebellar hemisphere (crus II). This study, like that of Schwartzman et al. 1981, suffers from the disadvantage of being a single set of measurements.

Visual perception

Described above in the discussions of signal detection, the unusual paper by Fox and associates (1987b) demonstrates the method for detecting subtle shifts in maximal activity associated with macular, perimacular, and peripheral visual stimuli (Figures 38, 39, and 40) (Table 2). Though CBF changes were only 20–30%, spatial localization of 0.5–15 mm was attained. This was accomplished with a tomograph having a spatial resolution of 18mm. With improved instrumentation, the ability to locate accurately changes below 1.0 mm should become commonly appreciated.

In an earlier paper, Fox and Raichle (1984) provide unambiguous physiological data regarding the coupling between rate of stimulation and rate of metabolic activity in the brain. Visual striate cortex rCBF, expressed as rCBF percentage of change from baseline unstimulated state, varied as a linear function of stimulus frequency between 0 and 7.8 Herz. Regional CBF declined with frequency increases beyond 7.8 Hz. This provides strong evidence regarding the use of PET in making neurophysiologically useful measurements, especially in the area of sensorimotor integration.

Using FDG, Schwartz and colleagues (1984) provide careful documentation of visual striate cortex activation using a complex visual stimulus. That stimulation activated a highly circumscribed cortical region in a unique pattern. This study indicates how an investigator may generate unique metabolic patterns in a subject by providing particular stimulus sets.

The primate study of Macko and coworkers (1982) reveals all cerebral areas that are strongly activated by retinal stimulation. Of the studies published, this is the most comprehensive in its directory of participant regions.

An early study in PET physiobehavioral research by Phelps and colleagues (1981a, 1981b) reports the metabolic response of the associative visual cortex to be more metabolically sensitive to image complexity than the primary visual cortex.

Somatosensory Stimulation

Strong correlations exist between rCBF and CMRoxy in the resting condition. Somatosensory vibratory stimulation was associated with a marked focal increase in CBF of the perirolandic cerebral cortex contralateral to the stimulated hand; a mean increase of 29% was observed. An equivalent local increase in CMRoxy was not present (Fox and Raichle 1986).

Using eight normal volunteers, Fox and colleagues (1987a) mapped the physiological activation of the first somatosensory region corresponding to lips, fingertips, and toes. Vibrotactile stimulation at a frequency of 130 Hz and amplitude of 2 mm was delivered with a hand-held vibrator beginning 30 to 60 seconds prior to isotope injection and halted at the end of the 40-second scan; 10 minutes elapsed before the beginning of the next stimulation period. A highly reliable test–retest pattern was obtained. Response magnitudes varied among the three response sites: fingertips—25% increase, lip—16%, toe—22%. Figures 43, 44, and 45 indicate the stereotaxic locations of activation foci.

The primate studies of Juliano and colleagues (1981) and Juliano and Whitsel (1985) provide a systematic mapping of metabolic activity patterns through the pericentral gyrus region. They are the metabolic equivalent of neurophysiological mapping.

In 21 normal adult controls, 30 minutes of 1/sec cutaneous stimulations, ranging in intensity from barely detectable to moderately noxious, administered to the right wrist, was associated with a significant left-hemispheric metabolic (FDG) enhancement. The entire left hemisphere glucose was higher than the right during shock and the right was higher than the left during rest. The left–right ratio was significantly different in the two conditions. Especially interesting is the difference in metabolic patterns between normal volunteers ($N = 21$) and schizophrenic patients

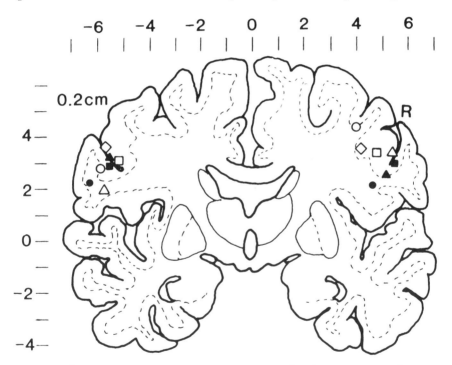

FIGURE 43. Human somatosensory cortex mapping by cutaneous vibratory stimulation and PET measurements of rCBF. Plot of stereotaxic coordinates of the first somatosensory cortex responses to lip vibration. Symbols indicate two responses, one per hemisphere, obtained for each subject from one bilateral (midline) stimulus trial. The mean right hemisphere response lay further from the midsagittal plane than did that of the left hemisphere (−5.6 cm vs. 4.8 cm; p < .001). This coronal brain section lies 0.2 cm anterior to the origin of the bicommissural coordinate system and corresponds to the mean anteroposterior axis coordinate of the lip responses. (Courtesy of Dr. P.T. Fox, McDonnell Center of Higher Brain Function and Department of Neurology, Neurosurgery, Radiology and Anatomy and Neurobiology, Washington University School of Medicine, St. Louis, Missouri; Journal of Neurosurgery 67:38–39, 1987)

($N = 17$). Whereas the former exhibited a robust left-greater-than-right sensory region difference, the latter group did not. Figures 46 and 47 illustrate the magnitude of this difference. Dark red pixels indicate a significant (p $<$ 0.05) left-greater-than-right difference in the respective groups (Buchsbaum et al. 1983a).

Lexical/Semantic and Auditory Stimulation

Heard in the right ear, either 500-Hz or 4-kHz monaural tones were presented to normal volunteers by Lauter and colleagues (1985). These

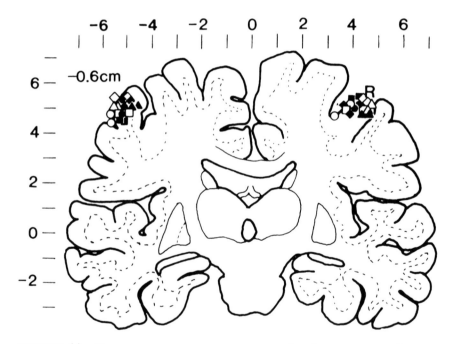

FIGURE 44. Human somatosensory cortex mapping by cutaneous vibratory stimulation and PET measurements of rCBF. Plot of the stereotaxic coordinates of the first somatosensory cortex responses to vibration of the fingers. Symbols indicate four responses, two per hemisphere, obtained for each subject from three stimulus trials: one bilateral trial and two unilateral trials. There was no significant asymmetry in response locale between hemispheres. This coronal brain section lies 0.6 cm posterior to the origin of the bicommissural coordinate system and corresponds to the mean anteroposterior axis coordinate of the finger responses. (Courtesy of Dr. P.T. Fox, McDonnell Center of Higher Brain Function and Department of Neurology, Neurosurgery, Radiology and Anatomy and Neurobiology, Washington University School of Medicine, St. Louis, Missouri; Journal of Neurosurgery 67:38–39, 1987)

investigators demonstrate unambiguous tonotopic, frequency-dependent areas of activation by pure tones. Not unlike the Washington University PET group's study of macular visual stimulation, this study maps those brain regions which respond best to these two different pure sounds. 500-Hz tones activate areas 6.7 cm lateral to the brain's midline (1.0 cm posterior to anterior–posterior, or AP, midpoint). In contrast, 4-kHz tones had their primary activating influence on areas 4.0 cm lateral to the brain midline (1.2 cm posterior to the AP midpoint). This study clearly points up the power of using within-subject multiple-study design and a standardized brain atlas system.

In an FDG study with 21 normals (Mazziota et al. 1982, 1984), visual versus verbal stimuli were presented. Bilateral activations of the thalamus

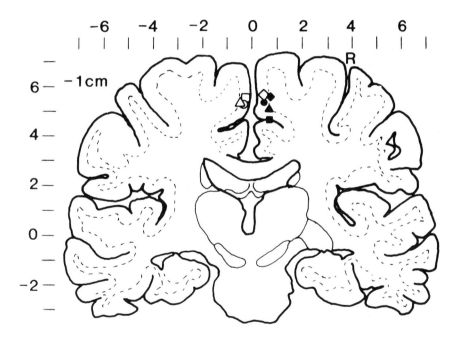

FIGURE 45. Human somatosensory cortex mapping by cutaneous vibratory stimulation and PET measurements of rCBF. Plot of the stereotaxic coordinates of the first somatosensory cortex responses to vibration of the toes. Symbols indicate the midline response obtained for each subject from a single bilateral stimulus trial. This coronal brain section lies 1.0 cm posterior to the origin of the bicommissural coordinate system and corresponds to the mean anteroposterior axis coordinate of the toe responses. (Courtesy of Dr. P.T. Fox, McDonnell Center of Higher Brain Function and Department of Neurology, Neurosurgery, Radiology and Anatomy and Neurobiology, Washington University School of Medicine, St. Louis, Missouri; Journal of Neurosurgery 67:38–39, 1987)

occurred with verbal stimuli; in contrast, the head of the left caudate was activated when subjects used visual imagery as a strategy to identify tone sequences.

During the unilateral presentation of a complex verbal story, normal subjects exhibited marked contralateral increases in temporal lobe metabolic activity (Reivich et al. 1983).

In a study by Petersen and associates (1988), four behavioral conditions are used to generate a three-level behavioral hierarchy related to single-word processing: 1) passive sensory processing, auditory or visual; 2) articulation and motor output programming; 3) and semantic associations. By using a series of tasks that add a small number of operations to those used in control state conditions, the investigator is able to subtract the stimulated from the control task condition. This subtractive data-

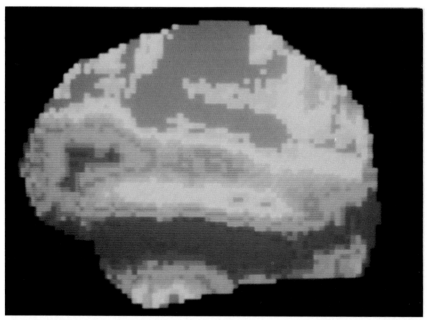

FIGURE 46. Left/right metabolic asymmetries in the brains of normal volunteers and schizophrenic patients receiving unilateral noxious cutaneous stimuli. Using normalized, group images, the authors show a consistent, topographically appropriate (somatosensory I), distribution of left > right differences in normal subjects receiving mildly noxious stimuli to the right wrist. Significant differences, left side greater than right, are indicated by dark red pixels. (Courtesy of Drs. M.S. Buchsbaum and H.H. Holcomb. These data were obtained at the National Institute of Mental Health, Section of Clinical Psychophysiology, Biological Psychiatry Branch, Bethesda, Maryland, 1981–1982)

analysis method permits rigorous comparisons of multivariate data in a small number of subjects.

In the first-level comparison the presentation of single words without a lexical task was compared to visual fixation without word presentation. No motor output or lexical processing is required in this primarily sensory state. In the second-level comparison, speaking each presented word was compared with word presentation without speech. In the third-level comparison the subject speaks a use for each presented word (shirt–wear). This third comparison targeted semantic processing.

Figure 48 summarizes the results of this study. First-level comparisons are represented by solid (visual) and open (auditory) triangles; second-level comparisons, by solid (visual) and open (auditory) circles; and third-level comparisons, by solid (visual) and open (auditory) squares. Whereas sensory comparisons activate mode-specific regions, with no overlap, motor and association comparisons generate foci in similar re-

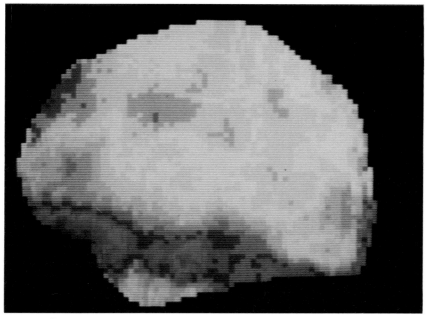

FIGURE 47.   Left/right metabolic asymmetries in the brains of normal volunteers and schizophrenic patients receiving unilateral noxious cutaneous stimuli. This normalized, group image indicates the absence of significant left > right differences in the schizophrenic patient population, in the somatosensory I area. (Courtesy of Drs. M.S. Buchsbaum and H.H. Holcomb. These data were obtained at the National Institute of Mental Health, Section of Clinical Psychophysiology, Biological Psychiatry Branch, Bethesda, Maryland, 1981–1982)

gions. Association tasks activated two areas of cerebral cortex for both auditory and visual presentation, the left inferior frontal areas and the anterior cingulate gyrus. From these findings the authors propose a general network of lexical processing.

Cognition

Using the Wechsler Adult Intelligence Scale, Chase and colleagues (1984) determined the association between IQ subtests and CMRgl, in a group consisting of 5 normal volunteers and 17 patients with Alzheimer's disease. Studied in the resting condition, the subjects exhibited strong correlations between the verbal IQ subtests and CMRgl in the left para-Sylvian region; scores on the performance subtests mainly localized to the right posterior parietal region.

Two groups of four normal subjects (all right-handed) participated in two cognitive studies, the Miller Analogies Test and spatial stimuli adapted from Benton's Line-Orientation Test. The verbal task produced greater CMRgl in Wernicke's area relative to the right-hemispheric

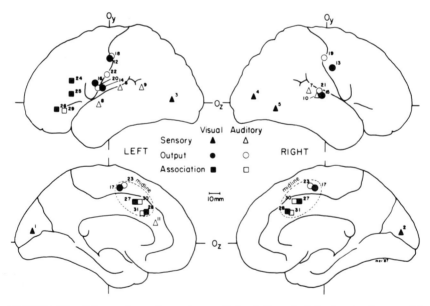

FIGURE 48. Schematic surface views of the left and right hemispheres with superimposed cortical activation foci. Note that no overlap in activation topography occurs in the sensory comparison, but that extensive overlap between visual and auditory modes occurs in the motor and association comparisons. (Courtesy of Dr. S.E. Petersen, Department of Neurology and Neurological Surgery, Washington University School of Medicine, St. Louis, Missouri; Nature 331:586, 1988)

homotopic region, whereas the spatial task produced greater metabolic activity in the right-hemispheric homotopic region (Gur RC et al. 1983a).

Aging and Cognitive Correlates

Using FDG scans in 23 healthy adults aged 27 to 78 years, Riege and associates (1985) determined the relationship between CMRgl and performances on 18 multivariate memory tests. Two of the five derived factors separated persons below age 42 from those above age 48 years, one reflecting secondary memory for material verbally processed together with Broca's metabolic ratio, the other defined by tests requiring sequential or organizational coding of information and metabolic measures of thalamic regions. Persons with high superior frontal and low caudate–thalamic metabolic measures were those who performed well in tests of memory for sentences, story, designs, and complex patterns.

Using FDG scans of subjects at rest in a sensory deprived state, Duara and colleagues (1984) studied CMRgl and various cognitive functions in 40 healthy men aged 21 to 83 years. Though age decrements were demonstrated in the error score on the Benton Revised Visual Retention Test and in the Performance Subtest of the WAIS, the cognitive test scores did not correlate with brain metabolic rates. Furthermore, CMRgl did not correlate with age.

Developmental Changes in CMRgl

FDG tomography performed in human infants during development revealed progressive changes in rCMRgl (Chugani and Phelps 1986) (Figure 49). In infants 5 weeks of age and younger, CMRgl was highest in the sensorimotor cortex, thalamus, midbrain–brainstem, and cerebellar vermis. By 3 months, CMRgl had increased in the parietal, temporal, and occipital cortices and in the basal ganglia; frontal and association regions increased in their CMRgl by 8 months. The interpretation of these studies is not uncomplicated; all of these children were studied by virtue of their having (or appearing to have) serious medical conditions. This is, nonetheless, the only group publishing PET CMRgl studies of human infants at this time.

Horowitz and coworkers (1986) analyzed intercorrelations between brain regional metabolic rates in 15 healthy young men ages 20 to 32 years, and 15 healthy elderly men ages 64 to 83 years. Elderly men had fewer statistically significant correlations; the most notable reductions observed were those between the parietal and frontal lobe regions. This group provides no immediate data that might help to determine the functional significance such a reduction might mean. Their review of the pertinent literature on parietal lobe function in the elderly is, however, revealing and useful.

Similar to that reported in the preceding study, de Leon and coworkers (1984) failed to find significant age-related changes in CMRgl. In their XCT measurements of young and old subjects they failed to find a relationship between normal brains' CT measurements and CMRgl activity. That is, though the normal brain undergoes structural change with age, it does not exhibit a corresponding reduction in CMRgl.

In contrast to the preceding studies, Kuhl and colleagues (1982a) found an age-associated reduction in mean overall cortex, caudate–thalamus, and white matter in their study of 40 normal subjects, aged 18 to 78. Importantly, no correction for cerebral atrophy was included in that analysis.

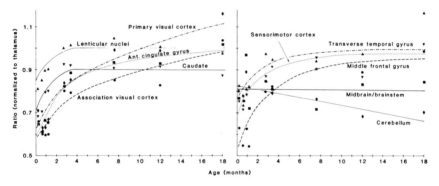

FIGURE 49. Regional brain metabolism rates (FDG) in normal infants during the first 18 months of life. LCMRgl is shown for several brain regions, expressed as a ratio to thalamic glucose utilization and plotted as a function of age for all nine infants. Because absolute glucose metabolic rates were not obtained in all subjects, the data were analyzed by several different approaches. The absolute values of LCMRgl were normalized to supratentorial global values of glucose utilization for all subjects with successful blood sampling. In subjects whose blood was not sampled, local tissue concentrations of radioactivity were normalized to average supratentorial global image counts to avoid errors intrinsic in absolute measurements and variable use of alternate substrates known to occur in early postnatal periods. In addition, local concentrations of radioactivity were normalized to values for the thalamus, a structure serving as a clear reference landmark in all our studies. Glucose utilization in the thalamus was well developed even in the youngest infant (5 days); preliminary data indicate that the absolute LCMRgl for this structure (26.97 micromoles per 100 grams per minute, mean ± standard error) does not undergo any significant change during the ensuing years. Both the global and thalamus reference yielded the same developmental trends, although the thalamus reference demonstrated less variability. (Courtesy of Dr. H.T. Chugani, UCLA School of Medicine, Los Angeles, California; Science 231:842, 1986)

Inactive/Resting Condition

Two studies by Mazziotta and colleagues (1981a, 1983) provide the first comprehensive directory of the resting human brain's CMRgl profile. In the initial study, this group demonstrates metabolic symmetry of the left and right hemispheres at rest. In the second study using 22 right-handed normal volunteers, this group describes CMRgl in three states consisting of selective or combined auditory or visual deprivation. A progressive decline in overall glucose metabolism occurs with reduced sensory input. The relative metabolism of the frontal cortex, compared to that of the parietal and occipital cortex, increased from the eyes-closed to the ears-closed to the both-closed states. A relative decrease in right-sided metabolism occurred in the combined audiovisual deprivation state. The most significant metabolic asymmetries occurred in the peri-Sylvian, inferior prefrontal, and lateral occipital cortex.

Sleep

Using FDG to assess brain CMRgl during sleep and dreaming, Heiss et al. (1985) studied four healthy male volunteers during wakefulness and sleep. Three of the subjects reported no dreaming, and during sleep stages I–IV of variable duration, exhibited a nonselective decrease in metabolic rates averaging 12.6% for the entire brain; in contrast, the fourth volunteer experienced an extended nightmare during his sleep study and he showed a generalized increase in cerebral glucose utilization ranging from 2.1% to 30%. Energy metabolism in the human brain is generally depressed during slow-wave sleep but may be especially active during dreaming. That reduction is consistent with an extensive primate study completed by Kennedy and coworkers (1982).

Metabolic Studies: Pathological Conditions

Epilepsy

In 80% of patients studied, discrete zones of hypometabolism in the interictal period are found; hypermetabolic cortical and subcortical regions are found during seizures (Engel et al. 1982a–d, 1983, 1985). Hypometabolic zones correspond with EEG recordings. These areas of depressed CMRgl coexisted with histopathologically verified lesions in 19 of 22 patients who exhibited this pattern in a 25-patient study. Figure 50, taken from Theodore et al. 1983, vividly illustrates the hypometabolic focus; electroencephalographic recordings taken from this subject's left hemisphere complement the functional image.

Temporal lobe epilepsy also appears to be characterized by marked disturbances in opiate-receptor distribution. Figure 51, from Frost et al. 1988, schematically indicates the large carfentanil-binding asymmetry associated with this disorder. The strong inverse correlation between glucose metabolism and carfentanil binding is particularly interesting (Figure 52). The physiological basis for this relationship is unknown at this time .

Parkinson's Disease (PD)

Patients with unilateral illness tend to have higher local CBF (LCBF) and local CMRoxy (LCMRoxy) in the basal ganglia contralateral to the symptomatic limbs. L-dopa given acutely tends to reduce LCBF and LCMRoxy but given chronically tends to enhance metabolic activity in the affected striatum (Leenders et al. 1983).

The number of significant cortical-to-cortical correlations was markedly reduced in PD patients compared to normals. PD patients show a loss of significant frontal–parietal and frontal–occipital region correlations. This loss of "statistical interconnectedness" may reflect reduced cortical functional integration (Metter et al. 1984a).

rCBF, rCMRoxy, and rCBV determinations in a man with strictly uni-

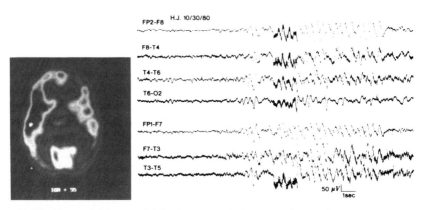

FIGURE 50.   Left temporal lobe hypometabolism (epileptic focus) and EEG recordings from the left hemisphere. *Left:* Interictal positron emission tomographic scan from a patient exhibiting a hypometabolic region of 28% over a wide area of the right hemisphere, maximal in the right frontal, superior temporal, and parietal areas. *Right:* Simultaneously recorded electroencephalogram showing bilateral irregular sharp waves and spikes and slow waves. (Courtesy of Dr. W.H. Theodore, Epilepsy Branch, Clinical Epilepsy Section, National Institute of Neurological and Communicative Disorders and Stroke, National Institutes of Health, Bethesda, Maryland; Annals of Neurology 14:434, 1983)

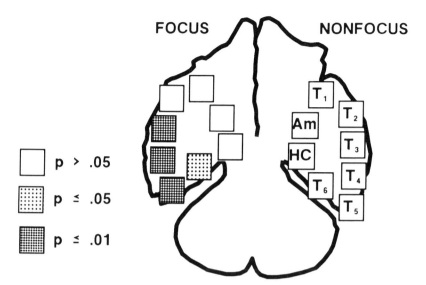

FIGURE 51.   Regional asymmetry in carfentanil binding, represented by a focus/nonfocus paired T-test map. Significantly elevated opiate receptor binding was observed only in regions of the temporal cortex ipsilateral to the seizure focus and not in the amygdala or hippocampus. (Courtesy of Dr. J.J. Frost, Nuclear Medicine Division, Department of Radiology, Johns Hopkins Medical Institutes, Baltimore, Maryland; Annals of Neurology 23:235, 1988)

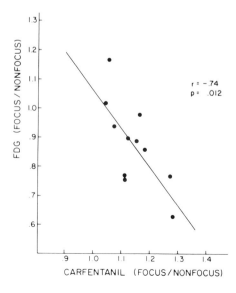

FIGURE 52. RCMRgl asymmetry versus carfentanil binding in the temporal lobes of epileptic patients. This graph plots the relationship between the mean asymmetry in [^{11}C]carfentanil specific binding and glucose utilization for regions T4 and T5 ($N = 11$), Figure 51. This highly significant inverse correlation between focus hypometabolism and opiate ligand binding may reflect selective neurotransmitter receptor upregulation secondary to opiatergic neuronal loss. (Courtesy of Dr. J.J. Frost, Nuclear Medicine Division, Radiology Department, Johns Hopkins Medical Institutes, Baltimore, Maryland; Annals of Neurology 23:235, 1988)

lateral PD symptoms revealed a normal CMRoxy for the entire brain. Precise, stereotaxically placed measurements of the affected globus pallidus indicated a marked increase in pallidal oxygen metabolism (48%), a finding consistent with extensive animal research (Raichle et al. 1984).

When compared with age-matched controls, PD patients exhibit a global cortical decrease in rCMRgL (18%). Follow-up studies indicate that rCMRgL is negatively correlated with the patient's severity of bradykinesia and dementia. No focal regions of hypo- or hypermetabolism were identified (Kuhl et al. 1984).

In four PD patients studied before and after L-dopa treatment, the rCMRgl of the lenticular nucleus and caudate nucleus was higher than in age/gender-matched controls (Rougemont et al. 1984).

The degree of pallidal rCMRgl hypermetabolism was proportional to severity of illness demonstrated on the contralateral side in four PD patients. Asymmetries in thalamus and cortex were not evident (Martin et al. 1984).

Mean CBF for the mesocortical regions contralateral to the patients' sympotomatic side was significantly lower than that measured in control subjects when studied in 11 hemiparkinsonian patients. After L-dopa treatment the contralateral mesocortical region CBF remained significantly less than that observed in normals (Perlmutter et al. 1985).

rCBF and rCMRoxy were determined in six normals, six hemiparkinsonian patients, and eight PD patients with bilateral illness. Consistent with previously cited studies, this report shows that the rCBF and rCMRoxy of the basal ganglia contralateral to the affected side were significantly greater than that found in either normal or bilaterally affected PD patients. Frontal cortex in hemiparkinsonian patients exhibited marked asymmetry in LCBF and LCMRoxy. Both were reduced in brain tissue ipsilateral to the hypermetabolic basal ganglia region (Wolfson et al. 1985).

Huntington's Disease

A study by Clark and colleagues (1986) finds that some patients at risk exhibit lower caudate metabolic rates than controls. When regional intercorrelations of standardized scores are examined with respect to caudate–thalamic activity, some at-risk subjects exhibit a marked disparity in predicted values. That is, in normals, metabolic activity in the right caudate predicts metabolic activity in the right thalamus. In patients with Huntington's disease this relationship is completely absent. Some patients at risk for developing HD fall outside a 2-standard-error boundary defined about the regression line for the normal controls. Using this regression line which relates thalamic to caudate activity, all 15 normal controls fell within 2 standard errors, none of the HD patients fell within 2 standard errors of prediction, and 6 of 18 at-risk subjects fell outside the 2 standard errors of prediction. This approach may become a powerful predictive tool for PET neuropathological studies.

In a combined FDG-XCT study (Hayden et al. 1986), the PET research group at the University of British Columbia makes a strong case for PET–FDG abnormalities preceding XCT-detectable tissue loss in the caudate. They demonstrate that caudate rCMRgL measurements are exceedingly sensitive and reliable in detecting HD. The lowest normal rCMRgl value for the left caudate was 6.96 mg/100 g/min, and the highest HD value for that region was 5.82. A similar finding for the right caudate was not shared by thalamic measurements. These 10 patients had a positive family history and neurological or psychiatric signs and symptoms, including chorea, a change in personality, or major psychiatric illness including depression or intellectual decline. No correlation between chorea score and caudate glucose metabolism was found.

In a paper from the University of Michigan PET research group (Young et al. 1986), 15 patients with early-to-midstage HD were evaluated with quantitative neurological examinations, scales for functional capacity, computed tomographic (XCT) scans, and PET–FDG/CMRgl. All patients had abnormal indices of caudate metabolism whereas in patients with early disease, indices of putamen metabolism and CT measures of caudate atrophy were normal. Caudate CMRgl correlated highly with the patients' overall functional capacity and bradykinesia/rigidity. Putamen CMRgl correlated highly with chorea, occulomotor abnormalities, and fine motor coordination. It is especially interesting that thalamic activity correlated with dystonia in a positive direction. Thalamic CMRgl was increased in HD patients compared to normal controls. Increased thalamic activity in this group may have a similar origin to that observed in animals treated with MPTP, a neurotoxin which induces parkinsonism. In both cases the loss of inhibitory input from caudate–putamen to the globus pallidus and substantia nigra may "permit" increased pallidal output to the ventrolateral (motor) thalamus.

In two studies (Mazziotta et al. 1985; Kuhl et al. 1982b) symptomatic Huntington's disease (SHD) ($N = 19$) and at-risk HD (ARHD) subjects were examined using FDG/PET. Initial studies demonstrated reductions in striatal CMRgl that preceded bulk tissue loss as determined by XCT. Three of the four ARHD subjects with the greatest reductions in CMRgl subsequently developed symptoms of the disease. In the follow-up study (Mazziotta et al. 1985) significant correlations were found between disease duration and the metabolic ratio of the caudate to the putamen in the SHD group ($r = 0.86$, $p < 0.005$). There were also significant correlations between the severity of occulomotor abnormalities (slowing of saccades, inability to maintain fixation) and the ratio of the caudate CMRgl to either the lenticular nuclei (r = −0.94, p < 0.01) or the thalamus (r = − 0.82, p < 0.01). No correlations were found between age, disease duration, or chorea and values for CMRgl in single structure or ratios of subcortical regions. The range of caudate CMRgl values in the ARHD group was greater than in controls. Five of the ARHD subjects had values for caudate metabolism that were within one standard deviation of the mean value of the SHD group, whereas no control subject had values in this range. The two ARHD subjects that had the lowest caudate CMRgl, had caudate–putamen ratios that were lower (> 2 SD) than controls. The authors suggest that the metabolic abnormality in the striatum begins in the caudate during the ARHD period and then progresses to involve the putamen during the symptomatic phase of the disease. Extrapolation of the caudate–putamen ratio curve indicates that a minimal value of 0.70 should be found at about the time of motor symptom onset.

Torticollis and Hemidystonia

Using FDG/PET measurements of regional CMRgl (rCMRgl), the University of British Columbia PET group (Stoessl et al. 1986) studied 16 patients with idiopathic *torticollis* and 11 normal subjects, all at rest (the normals did not rotate their heads as the patients were compelled to do). Regional CMRgl values in the two groups did not differ. When an interregional correlational analysis was performed using standardized scores, two different patterns emerged. Whereas normals exhibited high (p < 0.01) interregional correlations between ipsilateral and contralateral structures (caudate, lentiform, and thalamus), torticollis patients failed to exhibit significant caudate–thalamus or lentiform–thalamus intercorrelations.

In this single case study of *hemidystonia* using oxygen-15, the Washington University PET group (Perlmutter and Raichle 1984) point up the extreme sensitivity of this method in detecting focal abnormalities. A 50-year-old left-handed man suffered minor trauma to the right side of his head and neck. Within 20 minutes he developed paroxysmal intermittent dystonic posturing of his right face, forearm, hand, and foot with weaker contractions of the left foot, lasting several seconds and recurring every few minutes. Neurological findings between spells were normal. XCT scans were normal initially and four weeks later. Cerebral angiography was also unremarkable. In marked contrast, PET measurements revealed abnormalities in the left basal ganglion region, including decreased oxygen metabolism, decreased oxygen extraction, increased blood volume, and increased blood flow.

Schizophrenia

Introduction to the Problem: Neuropathology, CBF, and Neurological Abnormalities. Clinicians caring for patients with schizophrenia are often puzzled regarding the elusive origins of the illness. How can people with such profound behavioral disturbances have an illness that is so difficult to understand, so poorly localized. Neuropathological studies recently reported by Brown et al. (1986) indicate that when brains of schizophrenic patients were compared with brains of nonpsychiatric patients and patients with affective illness, the schizophrenic patients had brains that 1) were 6% lighter, 2) had larger lateral ventricles in the anterior and temporal horn cross section, and 3) had significantly thinner parahippocampal gyri, by 11%. These studies are consistent with XCT findings of enlarged ventricles in this group.

CBF studies, reviewed in this book, also suggest that patients with schizophrenia have severely abnormal patterns of neurophysiological activity in association with many behavioral challenges (Ingvar and Franzen 1974; Franzen and Ingvar 1975; Gur RE 1983; Gur RE et al. 1983, 1984, 1985; Weinberger et al. 1986; Berman et al. 1986; Guenther et al. 1986). *Generally, these studies suggest that the orderly transfer of programmatic information (especially the temporally contingent type) to and from various cortical, basal ganglia, and thalamic stations is severely impaired.*

Abnormal neurological functioning also characterizes patients with schizophrenia. Woods and his co-workers (Woods et al. 1986) recently published a carefully controlled analysis of neurological exams performed on various psychiatric diagnostic groups and normals. In their final analysis using only motor abnormalities of localizing significance (corticospinal, cerebellar, or unilateral extrapyramidal) the schizophrenic group was significantly more abnormal than either the normal or manic-depressive subjects.

PET: Glucose Metabolism and Blood Flow (Oxygen-15). PET studies of glucose metabolism and blood flow (oxygen-15) from the National Institute of Mental Health, New York University, the University of Pennsylvania, UCLA and Washington University, and England are reviewed below.

National Institute of Mental Health. This group's primary findings include a reduction in the frontal CMRgl/parieto-occipital CMRgl ratio, a nonphysiological cerebral metabolic pattern generated by unilateral noxious somatosensory stimulation, and neuroleptic enhanced CMRgl in left caudate and left temporal cortical regions.

Unmedicated schizophrenic ($N = 8$) and normal volunteers studied at rest with FDG exhibit significantly different anteroposterior gradients. Normal subjects have a higher front:back ratio than did schizophrenic patients (Buchsbaum et al. 1982).

Unmedicated schizophrenic ($N = 7$) and normal volunteers ($N = 10$) differ in their CMRgl response patterns to mildly noxious, cutaneous stimulation (electrical shocks ranging from 2–23 milliamps, one millisecond in duration, spaced one second apart, for 30 minutes, delivered to the right forearm area). Normal subjects exhibit a physiologically greater increase in the left postcentral cortex than the right; schizophrenic patients fail to generate that lateralized response (Figures 46 and 47) (Buchsbaum et al. 1983b).

Using the same experimental design described in Buchsbaum et al. (1983a), the authors show that right-sided cortical anteroposterior ratios were significantly higher in normal subjects than in either schizophrenic or affectively ill patients. More than a third of the patients had lower frontal than posterior rates of glucose use. No significant differences between affectives and schizophrenics were observed. Higher CMRgl levels in parietal–occipital regions of patients, especially those with affective illness, generated this abnormal pattern (Buchsbaum et al. 1984).

Using the same experimental design, these authors describe marked differences in the interregional correlation patterns observed in schizophrenic patients and normal volunteers. Normal subjects show a strong frontal coupling with left-sided regions, especially the left posterior frontal area. Schizophrenic patients, in contrast, exhibited few frontal correlations and no left-sided lateralization. This analysis of the data is consistent with the findings cited in Buchsbaum et al. (1983b), the failure of schizophrenic patients to generate metabolically lateralized activity patterns in response to somatosensory stimulation (Clark et al. 1984).

In this clinical correlation study (DeLisi et al. 1985a), the authors find no significant relationship between XCT-derived cortical atrophy measurements in the schizophrenic patients. Anteroposterior ratios did show a 0.59 correlation with emotional withdrawal on the Brief Psychiatric Rating Scale.

In their only test–retest study of patients, these authors found that schizophrenic patients treated with neuroleptics had significantly higher cortical CMRgl than the same subjects without medication; *left temporal lobe* regions were especially sensitive to the medication effect. Figure 53 illustrates enhanced rCMRgl in the frontal and cingulate cortex of a neuroleptic-treated patient (DeLisi et al. 1985b).

In one of the few reported PET/FDG/schizophrenia studies using a cognitively demanding task, Cohen and colleagues (1987) describe the distinguishing metabolic characteristics of normals and patients performing an auditory continuous-performance task (CPT), a strategy likely to emphasize group differences. This study is especially noteworthy for its use of an appropriate, neuropsychologically activating condition, and its reliance on conservative, multivariate statistical methodology. These investigators used 27 healthy volunteers and 16 drug-free patients. The CPT task employed a random series of 500-Hz tones, 1.0-second duration and 2.0-second inter-tone interval, with an intensity of 67, 75, or 86 decibels. Subjects were instructed to press a hand-held response button when the lowest volume tone was detected. After 30 minutes of this task (eyes were covered and the subjects were seated in a darkened room) 7 to 8 brain

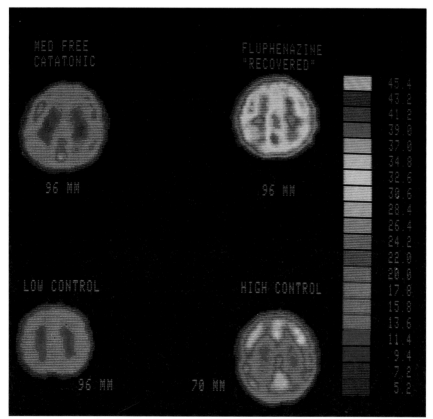

FIGURE 53. Neuroleptic treatment enhances regional CMRgl, especially in temporal lobe and basal ganglia regions. This set of images illustrates one patient's frontal cortex metabolic activity enhancement following treatment. Low and high control images are provided for comparison. (Courtesy of Dr. M.S. Buchsbaum. These data were obtained at the National Institute of Mental Health, Section on Clinical Psychophysiology, Biological Psychiatry Branch, Bethesda, Maryland, 1981–1982)

FDG/PET images were obtained. All subjects had learned the task satisfactorily (18 out of 20 correct responses) prior to the study (Figure 54) (Table 4).

Three sets of findings are described. First, the regions which differed most dramatically in the two groups (normal versus schizophrenic) were the left temporal cortex, 52 mm above the cantho-mental (CM) line (p = .02); and the middle frontal cortex, 65 mm and 52 mm above the CM line (p = .004, p = .04; respectively). These regions approximate Brodmann areas 10, 45, and 46.

Second, in normal controls performance and rCMRgl correlated highly in the medial, right anterior, and left anterior mid-prefrontal cortical regions. Schizophrenic patients exhibited no significant correlations with performance in the prefrontal cortex.

Third, both schizophrenic patients who scored as well as normals and patients who scored far below normals exhibited significantly lower rCMRgl in the middle prefrontal cortex than normal controls. The two patient subgroups did not differ from one another.

These findings are consistent with and extend those findings described in this review. It will be especially useful, in future studies, to characterize the regional brain metabolic changes in schizophrenic patients as they move from one set of tasks to another. By matching tasks and error rates against appropriate normals, investigators should gain useful information regarding brain function in this illness.

New York University. The principal strength of this group of reports, in contrast with studies cited from the NIMH group, is the use of a test–retest design. A second important methodologic feature is the use of

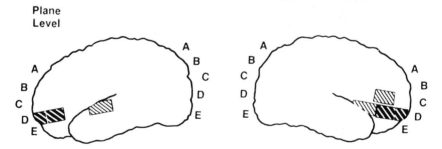

FIGURE 54. Schizophrenic patients performing an auditory continuous performance task exhibit marked cerebral glucose metabolism decrements, relative to normal controls, in the inferior frontal cortex and left anterior temporal lobe. Lightly hatched regions indicate p = .05 significance level; darkly hatched regions indicate p = .001 significance level. (Courtesy of Dr. R.M. Cohen, Clinical Brain Imaging Section, Laboratory of Cerebral Metabolism, National Institute of Mental Health, Bethesda, Maryland; Life Sciences 40:2035, 1987)

TABLE 4. Regional Glucose Metabolic Rate Differences Between Normal Controls and High and Low Scoring Schizophrenic Patients

Frontal Cortex

REGION	L. Posterior	L. Anterior	Medial	R. Anterior	R. Posterior
Plane					
A	+9.9* (−0.5)	+5.4 (+2.0)	+5.1 (+3.1)	+8.7* (+0.8)	+9.1** (+1.4)
B	+2.1 (+0.4)	+0.8 (−3.1)	+1.5 (−0.0)	−0.2 (−2.4)	+0.8 (+2.7)
C	−0.2 (+3.1)	−3.6 (−3.4)	−4.9 (−1.2)	−4.4 (−5.3+)	−3.5* (+1.4)
D	−6.4* (+0.2)	−7.2* (−7.7*)	−8.5+ (−7.8**)	−5.8* (−6.5**)	−9.0** (−1.7)
E	−2.2 (+7.2+)	+1.6 (−1.7)	−1.2 (−2.8)	+3.1 (−1.9)	−2.1 (+7.4+)

Temporal Cortex

	L. Posterior	L. Middle	L. Anterior	R. Anterior	R. Middle	R. Posterior
Plane						
D	−2.8 (−4.7)	−5.0 (+0.8)	−6.8* (−2.6)	−7.5* (−1.1)	−5.0 (+2.6)	−2.2 (−3.1)
E		−2.6 (+7.4*)			+1.4 (+5.0)	

Differences from normals and high-scoring patients are given outside of the parentheses; the differences from the low-scoring subgroup are given inside the parentheses. Differences between normal controls and all patients with schizophrenia is a weighted average of the two. Statistical significance (2 tailed t-test) for the high or low scoring subgroup comparisons to the normal group are represented by +, P = .06; *, P = .05; **, P = .01. Significance for all schizophrenic patients compared to normal controls is represented by single underline, P = .05; and double underline, P = .001. Values are uncorrected for the number of comparisons.

(Courtesy of Dr. R.M. Cohen, Clinical Brain Imaging Section, Laboratory of Cerebral Metabolism, National Institute of Mental Health, Bethesda, Maryland; Life Sciences 40:2035, 1987)

factor analysis (Volkow et al. 1986b) to reduce data redundancy. Generally, this group consistently found reduced CMRgl in frontal regions of schizophrenic patients. They also found higher temporal lobe CMRgl in schizophrenic patients treated with neuroleptics than in the same patients during their untreated phase. In both schizophrenics and normals amphetamine decreased frontal cortex CMRgl. Individual studies are summarized.

In a study of 13 schizophrenic patients (6 medicated, 7 unmedicated), Farkas and colleagues (1984) replicate Buchsbaum's first study which found a reduced anteroposterior ratio in patients compared with normals.

In this test–retest study of 10 schizophrenic patients and 8 normal volunteers, Wolkin and coworkers (1985) find significantly lower CMRgl in the left frontal and temporal cortical regions of schizophrenic patients than normals. In 8 patients scanned a second time (on medication), the *right temporal cortex* exhibited a marked elevation in CMRgl; the most impressive change was the marked decrease in relative frontality following treatment. That effect was dependent on a marked elevation in occipital cortex activity. They also noted no significant correlations between changes in CMRgl and clinical symptomatology. In this study, as in that by DeLisi et al. (1985b), normal subjects were scanned only once. This lack of parallelism prevents one from determining the "normal" measurement error expected for various regions on a test–retest schedule.

In an effort to better determine the metabolic impact of acute neuroleptic medication, Volkow and associates (1986a) administered 5 mg of intramuscular thiothixene 60 minutes prior to a second scan, the first scan having been obtained three hours prior to the second. A highly significant elevation in CMRgl was observed in the right caudate–putamen of the four schizophrenic subjects studied. Three of those four subjects had never received neuroleptic medication. When compared with 12 normal controls, the schizophrenic patients exhibited similar or slightly higher overall CMRgl activity patterns. No hypofrontality was found in this group of patients with relatively untreated illness. Plasma levels of neuroleptic were not determined.

The effects of d-amphetamine (0.5mg/kg p.o.) on CMRgl in 8 normal and 16 chronic schizophrenic patients was determined in a placebo-controlled, same-day, test–retest study using [^{11}C]-2DG (Brodie et al. 1986). A comparison of baseline scans demonstrated decreased cerebral metabolism in schizophrenic patients, especially the frontal areas, following amphetamine ingestion. Amphetamine-associated CMRgl reductions were highly correlated in both normal and schizophrenic groups with plasma drug levels.

Using [^{11}C]-2DG, Volkow and colleagues (1986b) studied 18 schizophrenic patients (stabilized with neuroleptic medication) and 12 normal volunteers (in both groups all were right-handed males) in a same-day test–retest design using a baseline condition consisting of eyes open, ears plugged, and a second eye-tracking visual task. They obtained four factor scores which characterized both groups and both conditions. Two factors, frontal and subcortical, clearly distinguished the two groups from one another. In both the baseline and the task condition normal subjects displayed higher factor scores for the frontal factor and lower factor scores for the subcortical factor. It is especially striking that the values for the factor scores rather than the organization of those factors discriminated between the two groups. No information is provided regarding the ability of the two groups to perform the visual task. The statistical methodology in this report was especially rigorous and clearly presented. When patients were characterized with respect to positive and negative symptoms, the authors found that during the visual task the patients with predominantly negative symptoms exhibited lower relative metabolic activity of the frontal regions and significantly lower activity in the right frontal lobe than did patients with predominantly positive symptoms.

University of Pennsylvania. Gur and coworkers (1987a) describe an FDG/PET study using 12 unmedicated schizophrenic patients and 12 normal volunteers. These were unactivated studies in which the subjects kept their eyes open and ears unoccluded. The main findings included an abnormally steep subcortical/cortical gradient in schizophrenic patients versus normal subjects and a highly significant correlation between left-hemispheric CMRgl and symptom severity. Highly anxious normal subjects had lower metabolism than normal subjects with low anxiety scores. This relative hypocortical/hypersubcortical CMRgl pattern is consistent with the study by Volkow et al. (1986a).

A second study by Gur and coworkers (1987b), rigorous and methodologically thorough, uses normals and schizophrenic patients in two scans (Figure 55). This double-measurement study permitted the authors to demonstrate a highly significant correlation between relative increase in right-hemispheric CMRgl and clinical improvement. Treated with various neuroleptics, the schizophrenic patients continued to show their characteristic pattern of high subcortical/cortical CMRgl activity in the second study. There were no significant main effects or interactions involving study number as a repeated measure. The authors did not, however, compare the factor structure associated with scan 1 against that of scan 2. At this time, this is the only study that used both patients and normals in a two-scan design.

UCLA and Washington University. A report by Kling and colleagues (1986) analyzes FDG/PET measurements made on 12 normal volunteers, 6 medicated schizophrenic patients, and 6 unmedicated patients with depression. Using XCT, the authors also determined ventricular size for the subjects in this study. Univariate, but not multivariate, analyses showed that the schizophrenic patients' metabolic rates were lower than those of the control subjects in the high frontal, right posterior inferior frontal, left posterior inferior frontal, and left posterior superior temporal. After adjustment for multiple comparisons, only the metabolic rates in the right posterior inferior frontal and left Wernicke regions differed from normals.

In a rare study of never previously treated patients with schizophrenia, Early et al. (1987) initially studied five patients in an exploratory, hypothesis-generating protocol. Using that group's topographic, stereotaxic analysis method, the investigators found a marked elevation in left pallidal CBF. A second group of five untreated patients was added. Pallidal analysis of the 10 patients affirmed a highly robust asymmetry on the left side (p = 0.00011, Figure 56). A recent postmortem anatomical study indicating reduced pallidal volume in patients previously diagnosed as schizophrenic further highlights the importance of this structure in schizophrenia research (Bogerts et al. 1985).

England. The study by Sheppard and coworkers (1983) was the first PET [^{15}O]-CMRgl study of schizophrenic patients published. The sample consisted of 12 predominantly never treated and unmedicated schizo-

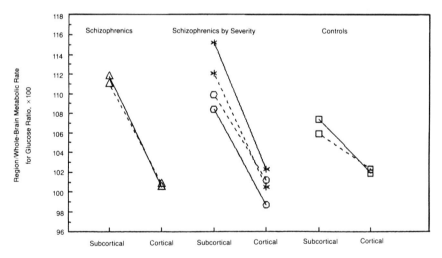

FIGURE 55. Local region/whole brain metabolic rates of glucose for left (solid lines) and right (broken lines) hemispheres in cortical and subcortical regions for the entire sample of schizophrenics, those with high (asterisks) and low (circles) severity, and controls. (Courtesy of Dr. Raquel E. Gur, Department of Psychiatry, University of Pennsylvania, Philadelphia, Pennsylvania; Arch Gen Psychiatry 44:123, 1987. Copyright 1987 American Medical Association)

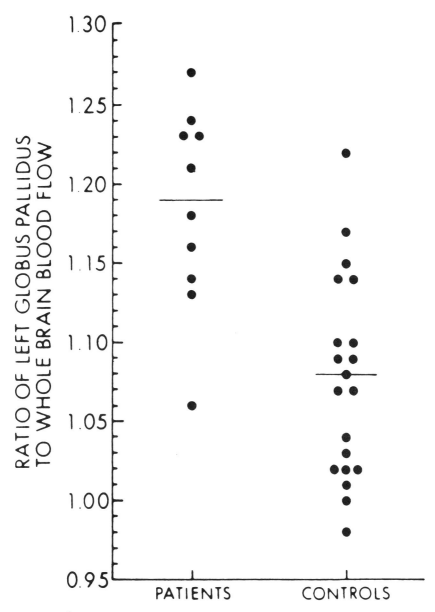

FIGURE 56. The ratio of left globus pallidus to whole brain blood flow in 10 never previously medicated schizophrenic patients and 20 normal control subjects. A horizontal line indicates the mean for each group. (Courtesy of Dr. T.S. Early, Department of Psychiatry, Washington University School of Medicine, St. Louis, Missouri; Proceedings of the National Academy of Sciences [USA] 84:562, 1987)

phrenic patients and 12 normal controls. Their eyes were closed and they were globally deprived of stimulation. Whereas normal subjects showed marked left–right asymmetry in CBF at every level, the schizophrenic patient group showed no asymmetry at any level. Since this patient group was relatively naive to drug treatment and institutionalization, it is difficult to compare this study with those cited above.

Conclusion. These studies provide an initial biological model which partially describes and accounts for the inattention and cognitive disorder associated with schizophrenia: 1) reduced frontal lobe CMRgl activity; 2) abnormal CMRgl patterns associated with physiological and cognitive challenges; and 3) a reversal in subcortical/cortical metabolic activity relationships. Schizophrenia may result from the brain's inability to regulate and monitor informational and programmatic traffic due to a deficit within the prefrontal cortex.

Affective Disorders

Using the somatosensory stimulation intervention described above in the schizophrenia section (Buchsbaum papers), Post and colleagues (1987) measured CMRgl in the temporal lobes of patients with affective illness ($N = 13$). In the moderately to severely depressed subgroup, the relative maximum-temporal lobe CMRgl was significantly reduced. That is, a ratio generated by dividing the maximum CMRgl measured in the right temporal pole by the maximum activity within the entire slice was significantly lower in the depressed patients than in controls. The maximum activity in the right temporal pole of depressed patients was higher than that of normal controls, but not statistically significant. In contrast, the maximum activity in the right temporal pole of schizophrenic patients was significantly higher than controls but not significantly higher than depressed patients. This suggests that depressed patients exhibit a more uniformly elevated CMRgl throughout basal brain regions than normals. No affectively ill patients were studied twice.

In another analysis of data which includes measurements of normal controls, schizophrenic patients, and affectively ill subjects, Buchsbaum and colleagues (1986) found that patients with bipolar illness have abnormal anteroposterior CMRgl activity patterns. The frontal/occipital ratio in normal controls ($N = 24$) is 1.09 whereas in bipolar patients the ratio = 1.02. Especially noteworthy is this group's observation concerning the basal ganglia of bipolar patients. When caudate and putamen CMRgl were expressed as ratios to the slice mean the basal ganglia activity was significantly lower (2-tailed t-test, $p < 0.05$) than that found in normal volunteers. Thalamic metabolic activity was not different from normal control values.

The most striking finding of the study by Baxter and colleagues (1985) is the reduced global CMRgl in bipolar depressed and mixed patients, compared to normal controls and unipolar depressed patients. In one case, a 48-hour rapid-cycling bipolar patient studied over a 10-day period exhibited a 36% higher CMRgl on hypomanic days than on depressed days which, in turn, were within 10% of one another. Brief Psychiatric Rating Scale (BPRS) measurements are plotted in Figure 57. CMRgl PET studies are shown in Figure 58 for this rapid-cycling bipolar.

Unlike Buchsbaum and colleagues' study, this report did not find abnormal anteroposterior gradients in patients with depression. Patients with unipolar depression exhibited significantly lower caudate/hemisphere CMRgl ratios than either normals or bipolar depressed patients (Figure 59); this finding replicates the observation by Buchsbaum described in the preceding reference.

Conclusion. These initial studies suggest that basal ganglia CMRgl is reduced in patients with depression and that marked changes occur in

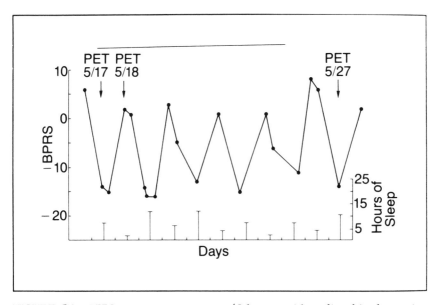

FIGURE 57. BPRS measurements on a 48-hour rapid cycling bipolar patient studied over a 10-day hospital period. She had been drug-free for 6 years. Brief Psychiatric Rating Scale (BPRS) scores are with items 8, 17, 19, 20, and 21, which relate to mania, scored as positive and all other items as negative. Hours of sleep were recorded 24 hours a day by nursing personnel checking every 30 mintues. Arrows indicate times and BPRS scores for 3 positron emission tomographic (PET) scans; see Figure 58. (Courtesy of Dr. L.R. Baxter, Department of Psychiatry, UCLA Neuropsychiatric Institute, Los Angeles, California; Arch Gen Psychiatry 42:444, 1985. Copyright 1985 American Medical Association)

global CMRgl in association with manic-depressive cycling. The left-sided caudate metabolic-rate reduction is especially provocative in light of the association between mood and movement disorders (Holcomb 1985). Starkstein and Robinson's studies linking left frontal strokes and depression are also consistent with these findings (Starkstein et al. 1988). Parkinsonian patients, who tend to exhibit reduced CMRgl in frontal cortex, exhibit an especially high predisposition toward depression; conversely, patients with depression frequently exhibit motoric retardation. In the context of motor-behavior tasks and manipulations, it will be useful to determine how patients with depression and Parkinsonism compare with one another and with normals in their CMRgl patterns.

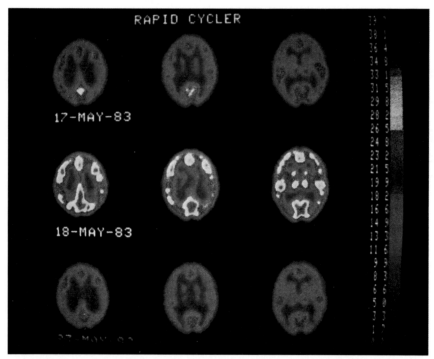

FIGURE 58. rCMRgl PET images of the same rapid cycling bipolar patient. Note the global shifts in metabolic rate. Colors of scans correspond to glucose metabolic rates which are indicated in color bar to right (in micromoles of glucose per minute per 100 g of brain; 1 mg of glucose = 5.56 micromoles). Whole brain metabolic rates of glucose were 36% higher on the hypomanic day than the average of depressed days, which were within 10% of each other. (Courtesy of Dr. L.R. Baxter, Department of Psychiatry, UCLA Neuropsychiatric Institute, Los Angeles, California; Arch Gen Psychiatry 42:444, 1985. Copyright 1985 American Medical Association)

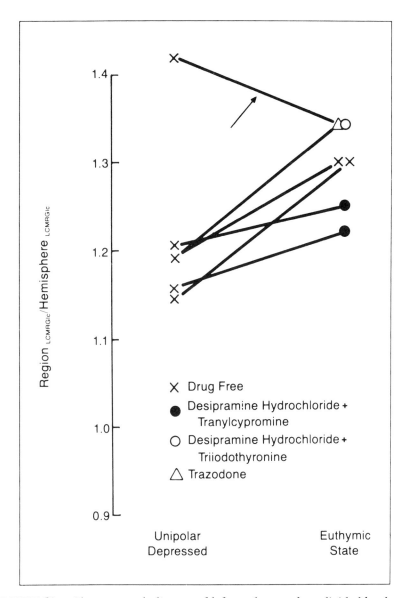

FIGURE 59: Glucose metabolic rate of left caudate nucleus divided by that of whole hemisphere in five patients with unipolar depression studied in the morbid state and again after recovery. The arrow indicates a unipolar patient whose value on this measure is more than 2.5 standard deviations greater than group mean. LCMRgl indicates local cerebral metabolic rate for glucose. (Courtesy of Dr. L.R. Baxter, Department of Psychiatry, UCLA Neuropsychiatric Institute, Los Angeles, California; Arch Gen Psychiatry 42:444, 1985. Copyright 1985 American Medical Association)

Anxiety and Panic Disorder

In an early study by Reivich and colleagues (1983), the importance of the right hemisphere in regulating anxiety and affect is addressed. From a series of FDG/PET experiments the authors calculated CMRgl for homotopic regions in the two cerebral regions that contain the primary cortical projections of the limbic system, the posterior fronto-orbital and the middle frontal regions. When these rates were evaluated as a function of trait and state anxiety, a curvilinear relationship between anxiety and frontocortical metabolic rates became evident. Metabolic rates in these regions increased as a function of anxiety up to a point and then decreased in association with progressively higher anxiety. That pattern was not observed in association with control regions. In order to evaluate the data with regard to hemispheric involvement the authors performed an ANOVA on the groups consisting of high anxious and low anxious subjects. The two groups did not differ in overall metabolic rates but the interaction between anxiety and metabolic rates in the two hemispheres was significant. High-anxiety subjects had higher metabolic rates in the right, relative to the left, hemisphere to a significantly greater extent than the low-anxiety group. The nonlinear, U-shaped relationship between anxiety level and frontal rCMRgl is further substantiated and described in a recent follow-up study by this group (Gur RC et al. 1987).

In two reports (Reiman et al. 1984, 1986) the Washington University PET research group uses [15]Oxygen-labeled water to assess abnormal CBF patterns in patients with panic disorder who are susceptible to lactate infusions (Pitts and McClure 1967). In patients responsive to lactate infusion the left–right parahippocampal CBF ratio is significantly lower than that of patients not responsive to lactate infusion or normals (Figure 60). In the follow-up study (Reiman et al. 1986) this observation is extended to indicate that parahippocampal blood flow, blood volume, and CMRoxy are abnormal in the lactate infusion-sensitive subgroup.

Conclusion.   These three studies consistently suggest that the right hemisphere is preferentially activated in subjects feeling anxious and that the parahippocampal gyrus is especially inactive in patients sensitive to the panic-inducing effects of lactate infusion (Pitts and McClure 1967).

Obsessive Compulsive Disorder (OCD)

FDG/PET studies performed on 14 patients with OCD were compared with 14 patients with unipolar depression and 14 normal controls (Baxter et al. 1987) (Figures 61 and 62). *In OCD patients the CMRgl rates were significantly increased in the left orbital gyrus and in the caudate*

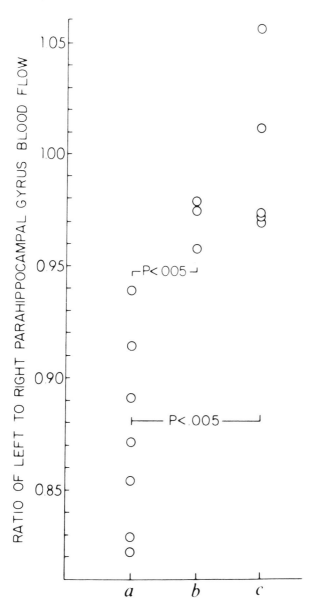

FIGURE 60. Left-to-right ratio of blood flow in the parahippocampal gyrus of: *(a)* patients with a history of panic disorder and a positive response to sodium lactate infusion (panic attack induced); *(b)* patients with a history of panic disorder and negative response to sodium lactate infusion; and *(c)* normal control subjects. These data were obtained in a quiet, resting state. (Courtesy of Dr. E.M. Reiman, Department of Psychiatry, Mallinckrodt Institute of Radiology, Washington University School of Medicine, St. Louis, Missouri; Nature 310:683, 1984)

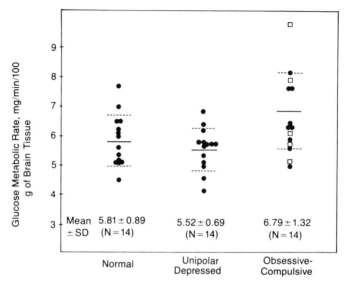

FIGURE 61. Glucose metabolic rates for head of right caudate nucleus. Rates for all subjects combined were significantly higher in patients with OCD than in subjects from either comparison group. Circles indicate drug-free subjects; squares, drug-taking subjects (p < .005). (Courtesy of Dr. L.R. Baxter, Department of Psychiatry, UCLA Neuropsychiatric Institute, Los Angeles, California; Arch Gen Psychiatry 44:213, 1987. Copyright 1987 American Medical Association)

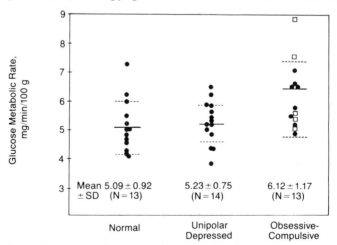

FIGURE 62. Glucose metabolic rates for right orbital gyrus. Metabolic rates were significantly higher in patients with OCD than in subjects from either comparison group. Circles indicate drug-free subjects; squares, drug-taking subjects (p < .02). (Courtesy of Dr. L.R. Baxter, Department of Psychiatry, UCLA Neuropsychiatric Institute, Los Angeles, California; Arch Gen Psychiatry 44:213, 1987. Copyright 1987 American Medical Association)

nuclei bilaterally. In those OCD patients who improved with drug therapy, the caudate–hemisphere CMRgl ratio increased uniformly and significantly bilaterally.

Alcoholism

Using FDG/PET, Samson and colleagues (1986) prospectively studied six neurologically unaffected chronic alcoholics. With respect to age-matched control values, cerebral metabolic rate was not significantly modified in the cortical, subcortical, and cerebellar regions of interest. The metabolic regional distribution index which reflects the distribution pattern of glucose utilization was selectively and significantly decreased in the *mediofrontal* area. This group did not observe significant widespread changes in CMRgl activity.

Anorexia Nervosa

Using FDG/PET, Herholz and coworkers (1987) measured CMRgl in 5 female anorectic patients during the anorectic state and after weight gain. Their measurements were compared with those of 15 young male normal controls. During the anorectic state significant caudate hypermetabolism was found bilaterally in the anorectic patients; this differed markedly from the patients' caudate CMRgl measurements in their fed state and also from the normal male volunteers. Bilateral measurements in the temporal cortex also showed elevated activity in the anorectic state as compared to the fed state. The authors suggest that these findings may reflect the hyperaroused state associated with stress. The investigators also invite comparisons with the Buchsbaum et al. (1986) and Baxter et al. (1985) reports cited above, specifically in regard to the differences in caudate metabolism.

Alzheimer's Disease

In the temporal and parietal cortical regions of patients with dementia of the Alzheimer's type (DAT), CMRgl is reduced (Haxby et al. 1985); this is evident in patients with mild illness severity as well as those with more advanced disease. Lateral asymmetry of CMRgl correlated significantly with asymmetry of language and visuospatial functions in AD patients but not in normal controls. Detailed analyses of CMRgl measurements in selected cerebral regions indicates that the reduced metabolism is not due to a partial volume inclusion of inert cerebrospinal fluid. In mild-to-moderate cases the principal finding may be a prominent right–left asymmetry rather than an absolute reduction in CMRgl rate.

Finally, neuropsychological testing suggests that patients with disproportionate failure of language function have markedly diminished metabolism in the left frontal, temporal, and parietal regions. Patients with predominantly visuoconstructive dysfunction show a hypometabolic focus in the right parietal cortex. Patients with memory failure as the most apparent feature have no significant metabolic asymmetry in cortical regions.

Down's Syndrome

Using FDG/PET, Schwartz and coworkers (1983) found that CMRgl in four healthy subjects with Down's syndrome (DS) was significantly higher than the mean rate in healthy young controls. Values in DS subjects were as much as 40% higher than the respective mean values in young controls. In contrast, CMRgl measurements of a 51-year-old DS subject did not differ from those of other middle-aged control subjects. The middle-aged patient was not demented. The authors suggest that the high CMRgl values in their four young patients may reflect dysfunction at the sodium-transport level of membrane activity.

Autism

An NIMH/NIH PET research group (Rumsey et al. 1985) studied 10 men with well-documented histories of infantile autism and 15 age-matched normal male controls with FDG/PET. Performed while the subjects were in an inactive, sensory-deprived condition, the PET studies generated CMRgl metabolic measurements in the patient group that were significantly more variable than their control counterparts. A greater number of outliers was seen in the autistic group when subjects were classified on the basis of presence versus absence of deviant (3 or more SDs from the normal mean) relative metabolic rates. No deficiencies in absolute resting cerebral metabolic rates for glucose either diffuse or focal were observed.

Neuroreceptor Studies

Sedvall et al. (1986) have reviewed the methodology and findings of PET receptor progress up through July 1986. Their monograph provides a useful guide to this new approach, explaining that the optimal selection of ligands is one of the crucial steps in the successful development of a receptor-imaging protocol. The following criteria for an appropriate ligand are listed:

1. High selectivity of binding in vitro
2. Stereoselectivity of binding in vitro

3. Nanomolar (10^{-9}) binding affinity for receptor in vitro
4. Rapid establishment of steady state over blood–brain barrier in vivo
5. Low in vivo accumulation of labeled or active ligand metabolites
6. Low degree of nonspecific binding in vivo
7. Saturability of binding in vivo
8. Tolerable side effects at saturating doses of ligand
9. The chemical structure of the ligand must allow for the rapid introduction of a positron-emitting isotope into the molecule

The autoradiographic and PET studies reviewed below use ligands that meet most of the requirements specified by Sedvall and his colleagues (1986). It is important to note that these groups are just beginning the difficult task of correlating receptor occupancy or number with physiologically relevant perturbations. That is, these papers represent the first stage of receptor research, the determination of how much tracer binds to particular brain regions in various diagnostic groups. Receptor studies using the tissue homogenate binding method are not discussed in this section; this selective focus is made to emphasize the similarity between autoradiography and PET. These methods provide anatomically specific neurochemical measurements.

Aging

In a study of 22 male and 22 female volunteers (Wong et al. 1984) the investigators used ^{11}C-labeled 3-N-methylspiperone (NMSP) to measure dopamine type 2 receptors (D2) in the caudate, putamen, and frontal cortex. Levels of NMSP binding in these regions declined over the age span studied (19 to 73 years).

Schizophrenia

Using ^{11}C-labeled raclopride, a D2 antagonist, Farde and colleagues (1986, 1987, 1988) (Figures 63 and 64) measured the receptor occupancy and receptor number in a group of four normal males and three patients with schizophrenia using various clinically effective doses of neuroleptic. The mean D2 receptor number (B_{max}) of normal subjects was 14.4 picomoles/cm^3. Seeman et al. (1984) found a B_{max} value of about 13 picomole/g for labeled spiperone binding to putamen from deceased human subjects. The schizophrenic patients were treated with haloperidol, sulpiride, and flupenthixol. When the drugs were given in clinically antipsychotic doses, the relative degree of ^{11}C raclopride binding to D2 dopamine receptors indicated an 84–90% blockade of these receptors in the putamen. That three chemically distinct neuroleptics produced the

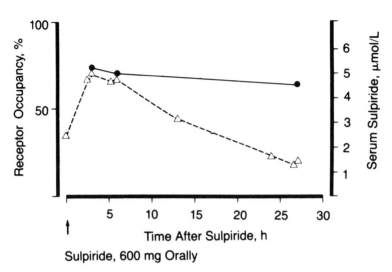

FIGURE 63. D_2 dopamine receptor occupancy in putamen, and sulpiride concentration in serum of a schizophrenic patient after withdrawal of sulpiride treatment. The solid line indicates receptor occupancy; the broken line indicates sulpiride concentration. (Courtesy of Dr. L. Farde, Department of Psychiatry, Karolinska Institute, Stockholm, Sweden; Arch Gen Psychiatry 45:71–76, 1988. Copyright 1988 American Medical Association)

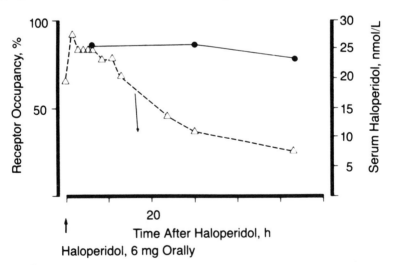

FIGURE 64. D_2 dopamine receptor occupancy in putamen and haloperidol concentration in serum of schizophrenic patient after withdrawal of haloperidol treatment. The solid line indicates receptor occupancy; the broken line indicates haloperidol concentration. (Courtesy of Dr. L. Farde, Department of Psychiatry, Karolinska Institute, Stockholm, Sweden; Arch Gen Psychiatry 45:71–76, 1988. Copyright 1988 American Medical Association)

same degree of D2 receptor blockade suggests that the antipsychotic effects of these drugs depend on their D2-blocking capacity. In a follow-up of that initial investigation (1988) these investigators studied the time course of D2-receptor occupancy. In subjects treated with sulpiride and haloperidol the D2-receptor occupancy remained above 65% for many hours despite a substantial reduction of serum drug concentration (Farde et al. 1986, 1988).

The group at the Karolinska Institute has also studied 15 young, completely drug-naive, first-admission schizophrenic patients (age, 24 ± 3.7 years) and 14 healthy normal volunteers (age, 29.1 ± 4.6 years). All the schizophrenic patients had been ill for more than six months and met *DSM-III* criteria for a schizophrenic disorder. The B_{max} and Kd values in the putamen were determined from individual Scatchard plots, based on two studies obtained from each person. Figure 65 indicates the pooled data from right and left putamen. The mean B_{max} values were 24.6 (± 6.0) pmol/mL in the controls and 25.1 (± 7.0) pmol/mL in the schizophrenic patients. The Kd values were 7.1 ± 1.3 nmol/L in

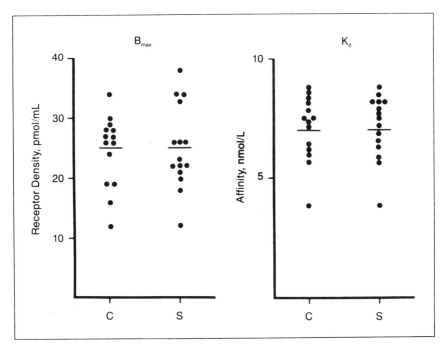

FIGURE 65. D_2 dopamine receptor density (B_{max}) and affinity (K_d) in healthy control subjects (C) and schizophrenic patients (S). (Courtesy of Dr. L. Farde, Department of Psychiatry and Psychology, Karolinska Institute, Stockholm, Sweden; Arch Gen Psychiatry 44:671, 1987. Copyright 1987 American Medical Association)

the controls and 7.1 ± 1.3 nmol/L in the patients. In 4 of the schizo-phrenic patients the B_{max} values in the putamen of the left side were 10% to 30% higher than those on the right side. This degree of asymmetry was not observed in any of the control subjects. This study does not confirm those findings of Wong et al. 1986c (Farde et al. 1987) (Figure 65).

Wong and colleagues (1986c) have studied drug-naive patients with schizophrenia using ^{11}C-labeled NMSP. In their comparison of caudate –putamen D2 B_{max} of normal volunteers, drug-naive, and drug-treated schizophrenics, they found higher D2-receptor densities in both patient groups (Figure 66). Their findings suggest that schizophrenia is itself associated with an increase in brain D2 receptors which is not due entirely to neuroleptic-induced hypersensitivity.

Seeman and colleagues (1984) have measured D2 receptors in au-topsy tissue specimens from normals and patients with schizophrenia. In their receptor measurements of the caudate, putamen, and accumbens they find a bimodal distribution of receptor densities in the three brain regions of patients with schizophrenia but only one, normally distributed, group of receptors in the controls. They argue that this indicates direct evidence for two distinct categories of schizophrenia. This suggestion is difficult to assess since little clinical data were available in the report.

Parkinson's Disease

Guttman and colleagues (1986) have provided a postmortem study of D2 dopamine receptor density in the caudate nucleus and putamen of 36 parkinsonian patients. In striking contrast with the aging study de-scribed above (Wong et al. 1984), this study found no change in B_{max} with age in this group whose ages ranged from 56 to 90 years. The average B_{max} was 10.1 ± 0.5 pmol/gm for the putamen and 8.1 ± 0.4 pmol/gm for the caudate. No correlation between disease duration of L-dopa treatment duration and B_{max} was observed. Postmortem studies such as this and Seeman's (1984) provide points of reference and contention for PET receptor studies.

In Uhl and colleagues' (1986) extensive autoradiographic receptor study of the substantia nigra, binding sites for somatostatin, neurotensin, mu-opiate, and benzodiazepines are measured in normal and parkinsonian patients. Uhl and coworkers (1986) describe marked peptidergic neuroreceptor abnormalities in this degenerative brain disorder. Somatostatin, neurotensin, mu-opiate, and kappa-opiate binding were substantially reduced in contrast to "modest" reductions in dopamine and benzodiazepine I binding. The receptors most severely reduced mediate the actions of peptides that modulate and modify striato-nigral dopamine activity. Loss of these receptors may have a profound impact on

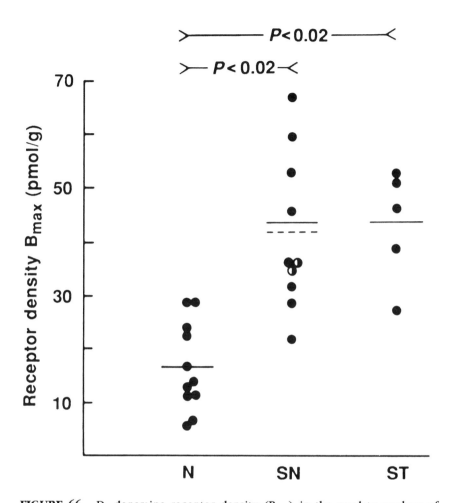

FIGURE 66. D_2 dopamine receptor density (B_{max}) in the caudate nucleus of normal volunteers (N), drug-naive (SN) and drug-treated (ST) schizophrenic patients. The solid horizontal lines are the mean values in each group. For the drug-naive group this line is the value for the eight subjects who had only a single 7.5 mg dose of haloperidol before their second pet scan (43.3 ± 5.7 pmol/g [SEM]). The dotted line below it is the mean of all 10 subjects, including the 2 who received more than a single dose of haloperidol before their second PET scan. The average receptor density of this group was $41.L7 \pm 4.6$ pmol/g. Mean receptor densities for the normal volunteers and the drug-treated group where 16.6 ± 2.5 and 4.3 ± 4.7 pmol/g, respectively. There was a significant difference between either the 8 or 10 drug-naive or the drug-treated schizophrenics and the normal subjects (T = test with Bonferroni correction for multiple inference). (Courtesy of Dr. D. Wong, Nuclear Medicine Division, Radiology Department, Johns Hopkins Medical Institutes, Baltimore, Maryland; Science 234:1561, 1986)

dopaminergic function and contribute to the affective, congnitive, and motoric symptoms of parkinsonism.

Alzheimer's Disease

Postmortem studies support the presumption of multiple, widespread neurochemical abnormalities in this common illness (Table 5). These studies rely on quantitative autoradiography for the detailed spatial resolution necessary to distinguish between subnuclei within brain regions. This method can significantly enhance the utility and validity of PET receptor measurements when similar ligands are used to map similar brain regions in the two methods. It is noteworthy that no published works have addressed receptor–metabolism relationships in this large, clinically important diagnostic group.

Huntington's Disease

Huntington's disease (HD) is biochemically characterized by decreases in gamma-aminobutyric acid (GABA), substance-P, and enkephalin in the following brain regions: striatum, substantia nigra, and lateral globus pallidus. In the late 1970s and early 1980s tritium-sensitive autoradiographic film became available for analysis of postmortem brain sections. The studies described here provide an indication of how neurobiol-

TABLE 5. Receptor Abnormalities in Postmortem Alzheimer Brain Tissue

Reference	Receptor	Tissue	% Difference from Control
Sparks et al. (1988)	NMSP	nuc. basalis of Meynert	66% reduction
Beale et al. (1985)	Somatostatin	frontal and temporal cortex	50% reduction
		hippocampus	40% reduction
		cingulate cortex	no change (nc)
		postcentral gyrus	nc
		temporal pole	nc
		superior temporal gyrus	nc
Lang and Henke (1983)	Muscarinic and nicotinic cholinergic	hippocampus	nc
		frontal cortex	nc
		temporal cortex	nc
		cingulate cortex	nc
Greenamyre et al. (1985)	Glutamate	cortex	reduced 50%
		caudate	nc
		putamen	nc
		claustrum	nc

ogists are using autoradiography to assess receptor distribution abnormalities in HD and other brain diseases. Future neuroreceptor studies with PET must be compared with these in vitro measurements. Those comparisons will help define PET sensitivity and specificity.

Penney and Young (1982) describe receptor autoradiographic findings in an HD patient. The pattern is consistent with the loss of GABA neurons in the caudate–putamen. GABA, benzodiazepine (BZ), and muscarinic cholinergic receptors (mACH) were depressed in caudate and putamen of the HD patient compared with a control patient. Binding to GABA and BZ receptors was increased in lateral and medial pallidum (which receive projections from the caudate and putamen) and depressed in ventrolateral thalamus (which receives projections from the pallidum). mACH receptors were markedly decreased in pallidum but not thalamus. These findings suggest that loss of striatal afferents to both segments of pallidum results in GABA and BZ receptor supersensitivity. Using the methodology described by Penney and Young, Greenamyre and colleagues (1985) reports reduced glutamate (one of the principal cortico–cortico and cortico–striate neurotransmitters) receptor density in the caudate–putamen of HD patients but not in Alzheimer patients.

Whitehouse et al. (1985) provide an extensive autoradiographic analysis of mACH, BZ, GABA, DA, and serotonin receptors in frontal cortex, parietal cortex, caudate, putamen, and globus pallidus in tissue sections from five HD patients and five controls matched for age, sex, and postmortem delay. This larger study agrees with Penney and Young (1982); reduced receptor number in the caudate–putamen and increased GABA and BZ receptors in the globus pallidus (external and internal segments) are confirmed. This group also finds an elevation in BZ receptors located in superficial cortical layers of the frontal cortex. Elevated cortical and pallidal BZ binding and reductions in various caudate–putamen receptors in HD patients provide a unique neurochemical profile that should prove useful to PET neuroreceptor investigators. Knowing that patients from this group have a particularly high or low receptor level in a given brain region, PET researchers can assess the sensitivity and resolution of the technology by comparing positron emission measurements against these postmortem studies.

Trifiletti et al. (1987) extend the Whitehouse study (1985) by completing a systematic cortical analysis of benzodiazepine receptor density, using homogenized tissue not autoradiography. [³H]RO-15-1788, a benzodiazepine antagonist now available as a positron-emitting radiotracer, exhibits higher binding levels only in the midfrontal region (A9/A10). Frontal pole, temporal pole, midparietal, cingulate, and occipital binding levels were not significantly different from controls. This study was unusual in its extensive biochemical characterization of the benzodiazepine binding site. The investigators further determined a marked reduction, localized to tissue from the midfrontal region, in the GABA and barbiturate stimulation of diazepam binding. Elevated benzodiazepine binding levels and abnormally low sensitivity to GABA/barbiturate stimulation of benziodiazepine binding characterize midfrontal cortical tissue in this patient group. Neither PET studies nor autoradiographic analyses of HD patients have provided clues regarding this cortical receptor abnormality. By combining morphologic, immunocytochemical, receptor, and track-tracing methodologies in selected patient autopsy material, on whom prior PET measurements were made, neuroscience groups will be able to provide complete analyses of cellular/neurochemical/metabolic derangements in this profound illness.

Is PET Useful in Making Clinical Decisions?

CT, MRI, and PET Comparisons in Various Clinical Problems

The principal advantages of PET metabolic imaging include its accuracy, sensitivity, and adaptability (receptors, metabolism, enzymes, and neurotransmitters). It is now scientifically safe to suggest that Alzheimer's disease, Huntington's disease, epilepsy, and hemiparkinsonism have characteristic metabolic patterns. Neither XCT, nor MRI can distinguish or identify these illnesses in their early stages. Severe depression, especially in the elderly, may resemble dementia. Metabolically, depression is associated with extremely high parietal CMRgl activity (Buchsbaum et al. 1985). Alzheimer's disease, however, is uniformly associated with hypometabolic parietal lobes. In the case of epilepsy, Engel (1982a, 1982b, 1982c, 1982d, 1983, 1985) and colleagues find exceptionally strong agreement between PET CMRgl activity profiles and histology of biopsy tissue from putative epileptogenic foci. Furthermore, several carefully executed studies compare the sensitivity and validity of XCT, MRI, and PET in epilepsy, brain trauma, and Alzheimer's disease (Latack et al. 1986; Langfitt et al. 1986; McGeer et al. 1986b, respectively). In an unusually thorough study of brain trauma, Langfitt and colleagues (1986) also compared PET with Xenon-133 measurements of CBF. These three reports are briefly summarized.

   In their triple-imaging study of patients with partial seizures, Latack and colleagues (1986) report that PET detected hypometabolic foci in 71% of the partial seizure patients whereas MRI detected signal abnormalities in 42%. Both MRI and PET exhibited significantly greater sensitivity than XCT.

   Langfitt and his colleagues (1986) at the University of Pennsylvania performed extensive evaluations of three head-trauma patients. Selected because they presented with intracranial hemorrhage on XCT, they were studied acutely and again approximately 6 months later (two out of three). In the acute stage MRI was superior to CT in identifying the precise location and extent of intracranial hemorrhage and associated edema. Small subdural hematomas diagnosed on MRI were missed with CT scanning. The extent of apparent encephalomalacia in the chronic stages of injury was also better defined with MRI. PET revealed disturbances of glucose metabolism that extended beyond the structural abnormalities demonstrated by MRI and CT; anterior temporal lobe dysfunction was particularly evident in all three patients. Regional CBF studies failed to detect a number of the abnormalities seen on MRI and CT, and even failed to detect the metabolic dysfunction apparent on PET. Neuropsychological studies localized frontal lesions, but did not suggest abnormalities attributable to the structural lesions and the reduced metabolism in the anterior temporal lobes.

McGeer and colleagues (1986b) at the University of British Columbia studied a patient with Alzheimer's disease prior to his death. PET (FDG), MRI, and XCT studies were performed 16 months before he died; the group then followed up their studies with histological autopsy analyses of the patient's brain. At autopsy the gross appearance of the brain correlated with MRI and CT, which showed some regional atrophy. PET, in marked contrast, correlated well with *microscopic* findings of neuronal loss and proliferation of glia. In areas of moderately impaired regional CMRgl, gliosis, primarily around numerous senile plaques, was observed. In areas of severely reduced metabolic activity there was a profound loss of neurons, extensive gliosis, and a diminished appearance of plaques. These investigators concluded that PET correlated most closely with neuronal pathology.

In summary, PET offers the most promising imaging modality for the classification, staging, and elucidation of neuropathology. When PET centers are able to selectively employ multiple intersecting tracer measurements, the clinical utility of this new imaging system is likely to grow significantly.

Where to Go for PET Imaging

The following list is adapted from Wolf and Fowler (1985); this list is changing each year and should not be considered definitive.

Northeast and Midatlantic
1. Massachusetts General Hospital, Boston, Massachusetts
2. New York University, New York City, using the Brookhaven National Laboratory, Upton, New York

3. Sloan-Kettering Cancer Center, New York
4. University of Pennsylvania, Philadelphia, Pennsylvania
5. Johns Hopkins University, Baltimore, Maryland
6. National Institutes of Health, Bethesda, Maryland

Southeast
7. Duke University, Durham, North Carolina (developing)
8. Oak Ridge and Associated Universities, Oak Ridge, Tennessee
9. Mt. Sinai Hospital, Miami Beach, Florida

Southwest
10. University of Texas Medical School, Houston, Texas

Midwest and Canada
11. University of Chicago, Chicago, Illinois
12. University of Michigan, Ann Arbor, Michigan
13. Washington University, St. Louis, Missouri
14. Case Western Reserve, Cleveland, Ohio
15. University of Wisconsin, Madison, Wisconsin
16. McMaster University, Hamilton, Ontario, Canada
17. McGill University, Montreal, Canada
18. University of Iowa, Iowa City, Iowa (developing)
19. University of Toronto, Toronto, Canada (developing)

Pacific Coast and British Columbia
20. University of British Columbia, Vancouver, Canada
21. University of Washington, Seattle, Washington
22. University of California, Berkeley, California
23. University of California, Los Angeles, California
24. University of California, Irvine, California

The easiest way to obtain access to those who manage, administer, and use these facilities is through the institutions' nuclear medicine departments.

Overall Assessment

Strengths

PET is unique in its capacity to provide high spatial resolution (4-millimeter FWHM resolution is now being delivered), high temporal resolution

(40-second scan periods are used at the Washington University PET center), and biochemical specificity (metabolic and neurochemical). Because of the recent advances in physics/electronics, nuclear chemistry, and biochemistry/physiology, physicians can systematically describe a wide spectrum of neurophysiological processes. This has permitted the neurometabolic characterization of Alzheimer's disease and epilepsy. Subtle physiological processes associated with sensory, motor, and cognitive phenomena are also being unraveled with this technology.

Limitations

The primary limitation has rapidly become the inability to generate interpretable experiments and clinical protocols. It is fair to suggest that clinical and experimental neurobiologists do not know enough about the brain to interpret changes in either neuroreceptor patterns or metabolic profiles in most instances. Only by generating progressively more carefully controlled, intersecting studies can the neuroscience community explicate the complex measurements it so readily generates.

Cost

The annual costs and logistics associated with maintenance of a PET facility are described in three recent publications: Wagner 1986; Hawkins and Phelps 1986; and Evens et al. 1983. Three components are required for PET operations: a medical cyclotron for radionuclide production, a chemistry unit for labeling radiopharmaceuticals, and a diagnostic imaging unit. Purchase and installation of a medical cyclotron requires a capital expenditure of about $1,650,000.00. Personnel required to operate a medical cyclotron are two cyclotron operators, one chemistry technician, one-half of an engineer, and one-quarter of a radiopharmacist. Various supplies for cyclotron operation average about $75,000 to $100,000 per year. The annual costs of a diagnostic imaging unit including personnel, supplies, maintenance, and equipment are approximately $644,000, including indirect costs. The top-of-the-line commercial unit and its installation will cost $1,500,000 to $2,000,000 (Scanditronix and CTI). Simpler units may be obtained for as little as $400,000. The optimal PET diagnostic unit would maintain one PET system for the brain and one for the heart and body. Estimated annual cost of two PET imaging units is about $900,000. Evens and colleagues (1983) estimate that the economic break-even cost on a charge per procedure basis for 1,000 studies per year is $826. Were one to perform 6 studies per day on 300 days of the year and generate 1,800 studies, the break-even cost would fall to about $500 per study. Irrespective of how one approaches the task of reducing PET costs,

Evens suggests, PET studies remain among the most costly of all diagnostic imaging procedures. Magnetic resonance studies now cost about the same as PET. At Johns Hopkins Hospital in 1987, the break-even, per study cost is about $1,500.

The manufacturers and suppliers of medical cyclotrons capable of producing ^{11}C, ^{15}O, ^{18}F, and ^{13}N are described in the following. Johns Hopkins Hospital installed the smallest of the Scanditronix cyclotrons, the MC16F, in 1981 for a cost of about one million dollars. Today, 1987, that radionuclide-production system with its cyclotron costs about 1.6 million dollars and routinely produces ^{11}C, ^{18}F, and ^{15}O. Maintenance costs on the Scanditronix unit are approximately $75,000 per year; that includes about $20,000 for parts. Scanditronix cyclotrons are now installed at the following institutions: Case Western Reserve in Cleveland, Ohio; University of Texas Medical School in Houston, Texas; Veterans Administration Hospital in Minneapolis, Minnesota; University of Washington, in Seattle, Washington; and (the first community hospital to have its own) North Shore University Hospital in Manhasset, New York. Japan Steel Works (JSW) has delivered its "baby cyclotron" to Brookhaven National Laboratory (June, 1982), National Institutes of Health (1984), and a third is being installed at the University of Pennsylvania. Sumitomo-CGR has installed medical cyclotrons in Kyoto, Japan, Italy, Belgium, and France. From the United States only Computer Technology and Imaging (CTI) of Knoxville, Tennessee, supplies cyclotrons. CTI has also built over 20 PET scanners and over 40 cyclotrons. A recent addition to the CTI list of installations is the NIH's second cyclotron, which is located in Bethesda, Maryland.

Future Directions

What Do We Want to Know? What Sort of Tools Are Required?

Improvements of Present Methods and Unresolved Questions

One unresolved conceptual problem that will require further investigation concerns receptor number (B_{max}) measurement. Because one cannot easily measure the binding dissociation constant (K_d) independent of the receptor number, it is especially important that tissue biopsy and postmortem in vitro receptor measurements be made to determine under what conditions one might expect a change in K_d. Significant changes in dissociation constants are not common. It is important to determine to what extent ligands that achieve temporary equilibrium (e.g., raclopride and carfentanil) can be used to determine B_{max} without additional studies to determine K_d.

Resolution and Sensitivity, Temporal and Spatial Limits

Advances in detector instrumentation will predictably reduce the spatial resolution of PET to 4 millimeters. Use of ^{15}O-labeled water in conjunction with dynamic scanning (Washington University uses this method) permits accurate assessment of physiological events that occur under 1 minute. The principal difficulty now becomes one of scientific foundations. That is, in order to use such impressive new limits one needs to ask the right question.

New Tracers, New Tricks

New candidates being developed and older tracers being modeled for PET technology include the following: Muscarinic receptors can now be measured with N-methyl-[^{11}C]-scopolamine (Frey et al. 1985) and (R)-3-quinuclidinyl-4-iodobenzilate [(R)-4-IQNB] (Eckelman et al. 1984). The former is an appropriate tracer for PET and the latter for SPECT. O'Tuama and Frost (O'Tuama et al. 1986) have completed animal studies that suggest alpha-1 adrenergic receptors may be labeled with I-125 2-Beta (4-hydroxyphenyl) ethylaminomethyl-tetralone (HEAT). This iodinated compound shows high specific binding in frontal cortex and thalamus and competitive displacement by prazosin. Labeled HEAT may be an appropriate ligand for imaging alpha-1 adrenergic receptors in humans using SPECT.

Two tracers advance PET imaging technology into the completely new areas of neurotransmitters and brain enzymes. 6-L-fluorodopa labeled with fluorine-18 provides an exciting opportunity to measure dopamine metabolism in vivo. Leenders and colleagues (1986a) recently used this tracer in a study of parkinsonian patients and normal volunteers. They found that the striatum's capacity to retain the labled DA precursor was severely impaired in parkinsonian patients and that patients showing the "on–off" phenomenon had an even greater decrease in striatal storage capacity. This group also studied the interaction between dietary amino acid loads and [^{18}F]-fluorodopa uptake in the striatum (Leenders et al. 1986b). Amino acid loading markedly impaired tracer uptake in a normal volunteer; this phenomenon may partially explain dietary interference with L-dopa therapy of parkinsonism. The initial studies by Garnett et al. (1983), Martin (1986), and Chiueh and Firnau (1986) also provide an optimistic picture for PET measurements of in vivo neurotransmitter (L-dopa/dopamine) activity.

Fowler et al. (1987) have provided a radical departure from the mainstream of PET tracer technology by labeling deprenyl and clorgyline (inhibitors of monoamine oxidase [MAO] A and monoamine oxidase B) with ^{11}C. With these enzymatic inactivators, researchers will be able to determine the in vivo rate of recovery (synthesis) of MAO B after a single therapeutic dose of L-deprenyl. This permits the measurement of the synthesis of a specific protein in vivo.

Mixing Methods in an Effort to Obtain Validation

Both dynamic cerebral blood flow and electrophysiology allow the clinical neurophysiologist to measure regional brain activity over brief periods of time. Correlations between brief behavioral states and transient physiological phenomena can be determined. It will be useful to determine to what extent changes in electrical activity (evoked potentials and EEG activity) correlate with rCBF and other dimensions of CMR. By combining methods, investigators will be better able to determine how to use the strengths of different technologies to characterize complex physiobehavioral relationships.

You Can't Get There from Here: The Need for More Powerful and Flexible Data-Analysis Systems

The analysis of image data is complex. As scanner resolution increases and more investigators use dynamic rCBF systems, the amount of data becomes increasingly more difficult to reduce and analyze. It is also likely that groups will use compound protocols involving multiple tracers and multiple conditions to evaluate subtle behaviors and disease states. An individual patient may well be analyzed with respect to blood flow, oxygen metabolism, glucose metabolism, neuroreceptor profiles, neurotransmitter activity, and enzyme levels. The task of using that data meaningfully is not straightforward. It is increasingly important that research groups have the means of generating complex statistical analyses and graphic displays of patient and group data in order to use the information they have acquired. Only then will they be able to describe the complex characteristics of brain function in the multidimensional, intersecting method that is required.

Generally speaking, investigators work with three types of image: 1) functional (e.g., PET 2DG); 2) structural (e.g., XCT); and 3) anatomical reference (e.g., stereotaxic brain atlas). Protocols are now being developed which will allow the image analyst to modify idealized atlas images with individual XCT scans and then to register conformed atlas images to fit functional PET scans. By drawing wire-frame boundaries onto the atlas image, the investigator can then transfer brain regions onto the functional image (Figure 67). Alternatively, the Washington University group has provided a means for mapping an individual's functional scan onto an idealized three-dimensional atlas. Both approaches permit three-dimensional reconstruction and analysis. Because the brain works as an ensemble of three-dimensional, interacting circuits, it is appropriate to analyze and order it as a three-dimensional matrix.

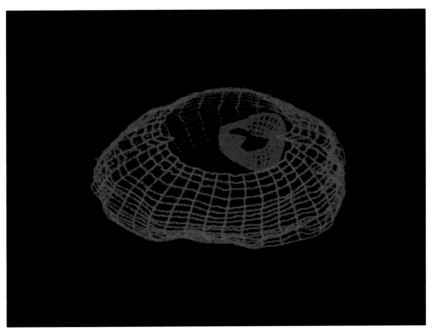

FIGURE 67.   Wire frame image generated from serial XCT images. This patient's tumor location, volume, metabolism, neuroreceptor characteristics, and response to treatment may all be mapped into this computer generated 3-D image. (Courtesy of H.L. Loats, Loats Associates, Westminster, Maryland)

References

Agranoff BW, Smith CB, Sokoloff L: Regional protein synthesis in rat brain after hypoglossal axotomy. Transactions of the American Society of Neurochemistry 11:95, 1980

Arnett CD, Wolf AP, Shiue CY, et al: Improved delineation of human dopamine receptors using [18F] N-methylspiroperidol and PET. J Nucl Med 27:1878-1882, 1986

Baxter LR Jr, Phelps ME, Mazziotta JC, et al: Cerebral metabolic rates for glucose in mood disorders: studies with positron emission tomography and fluorodeoxyglucose F-18. Arch Gen Psychiatry 42:441-447, 1985

Baxter LR, Phelps ME, Mazziotta JC, et al: Local cerebral glucose metabolic rates in obsessive-compulsive disorder, a comparison with rates in unipolar depression and in normal controls. Arch Gen Psychiatry 44:211-218, 1987

Beal MF, Mazurek MF, Tran VT, et al: Reduced numbers of somatostatin receptors in the cerebral cortex in Alzheimer's disease. Science 229:289-291, 1985

Bergstrom M, Litton J, Eriksson L, et al: Determination of object contour from projections for attenuation correction in cranial positron emission tomography. J Comput Assist Tomogr 6:365-372, 1982

Bergstrom M, Ericson K, Hagenfeldt L, et al: PET study of methionine accumulation in glioma and normal brain tissue: competition with branched chain amino acids. J Comput Assist Tomogr 11:208-213, 1987

Berman KF, Zec RF, Weinberger DR: Physiologic dysfunction of dorsolateral prefrontal cortex in schizophrenia, II: role of neuroleptic treatment, attention, and mental effort. Arch Gen Psychiatry 43:126-135, 1986

Bice AN, Wagner HN, Frost JJ, et al: Simplified detection system for neuroreceptor studies in the human brain. J Nucl Med 27:184-191, 1986

Bogerts B, Meertz E, Schonfeldt-Bausch R: Basal ganglia and limbic system pathology in schizophrenia, a morphometric study of brain volume and shrinkage. Arch Gen Psychiatry 42:784-791, 1985

Briere R, Sherwin AL, Robitaille Y, et al: Alpha-1 adrenoceptors are decreased in human epileptic foci. Ann Neurol 19:26-30, 1986

Brodie JD, Wolkin A, Angrist B, et al: Effects of amphetamine on local cerebral metabolism in normal and schizophrenic subjects as determined by positron emission tomography using [1-^{11}C]2-deoxy-D-glucose (^{11}C-2DG). J Nucl Med 27:901, 1986

Brooks RA, DiChiro G, Zukerberg BW, et al: Test–retest studies of cerebral glucose metabolism using fluorine-18 deoxyglucose: validation of method. J Nucl Med 28:53-59, 1987

Brown RM, Colter N, Corsellis JAN, et al: Postmortem evidence of structural brain changes in schizophrenia, differences in brain weight, temporal horn area, and parahippocampal gyrus compared with affective disorder. Arch Gen Psychiatry 43:36-42, 1986

Buchsbaum MS, Ingvar DH, Kessler R, et al: Cerebral glucography with positron tomography: use in normal subjects and in patients with schizophrenia. Arch Gen Psychiatry 39:251-259, 1982

Buchsbaum MS, Holcomb HH, Johnson J, et al: Cerebral metabolic consequences of electrical cutaneous stimulation in normal individuals. Hum Neurobiol 2:35-8, 1983a

Buchsbaum MS, Holcomb H, Kessler R, et al: Lateralized asymmetries in glucose uptake assessed by positron emission tomography in patients with schizophrenia and normal controls, in Laterality and Psychopathology. Edited by Flor-Henry P, Gruzelier J. New York, Elsevier Science Publishers, 1983b

Buchsbaum MS, DeLisi LE, Holcomb HH, et al: Anteroposterior gradients in cerebral glucose use in schizophrenia and affective disorders. Arch Gen Psychiatry 41:1159-1166, 1984

Buchsbaum MS, Wu J, DeLisi LE, et al: Frontal cortex and basal ganglia metabolic rates assessed by positron emission tomography with [18F]2 deoxyglucose in affective illness. J Affective Disord 10:137-152, 1986

Bunney WE Jr, Davis JM: Norepinephrine in depressive reactions. Arch Gen Psychiatry 13:483-494, 1965

Burns HD, Dannals RF, Langstrom B, et al: (3-N-[11C]methyl)spiperone, a ligand binding to dopamine receptors: radiochemical synthesis and biodistribution studies in mice. J Nucl Med 25:1222-1227, 1984

Bustany P, Henry JF, Rotrou JD, et al: Correlations between clinical state and positron emission tomography measurement of local brain protein synthesis in Alzheimer's dementia, Parkinson's disease, schizophrenia, and gliomas, in The Metabolism of the Human Brain Studied with Positron Emission Tomography. Edited by Greitz T, Ingvar DH, Widen L. New York, Raven Press, 1985

Buxton RB, Alpert NM, Ackerman RH, et al: Measurement of brain pH with positron emission tomography, in Positron Emission Tomography. Edited by Reivich M, Alavi A. New York, Alan R. Liss, Inc., 1985

Charnas L, Pyeritz RE: Neurologic injuries in boxers. Hosp Pract 30:21(5A), 30-31, 34-39, 1986

Chase TN, Fedio P, Foster NL, et al: Wechsler Adult Intelligence Scale performance: cortical localization by fluorodeoxyglucose F-18 positron emission tomography. Arch Neurol 41:1244-1247, 1984

Chiueh CC, Firnau G: Imaging of MPTP-induced change in turnover and damage to striatal dopamine. J Nucl Med 27:879, 1986

Chugani HT, Phelps ME: Maturational changes of glucose metabolic patterns in the human infant determined by 18F-2-fluorodeoxyglucose (FDG) positron emission tomography (PET). J Cereb Blood Flow Metab 5:S99-S100, 1985

Chugani HT, Phelps ME: Maturation changes in cerebral function in infants determined by 18FDG positron emission tomography. Science 231:840-843, 1986

Chugani DC, Ackerman RF, Phelps ME: [H-3] Spiperone and [F-18]2-fluoro-2-deoxyglucose studies of nigrostriatal stimulation in rats. J Cereb Blood Flow Metab 5 (suppl 1):S161-S162, 1985

Clark CM, Stoessl AJ: Glucose use correlations: a matter of inference. J Cereb Blood Flow Metab 6:511-512, 1986

Clark CM, Kessler R, Buchsbaum MS, et al: Correlational methods for determining regional coupling of cerebral glucose metabolism: a pilot study. Biol Psychiatry 19:663-678, 1984

Clark CM, Carson R, Kessler R, et al: Alternative statistical models for the examination of clinical positron emission tomography/fluorodexyglucose data. J Cereb Blood Flow Metab 5:142-150, 1985

Clark CM, Hayden MR, Stoessl AJ, et al: Regression model for predicting dissociations of regional cerebral glucose metabolism in individuals at risk for Huntington's disease. J Cereb Blood Flow Metab 6:756-762, 1986

Cohen RM, Semple WE, Gross M, et al: Dysfunction in a prefrontal substrate of sustained attention in schizophrenia. Life Sci 40:2031-2039, 1987

Comar D, Zarifian E, Verhas M, et al: Brain distribution and kinetics of 11C chlorpromazine in schizophrenics: positron emission tomography studies. Psychiatry Res 1:23-29, 1979

Cutler NR, Haxby JV, Duara R, et al: Brain metabolism as measured with positron emission tomography: serial assessment in a patient with familial Alzheimer's disease. Neurology 35:1556-1561, 1985

Dannals RF, Ravert HT, Frost JJ, et al: Radiosynthesis of an opiate receptor binding radiotracer: [^{11}C]carfentanil. Int J Appl Radiat Isot 36:303-306, 1985

Dannals RF, Ravert HT, Wilson AA, et al: An improved synthesis of (3-N-[11C]methyl)spiperone. Int J Rad Appl Instrum [A] 37:433-434, 1986

deLeon MJ, Ferris SH, George AE, et al: Computed tomography and positron emission transaxial tomography evaluations of normal aging and Alzheimer's disease. J Cereb Blood Flow Metab 3:391-394, 1983

deLeon MJ, George AE, Ferris SH, et al: Positron emission tomography and computed tomography assessments of the aging human brain. J Comput Assist Tomogr 8:88-94, 1984

DeLisi LE, Buchsbaum MS, Holcomb HH, et al: Clinical correlates of decreased anteroposterior metabolic gradients in positron emission tomography (PET) of schizophrenic patients. Am J Psychiatry 142:78-81, 1985a

DeLisi LE, Holcomb HH, Cohen RM, et al: Positron emission tomography in schizophrenic patients with and without neuroleptic medication. J Cereb Blood Flow Metab 5:201-206, 1985b

Des Rosiers MH, Sakurada O, Jehle J, et al: Functional plasticity in the immature striate cortex of the monkey shown by the [14C]deoxyglucose method. Science 200(4340):447-449, 1978

DiChiro G, Brooks RA, Bairamian D, et al: Diagnostic and prognostic value of positron emission tomography using [^{18}F] fluorodeoxyglucose in brain tumors, in Positron Emission Tomography. Edited by Reivich M, Alavi A. New York, Alan R. Liss, Inc., 1985

Dienel G, Nelson T, Cruz N, et al: Contaminants in inadequately purified glucose and incomplete recovery of metabolites are responsible for the erroneous conclusion of high glucose-6-phosphatase activity in rat brain. Soc Neurosci Abstr 12(part 2):1405, 1986

Duara R, Grady C, Haxby J, et al: Human brain glucose utilization and cognitive function in relation to age. Ann Neurol 16:703-713, 1984

Duell RK, Yue GM, Sherman WR, et al: Monitoring the time course of cerebral deoxyglucose metabolism by ^{31}P nuclear magnetic resonance spectroscopy. Science 228:1329-1331, 1985

Early TS, Reiman EM, Raichle ME, et al: Left globus pallidus abnormality in never-medicated patients with schizophrenia. Proc Natl Acad Sci USA 84:561-563, 1987

Eckelman WC, Reba RC, Rzeszotarski WJ, et al: External imaging of cerebral muscarinic acetylcholine receptors. Science 223:291-292, 1984

Engel J Jr, Brown WJ, Kuhl DE, et al: Pathological findings underlying focal temporal lobe hypometabolism in partial epilepsy. Ann Neurol 12:518-28, 1982a

Engel J Jr, Kuhl DE, Phelps ME: Patterns of human local cerebral glucose metabolism during epileptic seizures. Science 218:64-66, 1982b

Engel J Jr, Kuhl DE, Phelps ME, et al: Comparative localization of epileptic foci in partial epilepsy by PCT and EEG. Ann Neurol 12:529-537, 1982c

Engel J Jr, Kuhl DE, Phelps ME, et al: Interictal cerebral glucose metabolism in partial epilepsy and its relation to EEG changes. Ann Neurol 12:510-517, 1982d

Engel J Jr, Kuhl DE, Phelps ME, et al: Local cerebral metabolism during partial seizures. Neurology 33:400-413, 1983

Engel J Jr, Lubens P, Kuhl DE, et al: Local cerebral metabolic rate for glucose during petit mal absences. Ann Neurol 17:121-128, 1985

Evens RG, Siegel BA, Welch MJ, et al: Cost analyses of positron emission tomography for clinical use. AJR 141:1073-1076, 1983

Farde L, Ehrin E, Eriksson L, et al: Substituted benzamides as ligands for visualization of dopamine receptor binding in the human brain by positron emission tomography. Proc Natl Acad Sci USA 82:3863-3867, 1985

Farde L, Hall H, Ehrin E, et al: Quantitative analysis of D2 dopamine receptor binding in the living human brain by PET. Science 231:258-261, 1986

Farde L, Wiesel FA, Hall H, et al: No D2 receptor increase in PET study of schizophrenia [letter]. Arch Gen Psychiatry 44:671-672, 1987

Farde L, Wiesel FA, Halldin C, et al: Central D2-dopamine receptor occupancy in schizophrenic patients treated with antipsychotic drugs. Arch Gen Psychiatry 45:71-76, 1988

Farkas T, Ferris SH, Wolf AP, et al: 18F 2-deoxy 2-fluoro-D-glucose as a tracer in the positron emission tomographic study of senile dementia. Am J Psychiatry 139:352-353, 1982

Farkas T, Wolf AP, Jaeger J, et al: Regional brain glucose metabolism in chronic schizophrenia: a positron emission transaxial tomographic study. Arch Gen Psychiatry 41:293-300, 1984

Fishman RS, Karnovsky ML: Apparent absence of a translocase in the cerebral glucose-6-phosphastase system. J Neurochem 46:371-378, 1986

Ford I: Can statistics cause brain damage? J Cereb Blood Flow Metab 3:259-262, 1983

Ford I: Confounded correlations: statistical limitations in the analysis of interregional relationships of cerebral metabolic activity. J Cereb Blood Flow Metab 6:385-388, 1986

Foster NL, Chase TN, Mansi L, et al: Cortical abnormalities in Alzheimer's disease. Ann Neurol 16:649-654, 1984

Foster NL, Chase TN, Patronas NJ, et al: Cerebral mapping of apraxia in Alzheimer's disease by positron emission tomography. Ann Neurol 19:139-143, 1986

Fowler JS, Arnett CD, Wolf AP, et al: [11C]Spiroperidol: synthesis, specific activity determination and biodistribution in mice. J Nucl Med 23:437-445, 1982

Fowler JS, MacGregor RR, Wolf AP, et al: Mapping human brain monoamine oxidase A and B with 11C labeled suicide inactivators and PET. Science 235:481-485, 1987

Fox PT, Raichle ME: Stimulus rate dependence of regional cerebral blood flow in human striate cortex, demonstrated by positron emission tomography. J Neurophysiol 51:1109-1120, 1984

Fox PT, Raichle ME: Stimulus rate determines regional brain blood flow in striate cortex. Ann Neurol 17:303-305, 1985

Fox PT, Raichle ME: Focal physiological uncoupling of cerebral blood flow and oxidative metabolism during somatosensory stimulation in human subjects. Proc Natl Acad Sci USA 83:1140-1144, 1986

Fox PT, Fox JM, Raichle ME, et al: The role of cerebral cortex in the generation of voluntary saccades: a positron emission tomographic study. J Neurophysiol 54:348-369, 1985a

Fox PT, Perlmutter JS, Raichle ME: A stereotactic method of anatomical localization for positron emission tomography. J Comput Assist Tomogr 9:141-153, 1985b

Fox PT, Raichle ME, Thach WT: Functional mapping of the human cerebellum with positron emission tomography. Proc Natl Acad Sci USA 82:7462-7466, 1985c

Fox PT, Mintun MA, Raichle ME, et al: Mapping human visual cortex with positron emission tomography. Nature 323:806-809, 1986

Fox PT, Burton H, Raichle ME: Mapping human somatosensory cortex with positron emission tomography. J Neurosurg 67:34-43, 1987a

Fox PT, Miezin FM, Allman JM, et al: Retinotopic organization of human visual cortex mapped with positron emission tomography. J Neurosci 7:913-922, 1987b

Frackowiak RSJ, Lammertsma AA: Clinical measurement of cerebral blood flow and oxygen consumption, in Positron Emission Tomography. Edited by Reivich M, Alavi A. New York, Alan R. Liss, Inc. 1985

Frackowiak RS, Jones T, Lenzi GL, et al: Regional cerebral oxygen utilization and blood flow in normal man, using oxygen 15 and positron emission tomography. Acta Neurol Scand 62:336-344, 1980a

Frackowiak RS, Lenzi GL, Jones T, et al: Quantitative measurement of regional cerebral blood flow and oxygen, metabolism in man using 15O and positron emission tomography: theory, procedure, and normal values. J Comput Assist Tomogr 4:727-736, 1980b

Franzen G, Ingvar DH: Absence of activation in frontal structures during psychological testing of chronic schizophrenics. J Neurol Neurosurg Psychiatry 38:1027-1032, 1975

Frey KA, Hichwa RD, Ehrenkaufer RL, et al: Quantitative in vivo receptor binding, III: tracer kinetic modeling of muscarinic cholinergic receptor binding. Proc Natl Acad Sci USA 82:6711-6715, 1985

Friedland RP, Budinger TF, Ganz E, et al: Regional cerebral metabolic alterations in dementia of the Alzheimer type: positron emission tomography with [18F]fluorodeoxyglucose. J Comput Assist Tomogr 7:590-598, 1983

Friedland RP, Budinger TF, Brant ZM, et al: The diagnosis of Alzheimer type dementia: a preliminary comparison of positron emission tomography and proton magnetic resonance. JAMA 252:2750-2752, 1984

Friedland RP, Budinger TF, Koss E, et al: Alzheimer's disease: anterior posterior and lateral hemispheric alterations in cortical glucose utilization. Neurosci Lett 53:235-240, 1985

Frost JJ, Wagner HN Jr, Dannals RF, et al: Imaging opiate receptors in the human brain by positron tomography. J Comput Assist Tomogr 9:231-236, 1985

Frost JJ, Wagner HN Jr, Dannals RF, et al: Imaging benzodiazepine receptors in man with [11C]suriclone by positron emission tomography. Eur J Pharmacol 122:381-383, 1986

Frost JJ, Smith AC, Kuhar MJ, et al: In vivo binding of 3H-N-methylspiperone to dopamine and serotonin receptors. Life Sci 40:987-995, 1987

Frost JJ, Mayberg HS, Fisher J, et al: Mu-opiate receptors measured by positron emission tomography are increased in temporal lobe epilepsy. Ann Neurol 23:231-237, 1988

Gallagher BM, Ansari A, Atkins H, et al: 18F labeled 2-deoxy 2-fluoro-d-glucose as a radiopharmaceutical for measuring regional myocardial glucose metabolism in vivo: tissue distribution and imaging studies in animals. J Nucl Med 18:990-996, 1977

Garnett ES, Firnau G, Nahmias C: Dopamine visualized in the basal ganglia of living man. Nature 305:137-138, 1983

Garnett ES, Nahmias C, Firnau G: Central dopaminergic pathways in hemiparkinsonism examined by positron emission tomography. Can J Neurol Sci 11:174-179, 1984

Garnett ES, Nahmias C, Firnau G, et al: Patterns of local cerebral glucose metabolism in untreated schizophrenics. J Cereb Blood Flow Metab 5(Suppl 1):S179-S180, 1985

Ginsberg MD, Chang JY, Kelley RE, et al: Increases in both cerebral glucose utilization and blood flow during execution of a somatosensory task. Ann Neurol 23:152-160, 1988

Greenamyre JT, Penney JB, Young AB, et al: Alterations in L-glutamate binding in Alzheimer's and Huntington's diseases. Science 227:1496-1999, 1985

Greitz T, Bergstrom M, Boethius J, et al: Head fixation system for integration of radiodiagnostic and therapeutic procedures. Neuroradiology 19:1-6, 1980

Guenther W, Moser E, Mueller SF, et al: Pathological cerebral blood flow during motor function in schizophrenic and endogenous depressed patients. Biol Psychiatry 21:889-899, 1986

Gur RC, Reivich M: Cognitive task effects on hemispheric blood flow in humans: evidence, for individual differences in hemispheric activation. Brain Lang 9:78-92, 1980

Gur RC, Gur RE, Rosen AD, et al: A cognitive motor network demonstrated by positron emission tomography. Neuropsychologia 21:601-606, 1983

Gur RE: Hemispheric activation in schizophrenia: regional cerebral blood flow, in: Laterality and Psychopathology. Edited by Flor-Henry P, Gruzelier J. New York, Elsevier Science Publishers, 1983

Gur RE, Skolnick BE, Gur RC, et al: Brain function in psychiatric disorders, I: regional cerebral blood flow in medicated schizophrenics. Arch Gen Psychiatry 40:1250-1254, 1983

Gur RE, Skolnick BE, Gur RC, et al: Brain function in psychiatric disorders, II: regional cerebral blood flow in medicated unipolar depressives. Arch Gen Psychiatry 41:695-699, 1984

Gur RE, Gur RC, Skolnick BE, et al: Brain function in psychiatric disorders, III: regional cerebral blood flow in unmedicated schizophrenics. Arch Gen Psychiatry 42:329-334, 1985

Gur RC, Gur RE, Resnick SM, et al: The effect of anxiety on cortical cerebral blood flow and metabolism. J Cereb Blood Flow Metab 7:173-177, 1987a

Gur RE, Resnick SM, Alavi A, et al: Regional brain function in schizophrenia, I: a positron emission tomography study. Arch Gen Psychiatry 44:119-125, 1987b

Gur RE, Resnick SM, Gur RC, et al: Regional brain function in schizophrenia, II: repeated evaluation with positron emission tomography. Arch Gen Psychiatry 44:126-129, 1987c

Guttman M, Seeman P, Reynolds GP, et al: Dopamine D_2 receptor density remains constant in treated Parkinson's disease. Ann Neurol 19:487-492, 1986

Hand PJ: The 2-deoxyglucose method, in Neuroanatomical Track Tracing Methods. Edited by Heimer L, Robards M. New York, Plenum Press, 1981

Hatazawa J, Brooks RA, Di Chiro G, et al: Glucose utilization rate versus brain size in humans. Neurology 37:583-588, 1987

Hawkins RA, Miller DL: Loss of radioactive 2-deoxy-D-glucose-6-phosphate from brains of conscious rats: implications for quantitative autoradiographic determination of regional glucose utilization. Neuroscience 3:251-258, 1978.

Hawkins RA, Phelps ME: Clinical PET operational and cost considerations. Administrative Radiology April:20-26, 1986

Haxby JV, Duara R, Grady CL, et al: Relations between neuropsychological and cerebral metabolic asymmetries in early Alzheimer's disease. J Cereb Blood Flow Metab 5:193-200, 1985

Hayden MR, Martin WRW, Stoessl AJ, et al: Positron emission tomography in the early diagnosis of Huntington's disease. Neurology 36:888-894, 1986

Heiss WD, Pawlik G, Herholz K, et al: Regional cerebral glucose metabolism in man during wakefulness, sleep, and dreaming. Brain Res 327:362-366, 1985

Herholz K, Krieg JC, Emrich HM, et al: Regional cerebral glucose metabolism in anorexia nervosa measured by positron emission tomography. Biol Psychiatry 22:43-51, 1987

Herkenham M, Pert CB: In vitro autoradiography of opiate receptors in rat brain suggests loci of "opiatergic" pathways. Proc Natl Acad Sci USA 77:5532-5536, 1980

Herscovitch P, Raichle ME: Effect of tissue heterogeneity on the measurement of cerebral blood flow with the equilibrium $C^{15}O_2$ inhalation technique. J Cereb Blood Flow Metab 3:407-415, 1983

Herscovitch P, Raichle ME: What is the correct value for the brain blood partition coefficient for water? J Cereb Blood Flow Metab 5:65-69, 1985

Herscovitch P, Markham J, Raichle ME: Brain blood flow measured with intravenous $H_2{}^{15}O$, I: theory and error analysis. J Nucl Med 24:782-789, 1983

Herscovitch P, Mintun MA, Raichle ME: Brain oxygen utilization measured with oxygen 15 radiotracers and positron emission tomography: generation of metabolic images. J Nucl Med 26:416-417, 1985

Herscovitch P, Auchus AP, Gado M, et al: Correction of positron emission tomography data for cerebral atrophy. J Cereb Blood Flow Metab 6:120-124, 1986

Hichwa RD, Hutchins GD, Sackellares JC, et al: Determination of LCBF during the evolution of partial seizures in patients with temporal lobe epilepsy. J Nucl Med 27:902, 1986

Hoffman EJ, Phelps ME: Positron emission tomography: principles and quantitation, in Positron Emission Tomography and Autoradiography: Principles and Applications for the Brain and Heart. Edited by Phelps M, Mazziotta J, Schelbert H. New York, Raven Press, 1986

Hoffman EJ, Huang SC, Phelps ME, et al: Quantitation in positron emission computed tomography, 4: effect of accidental coincidences. J Comput Assist Tomogr 5:391-400, 1981

Hoffman EJ, Huang SC, Plummer D, et al: Quantitation in positron emission computed tomography, 6: effect of nonuniform resolution. J Comput Assist Tomogr 6:987-999, 1982

Hoffman EJ, Phelps ME, Huang SC: Performance evaluation of a positron tomograph designed for brain imaging. J Nucl Med 24:245-257, 1983

Hoffman EJ, van der Stee M, Ricci AR, et al: Prospects for both precision and accuracy in positron emission tomography. Ann Neurol 15 (Suppl):S25-S34, 1984

Hokfelt T, Smith CB, Peters A, et al: Improved resolution of the 2-deoxy-D-glucose technique. Brain Res 289:311-316, 1983

Hokfelt T, Smith CB, Norell G, et al: Attempts to combine 2-deoxyglucose autoradiography and tyrosine hydroxylase immunohistochemistry. Neuroscience 13:495-512, 1984

Holcomb HH: Parkinsonism and depression: dopaminergic mediation of neuropathologic processes in human beings, in The Catecholamines in Psychiatric and Neurologic Disorders. Edited by Lake CR, Ziegler MG. Boston, Butterworth Publishers, 1985

Holcomb HH, Loats HL, Tamminga C, et al: Registration of MRI-PET images, procedure and validation. J Nucl Med 29:853, 1988a

Holcomb HH, Loats HL, Tamminga CA, et al: Volume, shape, location, and gray/white tissue analysis of brain magnetic resonance images. CINP XVIth Congress, Munich, Germany, 1988b

Holden JE: Effects of blood flow on the positron emission tomographic determination of substrate transport rates. Circulation 72:72-76, 1985

Holman BL, Gibson RE, Hill TC, et al: Muscarinic acetylcholine receptors in Alzheimer's disease: in vivo imaging with iodine 123 labeled-3 quinuclidinyl-4 iodobenzilate and emission tomography. JAMA 254:3063-3066, 1985

Horwitz B, Duara R, Rapoport SI: Intercorrelations of glucose metabolic rates between brain regions: application to healthy males in a state of reduced sensory input. J Cereb Blood Flow Metab 4:484-499, 1984

Horwitz B, Duara R, Rapoport SI: Age differences in intercorrelations between regional cerebral metabolic rates for glucose. Ann Neurol 19:60-67, 1986

Huang M, Veech RL: The quantitative determination of the in vivo dephosphorylation of glucose 6-phosphate in rat brain. J Biol Chem 257:11358-11363, 1982

Huang SC, Phelps ME: Principles of tracer kinetic modeling in positron emission tomography and autoradiography, in Positron Emission Tomography and Autoradiography: Principles and Applications for the Brain and Heart. Edited by Phelps M, Mazziotta J, Schelbert H. New York, Raven Press, 1986

Huang SC, Hoffman EJ, Phelps ME, et al: Quantitation in positron emission computed tomography, 2: effects of inaccurate attenuation correction. J Comput Assist Tomogr 3:804-814, 1979

Huang SC, Hoffman EJ, Phelps ME, et al: Quantitation in positron emission computed tomography, 3: effect of sampling. J Comput Assist Tomogr 4:819-826, 1980a

Huang SC, Phelps ME, Hoffman EJ, et al: Noninvasive determination of local cerebral metabolic rate of glucose in man. Am J Physiol 238:E69-E82, 1980b

Huang SC, Carson RE, Phelps ME, et al: A boundary method for attenuation correction in positron computed tomography. J Nucl Med 22:627-637, 1981a

Huang SC, Phelps ME, Hoffman EJ, et al: Error sensitivity of fluorodeoxygucose method for measurement of cerebral metabolic rate of glucose. J Cereb Blood Flow Metab 1:391-401, 1981b

Huang SC, Carson RE, Hoffman EJ, et al: Quantitative measurement of local cerebral blood flow in humans by positron computed tomography and ^{15}O water. J Cereb Blood Flow Metab 3:141-153, 1983

Huang SC, Barrio JR, Phelps ME: Neuroreceptor assay with positron emission tomography: equilibrium versus dynamic approaches. J Cereb Blood Flow Metab 6:515-521, 1986a

Huang SC, Feng DG, Phelps ME: Model dependency and estimation reliability in measurement of cerebral oxygen utilization rate with oxygen 15 and dynamic positron emission tomography. J Cereb Blood Flow Metab 6:105-119, 1986b

Hubel DH, Wiesel TN: Receptive fields and functional architecture of monkey striate cortex. J Physiol 195:215-243, 1968

Hubel DH, Wiesel TN, LeVay S: Plasticity of ocular dominance columns in monkey striate cortex. Philos Trans R Soc Lond (Biol) 278:377-409, 1977

Hungerbuhler JP, Saunders JC, Greenberg J, et al: Functional neuroanatomy of the auditory cortex studied with [2-14C] deoxyglucose. Exp Neurol 71:104-121, 1981

Ido T, Wan CN, Casella V, et al: Labeled 2-deoxy-D-glucose analogs. ^{18}F-labeled 2-deoxy-2-fluoro-D-glucose, 2-deoxy-2-fluoro-D-mannose and ^{14}C-2-deoxy-2-fluoro-D-glucose. Journal Labeled Compounds and Radiopharmaceuticals 14:175-183, 1978

Ingvar DH, Franzen G: Abnormalities of cerebral blood flow distribution in patients with chronic schizophrenia. Acta Psychiatr Scand 50:425-462, 1974

Ingvar DH, Rosen I, Eriksson M, et al: Activation patterns induced in the dominant hemisphere by skin stimulation, in Sensory Functions of the Skin in Primates. Edited by Zotterman Y. New York, Pergamon Press, 1976

Ingvar MC, Maeder P, Sokoloff L, et al: Effects of ageing on local rates of cerebral protein synthesis in Sprague-Dawley rats. Brain 108:155-170, 1985

Jones SC, Alavi A, Christman D, et al: The radiation dosimetry of 2-[F-18]fluoro-2-deoxy-D-glucose in man. J Nucl Med 23:613-617, 1982a

Jones SC, Greenberg JH, Reivich M: Error analysis for the determination of cerebral blood flow with the continuous inhalation of ^{15}O labeled carbon dioxide and positron emission tomography. J Comput Assist Tomogr 6:116-124, 1982b

Jones SC, Robinson GD Jr, McIntyre E: Tandem van de Graaff accelerator production of positron labeled radiopharmaceuticals for routine clinical use. Int J Appl Radiat Isot 35:721-729, 1984

Jones T, Chessler DA, Ter-Pogossian MM: The continuous inhalation of oxygen-15 for assessing regional oxygen extraction in the brain of man. Br J Radiol 49:339-343, 1976

Juliano SL, Whitsel BL: Metabolic labeling associated with index finger stimulation in monkey SI: between animal variability. Brain Res 342:242-251, 1985

Juliano SL, Hand PJ, Whitsel BL: Patterns of increased metabolic activity in somatosensory cortex of monkeys macaca fascicularis subjected to controlled cutaneous stimulation: a 2-deoxyglucose study. J Neurophysiol 46:1260-1284, 1981

Kanno I, Miura S, Yamamoto S, et al: Design and evaluation of a positron emission tomograph: HEADTOME III. J Comput Assist Tomogr 9:931-939, 1985

Kato A, Menon D, Kiksic M, et al: Influence of the input function on the calcula-, tion of the local cerebral metabolic rate for glucose in the deoxyglucose method. J Cereb Blood Flow Metab 4:41-46, 1984

Kennedy C: Glucose use correlations. J Cereb Blood Flow Metab 5:619-621, 1985

Kennedy C, Des Rosiers MH, Sakurada O, et al: Metabolic mapping of the primary visual system of the monkey by means of the autoradiographic [14C]deoxyglucose technique. Proc Natl Acad Sci USA 73:4230-4234, 1976

Kennedy C, Sakurada O, Shinohara M, et al: Local cerebral glucose utilization in the normal conscious macaque monkey. Ann Neurol 4:293-301, 1978

Kennedy C, Miyaoka M, Suda S, et al: Local metabolic responses in brain accompanying motor activity. Transactions of the American Neurological Association 105:13-17, 1980

Kennedy C, Suda S, Smith CB, et al: Changes in protein synthesis underlying functional plasticity in immature monkey visual system. Proc Natl Acad Sci USA 78:3950-3953, 1981

Kennedy C, Gillin JC, Mendelson W, et al: Local cerebral glucose utilization in non-rapid eye movement sleep. Nature 297:325-327, 1982

Kessler RM, Ellis JR Jr, Eden M: Analysis of emission tomographic scan data: limitations imposed by resolution and background. J Comput Assist Tomogr 8:514-522, 1984a

Kessler RM, Goble JC, Bird JH, et al: Measurement of blood-brain barrier permeability with positron emission tomography and [68Ga]EDTA. J Cereb Blood Flow Metab 4:323-328, 1984b

Kety SS: The theory and applications of the exchange of inert gas at the lungs and tissues. Pharmacol Rev 3:1-41, 1951

Kety SS: Measurement of local blood flow by the exchange of an inert, diffusible substance. Methods of Medical Research 8:228-236, 1960

Kety SS: Basic principles for the quantitative estimation of regional cerebral blood flow. Res Publ Assoc Res Nerv Ment Dis 63:1-7, 1985

Kety SS, Schmidt CF: The nitrous oxide method for the quantitative determination of cerebral blood flow in man: theory, procedure and normal values. J Clin Invest 27:476-483, 1948

Kling AS, Metter EJ, Riefe WH, et al: Comparison of PET measurement of local brain glucose metabolism and CAT measurement of brain atrophy in chronic schizophrenia and depression. Am J Psychiatry 143:175-180, 1986

Kuhar MJ, Pert CB, Snyder SH: Regional distribution of opiate receptor binding in monkey and human brain. Nature 245:447-449, 1973

Kuhar MJ, Murrin LC, Malouf AT, et al: Dopamine receptor binding in vivo: the feasibility of autoradiographic studies. Life Sci 22:203-210, 1978

Kuhl DE, Metter EJ, Riege WH, et al: Effects of human aging on patterns of local cerebral glucose utilization determined by the [18F]fluorodeoxyglucose method. J Cereb Blood Flow Metab 2:163-171, 1982a

Kuhl DE, Phelps ME, Markham CH, et al: Cerebral metabolism and atrophy in Huntington's disease determined by 18FDG and computed tomographic scan. Ann Neurol 12:425-434, 1982b

Kuhl DE, Metter EJ, Riege WH: Patterns of local cerebral glucose utilization determined in Parkinson's disease by the [18F]fluorodeoxyglucose method. Ann Neurol 15:419-424, 1984

Lang W, Henke H: Cholinergic receptor binding and autoradiography in brains of non-neurological and senile dementia of Alzheimer-type patients. Brain Res 267:271-280, 1983

Langfitt TW, Obrist WD, Alavi A, et al: Computerized tomography, magnetic resonance imaging, and positron emission tomography in the study of brain trauma: preliminary observations. J Neurosurg 64:760-767, 1986

Latack JT, Abour Khalil BW, Siegel GJ, et al: Patients with partial seizures: evaluation by MR, CT, and PET imaging. Radiology 159:159-163, 1986

Lauter JL, Herscovitch P, Formby C, et al: Tonotopic organization in human auditory cortex revealed by positron emission tomography. Hear Res 20:199-205, 1985

Lear J: Principles of single and multiple radionuclide autoradiography, in Positron Emission Tomography and Autoradiography: Principles and Applications for the Brain and Heart. Edited by Phelps M, Mazziotta J, Schelbert H. New York, Raven Press, 1986

Leenders KL, Wolfson L, Gibbs J, et al: Regional cerebral blood flow and oxygen metabolism in Parkinson's disease and their response to L-dopa. J Cereb Blood Flow Metab 3(Suppl 1):S488-S489, 1983

Leenders KL, Palmer AJ, Quinn N, et al: Brain dopamine metabolism in patients with Parkinson's disease measured with positron emission tomography. J Neurol Neurosurg Psychiatry 49:853-860, 1986a

Leenders KL, Poewe WH, Palmer AJ, et al: Inhibition of L [18F]fluorodopa uptake into human brain by amino acids demonstrated by positron emission tomography. Ann Neurol 20:258-262, 1986b

Lewis ME, Mishkin M, Bragin E, et al: Opiate receptor gradients in monkey cerebral cortex: correspondence with sensory processing hierarchies. Science 211:1166-1169, 1981

Macko KA, Jarvis CD, Kennedy C, et al: Mapping the primate visual system with [2-14C]-deoxyglucose. Science 218:394-397, 1982

Martin WRW, Beckman JH, Calne DB, et al: Cerebral glucose metabolism in Parkinson's disease. Can J Neurol Sci 11(1 Suppl):169-173, 1984

Martin WRW, Stoessl AJ, Adam MJ, et al: Positron emission tomography in Parkinson's disease. J Nucl Med 27:936, 1986

Mazziotta JC, Phelps ME: Human sensory stimulation and deprivation: positron emission tomographic results and strategies. Ann Neurol 15 (Suppl):S50-S60, 1984

Mazziotta JC, Phelps ME, Miller J: Tomographic mapping of human cerebral metabolism: normal unstimulated state. Neurology 31:503-516, 1981

Mazziotta JC, Phelps ME, Carson RE, et al: Tomographic mapping of human cerebral metabolism: auditory stimulation. Neurology 32:921-937, 1982

Mazziotta JC, Phelps ME, Halgren E: Local cerebral glucose metabolic response to audiovisual stimulation and deprivation: studies in human subjects with positron CT. Hum Neurobiol 2:11-23, 1983

Mazziotta JC, Phelps ME, Carson RE: Tomographic mapping of human cerebral metabolism: subcortical responses to auditory and visual stimulation. Neurology 34:825-828, 1984

Mazziotta JC, Wapenski J, Phelps ME, et al: Cerebral glucose utilization and blood flow in Huntington's disease: symptomatic and at-risk subjects. J Cereb Blood Flow Metab 5(Suppl 1):S25-S26, 1985

McCulloch J, Savaki HE, Sokoloff L: Distribution of effects of haloperidol on energy metabolism in the rat brain. Brain Res 243:81-90, 1982

McGeer PL, Kamo H, Harrop R, et al: Positron emission tomography in patients with clinically diagnosed Alzheimer's disease (Review). Can Med Assoc J 134:597-607, 1986a

McGeer PL, Kamo H, Harrop R, et al: Comparison of PET, MRI, and CT with pathology in a proven case of Alzheimer's disease. Neurology 36:1569-1574, 1986b

Metter EJ, Riege WH, Kameyama M, et al: Cerebral metabolic relationships for selected brain regions in Alzheimer's, Huntington's and Parkinson's diseases. J Cereb Blood Flow Metab 4:500-506, 1984a

Metter EJ, Riege WH, Kuhl DE, et al: Cerebral metabolic relationships for selected brain regions in healthy adults. J Cereb Blood Flow Metab 4:1-7, 1984b

Mintun MA, Raichle ME, Kilbourn MR, et al: A quantitative model for the in vivo assessment of drug binding sites with positron emission tomography. Ann Neurol 15:217-27, 1984a

Mintun MA, Raichle ME, Martin WR, et al: Brain oxygen utilization measured with O-15 radiotracers and positron emission tomography. J Nucl Med 25:177-187, 1984b

Mitchell IJ, Cross AJ, Sambrook MA, et al: Neural mechanisms mediating 1-methyl-4-phenyl-1,2,3,6-tetrahydropyridine induced parkinsonism in the monkey: relative contributions of the striatopallidal and striatonigral pathways as suggested by 2-deoxyglucose uptake. Neurosci Lett 63:61-65, 1986

Mountz J, Curtis G, Santa C, et al: Alteration in regional cerebral blood flow in simple phobic anxiety demonstrated by O-15-H_2O positron emission tomograpy (PET). J Nucl Med 27:901, 1986

Mullani NA, Markham J, Ter Pogossian MM: Feasibility of time of flight reconstruction in positron emission tomography. J Nucl Med 21:1095-1097, 1980

Murugaiah K, Theodorou A, Mann S, et al: Chronic continuous administration of neuroleptic drugs alters cerebral dopamine receptors and increases spontaneous dopaminergic action in the striatum. Nature 296:570-572, 1982

Nelson T, Kaufman EE, Sokoloff L: 2-Deoxyglucose incorporation into rat brain glycogen during measurement of local cerebral glucose utilization by the 2-deoxyglucose method. J Neurochem 43:949-956, 1984

Nelson T, Lucignani G, Atlas S, et al: Reexamination of glucose-6-phosphatase activity in the brain in vivo: no evidence for a futile cycle. Science 229:60-62, 1985

Nelson T, Lucignani G, Goochee J, et al: Invalidity of criticisms of the deoxyglucose method based on alleged, glucose-6 phosphatase activity in brain. J Neurochem 46:905, 1986a

Nelson T, Lucignani G, Sokoloff L: Measurement of brain deoxyglucose metabolism by NMR. Science 232:776-777, 1986b

Nilsson A, Risberg J, Gustafson L: Regional cerebral blood flow in paranoid states before and during haloperidol treatment. J Cereb Blood Flow Metab 5 (Suppl 1):S195-S196, 1985

Oken BS, Chiappa KH: Statistical issues concerning computerized analysis of brainwave topography. Ann Neurol 19:493-497, 1986

O'Tuama LA, Frost JJ, Wilson AA, et al: In vivo labeling of alpha-1 adrenergic receptors with I-125 2-beta (4-hydroxyphenyl) ethylaminomethyl-tetralone (HEAT). J Nucl Med 27:969, 1986

O'Tuama LA, LaFrance ND, Dannals RF, et al: Quantitative imaging of neutral amino acid transport by human brain tumors. Paper presented at the XIII

International Symposium on Cerebral Blood Flow and Metabolism, Montreal, Canada, 1987

O'Tuama LA, Guilarte TR, Douglass KH, et al: Assessment of [11C]-L-methionine transport into the human brain. J Cereb Blood Flow Metab 8:341-345, 1988

Patlak CS, Blasberg RG, Fenstermacher JD: Graphical evaluation of blood-to-brain transfer constants from multiple-time uptake data. J Cereb Blood Flow Metab 3:1-7, 1983

Penney JB, Young AB: Quantitative autoradiography of neurotransmitter receptors in Huntington disease. Neurology 32:1391-1395, 1982

Perlmutter JS, Raichle ME: Pure hemidystonia with basal ganglion abnormalities on positron emission tomography. Ann Neurol 15:228-233, 1984

Perlmutter JS, Raichle ME: Regional blood flow in hemiparkinsonism. Neurology 35:1127-1134, 1985a

Perlmutter JS, Herscovitch P, Powers WJ, et al: Standardized mean regional method for calculating global positron emission tomographic measurements. J Cereb Blood Flow Metab 5:476-480, 1985b

Perlmutter JS, Larson KB, Raichle ME, et al: Strategies for in vivo measurement of receptor binding using positron emission tomography. J Cereb Blood Flow Metab 6:154-169, 1986

Persson A, Ehrin E, Eriksson L, et al: Imaging of [11C] labelled RO 15 1788 binding to benzodiazepine, receptors in the human brain by positron emission tomography. J Psychiatr Res 19:609-622, 1985

Pert CB, Danks JA, Channing MA, et al: 3-[18F]acetylcyclofoxy: a useful probe for the visualization of opiate receptors in living animals. Federation of European Biomedical Societies (FEBS) 177:281-286, 1984

Petersen SE, Fox PT, Posner MI, et al: Positron emission tomographic studies of the cortical anatomy of single-word processing. Nature 331:585-589, 1988

Phelps ME, Huang SC, Hoffman EJ, et al: Tomographic measurement of local cerebral glucose metabolic rate in humans with (F-18)2-fluoro-2-deoxy-D-glucose: validation of method. Ann Neurol 6:371-388, 1979

Phelps ME, Kuhl DE, Mazziota JC: Metabolic mapping of the brain's response to visual stimulation: studies in humans. Science 211:1445-1448, 1981a

Phelps ME, Mazziotta JC, Kuhl De, et al: Tomographic mapping of human cerebral metabolism visual stimulation and deprivation. Neurology 31:517-529, 1981b

Phelps ME, Huang SC, Hoffman EJ, et al: An analysis of signal amplification using small detectors in positron emission tomography. J Comput Assist Tomogr 6:551-565, 1982

Phelps ME, Barrio JR, Huang SC, et al: Criteria for the tracer kinetic measurement of cerebral protein synthesis in humans with position emission tomography. Ann Neurol 15(Suppl):S192-S202, 1984

Phelps ME, Barrio JR, Huang SC, et al: Measurement of cerebral protein synthesis in man with positron computerized tomography: model, assumptions and preliminary results, in The Metabolism of the Human Brain Studied with Positron Emission Tomography. Edited by Greitz T, Ingvar DH, Widen L. New York, Raven Press, 1985

Pitts FN Jr, McClure JN Jr: Lactate metabolism in anxiety neurosis. N Engl J Med 277:1329-1336, 1967

Post RM, DeLisi LE, Holcomb HH, et al: Glucose utilization in the temporal cortex of affectively ill patients: positron emission tomography. Biol Psychiatry 22:545-553, 1987

Raichle ME: Positron emission tomography. Ann Rev Neurosci 6:249-267, 1983

Raichle ME: Measurement of local brain blood flow and oxygen utilization using oxygen 15 radiopharmaceuticals: a rapid dynamic imaging approach, in Positron Emission Tomography. Edited by Reivich M, Alavi A. New York, Alan R. Liss, Inc., 1985

Raichle ME, Martin WRW, Herscovitch P, et al: Brain blood flow measured with intravenous $H_2^{15}O$, II: implementation and validation. J Nucl Med 24:790-798, 1983

Raichle ME, Permutter JS, Fox T: Parkinson's disease: metabolic and pharmacological approaches with positron emission tomography. Ann Neurol 15(Suppl): S131-S132, 1984

Reiman EM, Raichle ME, Butler FK, et al: A focal brain abnormality in panic disorder, a severe form of anxiety. Nature 310:683-685, 1984

Reiman EM, Raichle ME, Robins E, et al: The application of positron emission tomography to the study of panic disorder. Am J Psychiatry 143:469-477, 1986

Reivich M, Kuhl D, Wolf A, et al: The [18F]fluorodeoxyglucose method for the measurement of local, cerebral glucose utilization in man. Circ Res 44:127-137, 1979

Reivich M, Alavi A, Wolf A, et al: Use of 2-deoxy-D[1-^{11}C]glucose for the determination of local cerebral glucose metabolism in humans: variation within and between subjects. J Cereb Blood Flow Metab 2:307-319, 1982

Reivich M, Gur R, Alavi A: Positron emission tomographic studies of sensory stimuli, cognitive processes and anxiety. Hum Neurobiol 2:25-33, 1983

Reivich M, Alavi A, Wolf A, et al: Glucose metabolic rate kinetic model parameter determination in humans: the lumped constants and rate constants for [18F]fluorodeoxyglucose and [11C]deoxyglucose. J Cereb Blood Flow Metab 5:179-192, 1985

Riege WH, Kuhl DE: Correlation of memory and brain glucose metabolism in depression and probably Alzheimer's disease. J Cereb Blood Flow Metab 5 (Suppl 1):S125-126, 1985

Riege WH, Metter EJ, Kuhl DE, et al: Brain glucose metabolism and memory functions: age decrease in factor scores. J Gerontol 40:459-467, 1985

Rougemont D, Baron JC, Collard P, et al: Local cerebral glucose utilization in treated and untreated patients with Parkinson's disease. J Neurol Neurosurg Psychiatry 47:824-830, 1984

Rumsey JM, Duara R, Grady C, et al: Brain metabolism in autism: resting cerebral glucose utilization rates as measured with positron emission tomography. Arch Gen Psychiatry 42:448-455, 1985

Sacks W, Sacks S, Fleischer A: A comparison of the cerebral uptake and metabolism of labeled glucose and deoxyglucose in vivo in rats. Neurochem Res 8:661-685, 1983

Sakurada O, Kennedy C, Jehle J: Measurement of local cerebral blood flow with iodo[^{14}C]antipyrine. Am J Physiol 234:H59-H66, 1978

Samson Y, Hantraye P, Baron JC, et al: Kinetics and displacement of [11C]RO 15-1788, a benzodiazepine antagonist, studied in human brain in vivo by positron tomography. Eur J Pharmacol 110:247-251, 1985

Samson Y, Baron JC, Feline A, et al: Local cerebral glucose utilization in chronic alcoholics, a positron tomographic study. J Neurol Neurosurg Psychiatry 49:1165-1170, 1986

Schaltenbrand G, Wahren W: Atlas for Stereotaxy of the Human Brain. Chicago, Year Book Medical Publishers, Inc., 1977

Schildkraut JJ: The catecholamine hypothesis of affective disorders: a review of supporting evidence. Am J Psychiatry 122:509-522, 1965

Schwartz M, Duara R, Haxby J, et al: Down's syndrome in adults: brain metabolism. Science 221:781-783, 1983

Schwartz EL, Christman DR, Wolf AP: Human primary visual cortex topography imaged via positron tomography. Brain Res 294:225-230, 1984

Schwartzman RJ, Greenberg J, Reivich M, et al: Functional metabolic mapping of a conditioned motor task in primates utilizing 2-[14C]deoxyglucose. Exp Neurol 72:153-163, 1981

Sedvall G, Farde L, Persson A, et al: Imaging of neurotransmitter receptors in the living human brain. Arch Gen Psychiatry 43:995-1005, 1986

Sedvall G, Farde L, Wiesel FA: Quantitative determination of D2 dopamine receptor characteristics in healthy subjects and psychiatric patients. Life Sci 41:813-816, 1987

Seeman P, Ulpian C, Bergeron C, et al: Bimodal distribution of dopamine receptor densities in brains of schizophrenics. Science 225:728-731, 1984

Sheppard G, Manchanda R, Gruzelier J, et al: 15O positron emission tomographic scanning in predominantly never-treated acute schizophrenic patients. Lancet 2:1448-1452, 1983

Smith CB, Davidsen L, Deibler G, et al: A method for the determination of local rates of protein synthesis in brain. Transactions of the American Society Neurochemistry 11:94, 1980

Smith CB, Crane AM, Kadekaro M, et al: Stimulation of protein synthesis and glucose utilization in the hypoglossal nucleus induced by axotomy. J Neurosci 10:2489-2496, 1984

Sokoloff L: The radioactive deoxyglucose method, theory, procedure and applications for the measurement of local glucose utilization in the central nervous system, in Advances in Neurochemistry, vol 4. Edited by Agranoff BW, Aprison MH. New York, Plenum Publishing Corporation, 1982

Sokoloff L, Reivich M, Kennedy C, et al: The [14C]deoxyglucose method for the measurement of local cerebral glucose utilization: theory, procedure, and normal values in the conscious and anesthetized albino rat. J Neurochem 28:897-916, 1977

Sparks DL, Markesbery WR, Slevin JT: Alzheimer's disease: monoamines and spiperone binding reduced in nucleus basalis. Ann Neurol 19:602-604, 1986

Starkstein SE, Robinson RG, Price TR: Comparison of patients with and without poststroke major depression matched for size and location of lesion. Arch Gen Psychiatry 45:247-252, 1988

Stoessl AJ, Martin WRW, Clark C, et al: PET studies of cerebral glucose metabolism in idiopathic torticollis. Neurology 36:653-657, 1986

Talairach J, Szikla G, Tournoux P, et al: Atlas d'Anatomie Stereotaxique du Telecephale. Paris, Masson, 1967

Ter-Pogossian MM, Phelps ME, Hoffman EJ, et al: A position emission transaxial tomograph for nuclear imaging (PETT). Radiology 114:89-98, 1975

Ter-Pogossian MM, Mullani MA, Hood J, et al: A multislice positron emission computed tomograph (PETT IV) yielding transverse and longitudinal images. Radiology 18:477-484, 1978a

Ter-Pogossian MM, Mullani NA, Hood J, et al: Design considerations for a positron emission transverse tomograph (PETT V) for imaging of the brain. J Comput Assist Tomogr 2:539-544, 1978b

Ter-Pogossian MM, Mullani NA, Ficke DC, et al: Photon time of flight assisted positron emission tomography. J Comput Assist Tomogr 5:227-239, 1981

Ter-Pogossian MM, Ficke DC, Hood JT Sr, et al: PETT VI: A positron emission tomograph utilizing cesium fluoride scintillation detectors. J Comput Assist Tomogr 6:125-133, 1982

Tewson TJ, Welch MJ, Raichle ME: [18F] labeled 3-deoxy-3-fluro-D-glucose: synthesis and preliminary biodistribution data. J Nucl Med 19:1339-1345, 1978

Theodore WH, Newmark ME, Sato S, et al: [18F]fluorodeoxyglucose positron emission tomography in refractory complex seizures. Ann Neurol 14:429-437, 1983

Theodore WH, Brooks R, Margolin R, et al: Positron emission tomography in generalized seizures. Neurology 35:684-690, 1985

Theodore WH, Dorwart R, Holmes M, et al: Neuroimaging in refractory partial seizures: comparison of PET, CT, and MRI. Neurology 36:750-759, 1986

Trifiletti RR, Snowman AM, Whitehouse PJ, et al: Huntington's disease: increased number and altered regulation of benzodiazepine receptor complexes in frontal cerebral cortex. Neurology 37:916-922, 1987

Uhl GR, Hackney GO, Torchia M, et al: Parkinson's disease: nigral receptor changes support peptidergic role in nigrostriatal modulation. Ann Neurol 20:194-203, 1986

Volkow ND, Brodie JD, Wolf AP, et al: Brain metabolism in patients with schizophrenia before and after acute neuroleptic administration. J Neurol Neurosurg Psychiatry 49:1199-1202, 1986a

Volkow ND, Brodie JD, Wolf AP, et al: Brain organization in schizophrenia. J Cereb Blood Flow Metab 6:441-446, 1986b

Volkow ND, Wolf AP, Van Gelder P, et al: Phenomenological correlates of metabolic activity in 18 patients with chronic schizophrenia. Am J Psychiatry 144:151-158, 1987

Wagner HN: Setting up a clinical PET center. Diagnostic Imaging 8:82-91, 1986

Wagner HN Jr, Burns HD, Dannals RF, et al: Imaging dopamine receptors in the human brain by positron tomography. Science 221:1264-1266, 1983

Weinberger DR, Berman KF, Zec RF: Physiologic dysfunction of dorsolateral prefrontal cortex in schizophrenia, I: regional cerebral blood flow evidence. Arch Gen Psychiatry 43:114-125, 1986

Whitehouse PJ, Trifiletti RR, Jones BE, et al: Neurotransmitter receptor alterations in Huntington's disease, autoradiographic and homogenate studies with special reference to benzodiazepine receptor complexes. Ann Neurol 18:202-210, 1985

Wolf AP, Fowler JS: Positron emitter-labeled radiotracers—chemical considerations, in Positron Emission Tomography. Edited by Reivich M, Alavi A. New York, Alan R. Liss, Inc., 1985

Wolfson LI, Leenders KL, Brown LL, et al: Alterations of regional cerebral blood flow and oxygen metabolism in Parkinson's disease. Neurology 35:1399-1405, 1985

Wolkin A, Jaeger J, Brodie JD, et al: Persistence of cerebral metabolic abnormalities in chronic schizophrenia as determined by positron emission tomography. Am J Psychiatry 142:564-571, 1985

Wong DF, Wagner HN Jr, Dannals RF, et al: Effects of age on dopamine and serotonin receptors measured by positron tomography in the living human brain. Science 226:1393-139, 1984

Wong DF, Gjedde A, Wagner HN Jr: Quantification of neuroreceptors in the living human brain, I: irreversible binding of ligands. J Cereb Blood Flow Metab 6:137-146, 1986a

Wong DF, Gjedde A, Wagner HN Jr, et al: Quantification of neuroreceptors in the living brain, II: inhibition studies of receptor density and affinity. J Cereb Blood Flow Metab 6:147-153, 1986b

Wong DF, Wagner HN, Tune LE, et al: Positron emissin tomography reveals elevated D2 dopamine receptors in drug-naive schizophrenics. Science 234:1558-1563, 1986c

Woods BT, Kinney DK, Yurgelun-Todd D: Neurologic abnormalities in schzophrenic patients and their families. Arch Gen Psychiatry 43:657-668, 1986

Young AB, Penney JB, Starosta-Rubinstein S, et al: PET scan investigations of Huntington's disease: cerebral metabolic correlates of neurological features and functional decline. Ann Neurol 20:296-303, 1986

Younkin DP, Reivich M, Jaggi J, et al: Noninvasive method of estimating human newborn regional cerebral blood flow. J Cereb Blood Flow Metab 2:415-420, 1982

Index